Shaping Health Policy
Through
Nursing Research

Ada Sue Hinshaw, PhD, RN, FAAN, is Dean and Professor of the Graduate School of Nursing at the Uniformed Services University of the Health Sciences and Emeritus Dean and Professor at the University of Michigan School of Nursing, where she served as Dean from 1994 to 2006. Dr. Hinshaw was selected as an American Academy of Nursing/American Foundation of Nursing/Institute of Medicine Senior Nurse Scholar from 2006 to 2007.

Before her appointment as Dean at the University of Michigan, Dr. Hinshaw served as the first permanent Director of the National Center of Nursing Research and the first Director of the National Institute of Nursing Research at the National Institutes of Health (NIH). During her tenure at NIH, Dr. Hinshaw was responsible for promoting research in the areas of disease prevention, health promotion, acute and chronic illness, and investigating environments that enhance nursing care patient outcomes. Other positions at academic institutions include University of Arizona College of Nursing, UCSF College of Nursing and University of Kansas College of Nursing. She has conducted research in quality of care, patient outcomes, measurement of outcomes, and building positive work environments to enhance patient safety. She is the recipient of many awards for her work, including the MNRS Lifetime Achievement Award, the U.S. Public Health Service Health Leader of the Year award, Award for Excellence in Nursing Research (STT), Nurse Scientist of the Year award (ANA Council of Nurse Researchers), and the IOM Walsh McDermott award. She has received 13 honorary doctorates.

Patricia A. Grady, PhD, RN, FAAN, has been associated with the National Institutes of Health (NIH) since 1988, first as an extramural research program administrator in the areas of stroke and brain imaging at the National Institute of Neurological Disorders and Stroke (NINDS), then as a member of the NIH Task Force for Medical Rehabilitation Research, and as Assistant Director of NINDS until 1995, when she was appointed as Director of the National Institute of Nursing Research (NINR). Under her leadership, the Institute has more than doubled its budget and significantly increased the number of research and training grants awarded. Dr. Grady also is an internationally recognized researcher, whose focus has been on the topic of stroke. Before her work at NIH, she served as faculty at University of Maryland School of Nursing and School of Medicine. She has coauthored numerous articles and serves on many editorial journal boards, including *Stroke; Stroke and Cerebral Vascular Diseases;* and *Neurotherapeutics, the Journal of the American Society for Experimental Neuro Therapeutics.* Dr. Grady is a member of the American Academy of Nursing and is the recipient of a number of prestigious awards. Her most recent notable awards include the Second Century Award for Excellence in Health Care from Columbia University School of Nursing and the Honorary Doctor of Science degree from Thomas Jefferson University and the Medical University of South Carolina.

Shaping Health Policy
Through
Nursing Research

Ada Sue Hinshaw, PhD, RN, FAAN

Patricia A. Grady, PhD, RN, FAAN

Editors

SPRINGER PUBLISHING COMPANY

NEW YORK

Springer Publishing Company, LLC
11 West 42nd Street
New York, NY 10036
www.springerpub.com

Acquisitions Editor: Margaret Zuccarini
Production Editor: Gayle Lee
Cover Design: Steven Pisano
Composition: The Manila Typesetting Company

ISBN: 978-0-8261-1069-5

E-book ISBN: 978-0-8261-1070-1

10 11 12 13 14/ 5 4 3 2 1

The author and the publisher of this Work have made every effort to use sources believed to be reliable to provide information that is accurate and compatible with the standards generally accepted at the time of publication. Because medical science is continually advancing, our knowledge base continues to expand. Therefore, as new information becomes available, changes in procedures become necessary. We recommend that the reader always consult current research and specific institutional policies before performing any clinical procedure. The author and publisher shall not be liable for any special, consequential, or exemplary damages resulting, in whole or in part, from the readers' use of, or reliance on, the information contained in this book. The publisher has no responsibility for the persistence or accuracy of URLs for external or third-party Internet Web sites referred to in this publication and does not guarantee that any content on such Web sites is, or will remain, accurate or appropriate.

Library of Congress Cataloging-in-Publication Data

Shaping health policy through nursing research/[edited by] Ada Sue Hinshaw, Patricia A. Grady.
    p. ; cm.
  Includes bibliographical references and index.
  ISBN 978-0-8261-1069-5—ISBN 978-0-8261-1070-1 (e-book) 1. Medical policy. 2. Nursing—Research. I. Hinshaw, Ada Sue. II. Grady, Patricia A.
  [DNLM: 1. Health Policy. 2. Nursing Research. 3. Nursing Care. 4. Policy Making. WY 20.5]
  RA395.A3S45 2011
  362.1072—dc22
                                                                                      2010025862

Special discounts on bulk quantities of our books are available to corporations, professional associations, pharmaceutical companies, health care organizations and other qualifying groups.

If you are interested in a custom book, including chapters from more than one of our titles, we can provide that service as well.

For details, please contact:
Special Sales Department, Springer Publishing Company, LLC
11 West 42nd Street, 15th Floor, New York, NY 10036-8002
Phone: 877–687-7476 or 212-431-4370; Fax: 212-941-7842
E-mail: sales@springerpub.com

Printed in the United States by Hamilton Printing.

To nurse researchers,
past, present and future,
for their successes in confronting and reordering the status quo.
These pioneers' creativity and systematic efforts
have created the foundation for evidence-based practice
and data-based health policy
to provide for a healthier future.

Contents

SECTION III: CONCLUSIONS

Contributors

Linda H. Aiken, PhD, RN, FAAN
Trustee Professor of Nursing and Sociology, University of Pennsylvania, Philadelphia, Pennsylvania

Rhonda G. Cady, MS, RN
University of Minnesota, Minneapolis, Minnesota

Angela A. Crowley, PhD, APRN, PNP-PC, FAAN
Associate Professor, School of Nursing, Yale University, New Haven, Connecticut

David F. Dinges, PhD
Professor of Psychology in Psychiatry, Chief, Division of Sleep and Chronobiology, University of Pennsylvania, School of Medicine, Philadelphia, Pennsylvania

Lois K. Evans, PhD, RN, FAAN
van Ameringen Professor in Nursing Excellence, School of Nursing, University of Pennsylvania, Philadelphia, Pennsylvania

Suzanne L. Feetham, PhD, RN, FAAN
Visiting Professor, College of Nursing, University of Wisconsin, Milwaukee, Wisconsin, Nursing Research Consultant, Children's National Medical Center, Washington, DC

Stanley M. Finkelstein, PhD
Professor of Laboratory Medicine and Pathology, Director of the Schmitt Center for Home Telehealth, Division of Health Informatics, University of Minnesota School of Medicine, Minneapolis, Minnesota

Deborah Gross, DNSc, RN, FAAN
Leonard and Helen Stulman Professor in Mental Health and Psychiatric Nursing, Johns Hopkins University School of Nursing and School of Medicine, Baltimore, Maryland

Laureen Hayes, RN, EdD
Lawrence S. Bloomberg Faculty of Nursing, University of Toronto, Toronto, Ontario, Canada

Janet Heinrich, PhD, RN, FAAN
Associate Administrator, Bureau of Health Professions, Health Resources and Services Administration, Director, Health Care, Government Accountability Office, Washington, DC

William L. Holzemer, PhD, RN, FAAN
Dean and Professor, College of Nursing, Rutgers, The State University of New Jersey, Newark, New Jersey

Loretta S. Jemmott, PhD, FAAN
Professor and van Ameringen Professor in Psychiatric Mental Health Nursing, Director, Center for Health Disparities Research, University of Pennsylvania, Philadelphia, Pennsylvania

Ellen T. Kurtzman, MPH, RN, CPNP/PMHNP, FAAN
Assistant Research Professor, School of Nursing, The George Washington University, Washington, DC

Bernadette Mazurek Melnyk, PhD, RN, CPNP/PMHNP, FAAN
Dean and Distinguished Foundation Professor in Nursing, College of Nursing and Healthcare Innovation, Arizona State University, Phoenix, Arizona

Norma A. Metheny, PhD, RN, FAAN
Professor and Dorothy A. Votsmier Endowed Chair in Nursing, Associate Dean for Research, School of Nursing, Saint Louis University, St. Louis, Missouri

Mary D. Naylor, PhD, RN, FAAN
Marian S. Ware Professor in Gerontology, Director, New Courtland Center for Transitions and Health, School of Nursing, University of Pennsylvania, Philadelphia, Pennsylvania

Linda O'Brien-Pallas, RN, PhD, FCAHS
Professor, Lawrence S. Bloomberg Faculty of Nursing, Director and Co-Principal Investigator, Nursing Health Services Research Unit, CHSRF/CIAR Chair in Nursing/Health Human Resources, University of Toronto, Toronto, Ontario, Canada

Carolyn M. Sampselle, PhD, RN, FAAN
Carolyne K. Davis Collegiate Professor of Nursing, School of Nursing, Professor of Women's Studies, College of Literature, Science, and the Arts, Professor of Obstetrics & Gynecology, Medical School, University of Michigan, Ann Arbor, Michigan

Judith Shamian, PhD, RN, FAAN
President and CEO, VON Canada, Ottawa, Ontario, Canada
Lawrence Bloomberg Faculty of Nursing, University of Toronto, Toronto, Ontario, Canada

Moriah Shamian-Ellen, PhD, MBA
McMaster University, Hamilton, Ontario, Canada

Neville E. Strumpf, PhD, RN, FAAN
Edith Clemmer Steinbright Professor Emerita, University of Pennsylvania, Philadelphia, Pennsylvania

Virginia P. Tilden, DNSc, RN, FAAN
Dean and Professor, College of Nursing, University of Nebraska Medical Center, Omaha, Nebraska

Antonia M. Villarruel, PhD, RN, FAAN
Professor and Nola J. Pender Collegiate Chair, Associate Dean for Research and Global Affairs, School of Nursing, University of Michigan, Ann Arbor, Michigan

Kathleen M. Williamson, PhD, RN
Associate Director, Center for the Advancement of Evidence-Based Practice, College of Nursing and Healthcare Innovation, Arizona State University, Phoenix, Arizona

Foreword

With *Shaping Health Policy Through Nursing Research*, Ada Sue Hinshaw and Patricia Grady are changing the game. And the game desperately needs changing.

For far too long, nurses and nurse researchers have been overlooked and undervalued in the decision-making circles that inform and determine our nation's health policies. Nursing is greatly valued in our society as a whole: opinion polls and personal testimony continually confirm how much we need nurses, and how much we esteem their work. We know that nurses are at the core of our healthcare system, yet nursing is too often relegated to the margins of health policy making. This needs to change.

Change in health policy making will only come when nurses and nurse researchers themselves become policy leaders. Nursing professionals have for too long assumed that their work spoke for itself. Nursing has widespread credibility and respect: the importance of nursing is obvious. It was easy to assume that nurses did not need to be policy leaders: just get on with the work of nursing and leave the policy to others. But that is not how policy works. That is not how change happens in our society.

Policy is made by people who see themselves—and put themselves forward—as leaders. Policy is made by people who can talk the talk of policy making, who take a seat at the table having mastered the art, as well as the science, of decision making. Policy leaders who make a difference have mastered decision making informed by the best available evidence (especially when, as is often the case, the evidence base is incomplete), and have mastered the art of decision making that honors diverse values, is rooted in consensus, and subject to ongoing public scrutiny and debate.

Shaping Health Policy Through Nursing Research will speed the day when every student of nursing is ready, willing, and eager to assume a leadership role in creating health policy for our nation, and for the world. The rest of us—all of us who rely on nurses, trust nurses, admire and know how much we need nurses—eagerly await you!

Mary Woolley
President, Research!America

Preface

This book, *Shaping Health Policy Through Nursing Research,* is intended to help stimulate the reader to embrace the idea of shaping health policy through nursing research. It provides both a conceptual orientation to science/research shaping health policy as well as an operational approach to strategies for linking research to policy and influencing policy makers at the organizational, community, state, national, and international levels.

As the first compilation of information linking health policy and nursing research, this book will serve as a resource for undergraduate and graduate students, faculty, and professional nurses on how nursing research can shape and guide health policy decisions and programs. There are several strong health policy and politics textbooks that have a limited focus on research as related to health policy, but this text is unique in that it primarily addresses the interrelationship of health policy and nursing research. This text will also provide examples that will inspire an awareness among nurses in all settings to consider participating in shaping policy. This resource includes information on science shaping health policy in general, models and strategies for linking research and health policy, ways in which nursing research is shaping health policy, and multiple examples illustrating how major nursing research programs have influenced health policy as told by the investigators. The text also presents perspectives and frameworks within which to understand the processes bridging research and health policy, multiple factors influencing the processes, and actual examples of nursing research programs that have influenced health policy programs.

Historically, this is an ideal time to examine the effect of research on health policy. After some 25 years of stable funding for nursing research, substantial growth has occurred in both the breadth of the science and the research workforce, and emerging trends are evident. A growing body of knowledge is amassing, which forms the basis for evidence-based practice and leads to a better understanding of what we can accomplish in the broader goal of improving the public's health. The science has grown from the early efforts of individual researchers doing single studies to scientists developing programs of research that can be replicated by others and generalized into a variety of settings and environments. Researchers can now represent their substantive areas at policy tables at local, state, and federal levels as well as in their universities and communities.

Becoming leaders in this new role of shaping health policy is an important opportunity to capture. It is time to effectively put all of the newly discovered knowledge to work, with as broad a reach as possible. For the most part, moving research into practice is a change that is being successfully implemented. Moving research into policy, however, has proven to be more of a challenge. Since health policy occurs at multiple levels, affecting the process can also occur at multiple levels. There is no single best approach. This book is meant to address methods to think about and methods to approach the process of shaping health policy through research, using real examples of successful excursions in the process.

From practitioners changing policy in specific work settings to those walking the halls of Congress, any citizen has a potential role in shaping policy. Health policy can be influenced at home, in communities, schools, and day care; in evidence-based practice in healthcare organizations, including acute and long-term settings; or within community, state, national and international level policies. All of these areas provide opportunities to make modifications in policy, large or small, that will change people's lives. With the backdrop of healthcare reform, many issues are emerging and reemerging that can be informed, in fact, need to be informed, by nursing science. The process of informing health reform through nursing research also provides an opportunity for the assessment of what has been accomplished and highlights the challenge of what the future brings. Our work is defined for us. With nearly three million registered nurses available to participate in generating a body of knowledge, individually or in teams, and translate those results, there is great potential to make change.

Book Sections

Shaping Health Policy Through Nursing Research is organized in three sections. First, a set of chapters provide a context for science shaping policy, an introduction to models and strategies through which research can inform policy making, and an examination of the relationship of science policy to health policy. Second, a series of nursing research programs are outlined that have had an impact on health policy at multiple levels. The third section summarizes the valuable lessons learned from senior nurse investigators recounting their experiences and addresses future directions for nursing research in shaping health policy.

The first section consists of six chapters that provide diverse perspectives on how research informs health policy. The first chapter, "Science Shaping Health Policy: How is Nursing Research Evident in Such Policy Changes?" outlines informal discussions examining what national health policy influencers consider important research characteristics for gaining decision makers' attention. In addition, an exploratory study identifies the major research characteristics that nursing investigators judge valuable in enabling research programs, and the findings to shape policy makers' decisions. The second chapter, "Research: A Foundation for Health Policy," articulates how to influence policy, ways in which nursing research is useful in health policy processes and the successful application of research strategies in influencing health policy.

The third chapter, "Shaping Health Policy: The Role of Nursing Research—Three Frameworks and Their Application to Policy Development," suggests several models that can be used to understand and facilitate the transfer of research results into health policy. The author explains a model developed over a number of years while influencing health policy in Canada. The model is titled "From Talk to Action." Chapter 4, "The Role of Science Policy in Programs of Research and Scholarship," addresses the processes through which science policy shapes health policy from a general perspective. As national science policies change, how does this influence the information available for considering health policy decisions? In chapter 5, "Changing Science Policy: The Establishment of the National Institute of Nursing Research at the National Institutes of Health," the "From Talk to Action" model is used to examine the creation of the National Institute of Nursing Research (NINR) in the late 1980s. The founding of the NINR was a major national science policy decision that has influenced health policy over the ensuing years as evidenced in the experiences related in section 2 of this book. The final chapter in section 1, "Using Evidence-Based Practice to Enhance Organizational Policies, Healthcare Quality, and Patient Outcomes," speaks to the influence of research results being converted to evidence-based practice, shaping not only nursing policies but organizational policies concerning patient care.

In section 2, there are 12 chapters that examine the experiences of senior nurse scientists, funded for a series of studies, and the influence of their research program results on informing health policy. These experiences illustrate positive shaping for practice policies in healthcare organizations to inclusion of results in national guidelines for health improvements. The findings from these research experiences provide strong recommendations for work environments of nurses that, in turn, influence patient outcomes. Several of the experiences show change in community and state programs that enhance health for children or for older adults. Chapters 7 and 8 focus on the shaping of organizational policies and procedures resulting from major nursing research programs: "From Bedside to Bench to Practice" and "Translating Personal Challenges to Public Policy." Two chapters illustrate nursing research programs that have influenced community, state and national programs and policies for children and adolescents: "Shaping HIV/AIDS Prevention Policy for Minority Youth" and "Health Promotion and Prevention in Early Childhood." Nursing research has been influential across the life span. The chapter on "Research on Human Sleep: Need to Inform Public Policies" addresses sleep issues for working adults while the two chapters, "Influencing Policy for Improving End-of-Life Care" and" Two Decades of Research on Physical Restraint: Impact of Practice and Policy," address state- and national-level policy issues at the nursing facility for older adults. Four chapters relate to informing health policy for organizational work environments and the use of telehealth to address home care: "Transitional Care: Improving Health Outcomes and Decreasing Costs for At-Risk Chronically-Ill Older Adults," "Nursing: Saving Lives, Improving Patient Care Outcomes," "Nursing Workforce and Health Policy" and "Research Technology: Home Telehealth and Remote Monitoring." The last chapter addresses how experienced nurse investigators use their expertise to shape national and international health policies regarding HIV/AIDS.

The third section consists of a final chapter that summarizes the models, strategies and processes used by the nurse scientists to shape health policy based on their research programs. Many lessons were learned in these early years of stable, extramural funding for nursing investigations programs. Which are now explicitly understood as successful approaches for informing health policy from research findings? What are future directions for being more explicit in generating research that will address major public health issues or health reform concerns?

As is evident from the descriptions of the three sections, several unique features characterize this book:

- Several perspectives, models and strategies are examined for deliberately using nursing research in informing health policy.
- The current state of the science is delineated in terms of how nursing research is shaping health policy, thus addressing the knowledge foundation generated through two-and-a-half decades of stable funding of the discipline's science.
- Multiple experiences are shared by senior nursing investigators to show how nursing research is shaping health policy at the organizational, community, state, national and international levels.

Ada Sue Hinshaw
Patricia A. Grady

Acknowledgments

The authors are profoundly grateful to the many senior colleagues who have also been committed to the concept of producing a historical text that would chronicle the state of the science in terms of nursing research shaping health policy after the first 25 years of stable, substantial extramural funding. The nurse investigators sharing and analyzing the influence of their research on health policy in this book are truly pioneers; not only in terms of the long-term research programs they have built and sustained, but also in their concerted efforts to influence both health practice and policy at all levels. Several interdisciplinary colleagues also understood the book's vision and focus and, as they have conducted and supported nursing research, were willing to contribute to this historical endeavor. The interdisciplinary colleagues brought expertise and new perspective. A special thank you to all of this book's authors!

This historical book was made possible by the nursing leaders in the mid-1980's, and their professional organizations, who believed in the nursing research community of scholars and dared to strive for a scientific entity for nursing "within the mainstream" of health science. Thus, the National Center for Nursing Research, now the National Institute of Nursing Research, was born. Many thanks to the Division of Nursing at the Health Resources Service Administration, for a solid early foundation in research training and to the numerous nursing leaders who followed the dream of an institute at the National Institutes of Health.

The authors especially want to acknowledge the incredible expertise, valuable advice, and consistent support and nudging provided by Ms. Margaret Zuccarini, Executive Acquisitions Editor, at Springer Publishing Company.

The authors would also like to thank Mary Wooley, President, Research!America, for writing the foreword for this text and for her keen understanding of and consistent, strong support for nursing science. Mary's strong advocacy for biomedical and behavioral science and her ability to articulate the link between research and policy is a gift to the entire scientific community.

Ada Sue Hinshaw
Patricia A. Grady

1

Science Shaping Health Policy: How Is Nursing Research Evident in Such Policy Changes?

Ada Sue Hinshaw

INTRODUCTION

Shaping Health Policy Through Nursing Research focuses on the progress and challenges in the generation of the science of nursing as it has begun to inform health policy. The ability to inform such policy is based on a foundation of knowledge developed primarily over the past two-and-a-half decades of substantial financial, federal support. The establishment of the National Center of Nursing Research (NCNR) in 1986, which was redesignated as the National Institute of Nursing Research (NINR) in 1993, provided the stable, steadily increasing base needed for the nursing discipline's research programs. The current, strong emphasis on evidence-based practice within the profession shows the impact of the growing knowledge base on the nursing profession (Dickson & Flynn, 2009; Melynk & Fineout-Overholt, 2005). However, less well understood is the influence of the evolving body of nursing science on informing health policy. Nursing research's potential to shape health policy was evident early in the knowledge base development, with the *New York Times* article by Brody in 1991, "Beyond Tender Loving Care, Nurses Are a Force in Research." However, it was clear in the 2000 Gebbie, Wakefield, and Kerfoot study that nursing leaders involved in health policy positions and activities did "not report significant use of nursing research or information in policy making" (p. 307). Over the past decade, how has the evolving knowledge base for nursing begun informing health policy? What are the characteristics that make it relevant to policy makers and what are the different areas in which health policy is being informed through nursing research?

The information reported in this chapter represents the informal experiences and the findings of an exploratory study conducted while I was a Senior Nurse Scholar at the Institute of Medicine (IOM) from 2006 to 2007. The purpose of the scholarly period was, in general, to gain an understanding of how science shapes health policy and, in particular, to explore how nursing research was informing health policy.

I

This chapter will do the following:

- Examine the concept, models, and processes for science shaping health policy.
- Identify why national health policy influencers judge that research is used or not used by policy makers.
- Explore the nursing research characteristics that long-term research principle investigators (PIs) judge make it possible for policy makers to relate to their research, the external factors that facilitate nursing research informing health policy, the barriers that seem to exist in using their research for policy, and the various areas in which they have been successful in informing health policy.

SCIENCE SHAPING HEALTH POLICY

In his article "The Science of Good Government," Mecklin (2009) addresses the importance of science in shaping public policy. He suggests that some governmental administrations are more open and receptive to research as a major foundation to decision making in policy. Policy is defined as statements (documents) that reflect the "standing decisions" of an organization about a given problem, issue, or situation. These statements identify a series of actions or programs that articulate a desired set of conditions for society (Milstead, 2004). Block (2004) defines policies in several ways, including statements and principles that govern programs and the distribution of resources toward desired goals. More specifically, Block (2004, p. 7) defines health policy as "The collection of authoritative decisions made within government that pertain to health and to the pursuit of health." Part of the latter definition is attributed to Longest (1998), but Block elaborates the definition to include the private sector and the government.

Science is only one of many factors that influence health policy. Other influencers include constituent's opinions, policy maker beliefs and values, and politics, to cite a few (Leavitt, Chaffee, & Mason, 2006; Shamain, Skelton-Green, & Villeneuve, 2003). However, research can still be quite influential in two situations: (1) in times of new or controversial events and (2) in identification of the policy problem(s), as Milio (1984) suggested in her early, classic paper "Nursing Research and the Study of Health Policy."

Several types of research influence health policy: policy research, policy analysis, and disciplinary studies. These include the following:

- Policy research: This type of research involves the evaluation of a particular health policy's translation and implementation in specific situations to estimate effectiveness as well as efficiency.
- Policy analysis: Such studies are contracted by particular policy bodies in order to estimate the effect of potential policies on desired social programs, usually prior to implementation.
- Disciplinary studies: These are studies conducted to generate knowledge within various fields such as nursing, medicine, dentistry, and public health, from which findings can also shape health policy (Hinshaw, 1992).

Disciplinary research is the focus of this chapter in terms of science shaping health policy. Science from multiple disciplinary fields impacts health policy. Some fields are better represented than others in terms of informing policy (Mecklin, 2009). The intent of this chapter is to better understand how science from nursing investigators shapes health policy.

In an early article on nursing research and health policy, Hinshaw (1988) outlined multiple levels at which health policy occurs. Fawcett's (2001) model of Health Policy Foci and Outcomes delineates a similar set of five levels for health policy. Often, policy writers speak primarily of health policy at the state or national level. But given the earlier definition that stipulates an organization as the locus of policy, health policy can be considered at all levels of "organizations." Multiple levels of health policy can relate to a healthcare agency, such as a hospital or a community agency, as well as state, national, and international policies for societal health. Examples of health policies in a hospital are statements and processes promoting patient safety, whereas programs for nutrition and exercise are examples of community, school-based policies to prevent childhood obesity. State workforce laws such as mandated ratios for the number of nurses needed for patient care, preschool programs for the children of low-income families, and prevention programs for individuals with HIV/AIDS reflect well-known state, national and international health policies.

A number of models have been developed for understanding the policy process, most of which have an obvious stage that involves the integration of science. Block's (2004) Model for the Making of Public Policy is exemplary of most of those that are process based. The six stages include agenda setting, policy formulation, policy adoption, policy implementation, policy assessment, and policy modification. According to Birkland (2005), the Systems Model approach is also very popular in explaining the policy process. Such models include input and output states, with little understanding of the "black box" surrounding these two major stages (Birkland, 2005). For example, the input and output factors need to be identified; measurements, developed; and policy outcomes, more systematically studied (Mecklin, 2009).

Several models have been used in nursing to explain research integration into the policy process: the Richmond and Kotelchuck Model for Shaping Health Policy (Feetham & Meister, 1999; Richmond & Kotelchuck, 1983) and the model of Shamain, Skelton-Green, and Villeneuve (2003) entitled, From Talk to Action. The Model for Shaping Health Policy consists of three major stages: knowledge and information, political will, and social action. Policy results from the outcome of changes in and the interaction of the three components. The basic explanation is that relevant knowledge and information, combined with political will, lead to social action, which is the initiation of new health policy and policy programs. The model, From Talk to Action, encompasses two major stages, with multiple steps within each one. The model is dynamic and, thus, not linear in nature, with stages and steps interacting and science being utilized within multiple steps, although one step focuses explicitly on the accumulation of knowledge to address the problem or issue that is the focus of the policy process. The two stages are getting to the policy agenda and moving into action. This model acknowledges the preparation necessary for defining the policy problem or issue and accumulating the knowledge and research needed to address it adequately.

Mecklin (2009) attests to the importance of science in "good" government or policy. He is quoting the work of a mentor and colleague, Dr. Ken Prewitt, who is the Vice President for Global Centers and the Carnegie Professor of Public Affairs at Columbia University. Prewitt asserts, "Although the government consumes a huge amount of research into society's workings, no one, it seems, has documented clearly how the officials charged with solving our problems acquire, weigh and then use the research that comes before them" (Mecklin, 2009, p. 9). The scholarly experience at the IOM focused on part of this issue; that is, why is some science relevant to health policy makers and other research is never used? What are the characteristics of research that seem to be important to health policy makers?

SENIOR NURSE SCHOLAR EXPERIENCE AT THE IOM

The senior nurse scholar experience at the IOM was sponsored by the American Academy of Nursing (AAN), the American Nurses' Foundation, and the IOM. The program was partially planned and implemented with the Robert Wood Johnson Health Policy program. In essence, the experience represented an executive program in national health policy. As advisor for the nation's health, the environment of the IOM promotes the accumulation and synthesis of science for the purpose of informing health policy.

The purpose of the American Academy of Nursing/American Nurses' Foundation/ IOM scholar experience was to explore how science shaped health policy and, more specifically, to conduct an exploratory study focusing on how nursing research informs health policy. Prewitt (Mecklin, 2009) encourages this line of investigation, as is obvious from the earlier quote. The general questions of interest were the following:

- When are science and research most valuable for health policy makers?
- When are science and research least likely to be used in policy making?
- What are the research characteristics that facilitate health policy makers' use of such information?
- What are the facilitating factors and barriers to the use of research in policy?

These questions were asked in slightly different terms with two groups of individuals, i.e., informal discussions with national health policy influencers and senior nurse scientists with long-term research programs.

The model of Shamain et al. (2003, p. 92), "From Talk to Action," provided a conceptual perspective for understanding research in the context of the policy process. The model's two stages include multiple steps in a circular, dynamic approach. Stage 1, getting to a policy agenda, involves values and beliefs, problem or issue emerging, knowledge development and research, and public awareness. The second stage, moving into action, encompasses political engagement, interest group activation, public policy deliberation and adoption, and regulation, experience, and revision.

This model was valuable in illustrating how research is involved with the health policy process. The model teaches several lessons, for example:

- Research and knowledge development are explicit, valuable aspects of the health policy process.
- Research and knowledge are interactive with every step of the health policy process, from its beginning with values and beliefs to the final steps of regulation, experience, and revision.
- Science is active in moving issues into action by being relevant to policy problems or issues.

- Integrating science into health policy makes it a "lever for effecting change" (Shamain et al., 2003, p. 93).

Thus, science and research become integral aspects of the health policy process. The degree of integration and attention paid to science depends partly on the health policy makers' values and beliefs.

Informal Interviews With National Health Policy Influencers

A series of informal interviews with individuals who are experts in health policy and influencing health policy was an integral aspect of the IOM experience. The national health policy influencers were Executive Directors and Senior Staff who were with health foundations and think tanks in the Washington, DC, area. These individuals viewed their organizational mission as providing factual information, systematically surveyed public opinion, and evidence-based recommendations for health policy decision makers, e.g., the PEW Foundation. Fifteen well-known, recognized health policy influencers took part in these informal discussions.

The focus of these discussions was how they perceived science-shaped health policy and why policy makers would or would not choose to use research as part of their decision-making process. The discussions involved essentially three questions:

- When in the policy-making process are science and research most useful?
- What characteristics of science and research make them most useful?
- When are science and research least likely to be useful in policy making?

In response to the question "When in the policy-making process are science and research *most* useful?" the policy influencers suggested four situations:

- Times of disagreement to resolve conflict and "save face"
- Times of chaos when there is a need to solve a major problem and provide direction
- When the policy maker is "looking for" substantiation for a previously held position
- When there is a "window of opportunity" or policy receptor for the results

The health policy influencers almost all stated that research became a factor when policy makers were in conflict about a situation or did not have a clear definition of the policy problem, much less possible solutions. They sought knowledge to understand both the problem they were confronted with and how to handle it. Another aspect of this situation was that, sometimes, policy makers would take a stand without good information and then needed to change their stance on an issue. Using research provided a socially acceptable way to make such a change and *save face*, a term used by several of the health policy influencers.

Consistent with Milio's (1984, 1989) early writings on health policy, a time of chaos with a policy situation that has many unknowns is an opportunity for research to be valuable in the policy-making process. One of the health policy influencers cited the 9/11 situation as one of chaos. Research relating to disaster response was valuable while new policies following this situation funded new university centers and other entities on disaster preparedness.

Birkland (2005) suggests that, often, policy is driven by the values and biases of the decision makers or their constituents. However, the policy makers wish their decisions and policies to be creditable. Thus, using research to substantiate a previously-held position is understandable.

A number of policy scholars (Block, 2004; Harrington & Estes, 2004; Milstead, 2004) address the relationship between a policy window of opportunity and research. The creation of the NINR was an excellent example of a window of opportunity policy and subsequent new science program. The legislation for the NINR (then the NCNR) was passed in the Fall of 1985, and the national center was established in April 1986 at the National Institutes of Health. The middle of the 1980s was a time for health policy makers to be supportive of women's issues and legislation for women. The NCNR legislation provided an opportunity to vote for a positive women's issue; in addition, it involved health, science, and nursing, all positive attributes for the Congress men and women. How much the Congressional voters understood about nursing research was debatable, but the window of opportunity was there for nursing research to move into the mainstream of science at the National Institutes of Health. Planning a research program to provide information and data for windows of opportunity is one of the most challenging issues for investigators. L. H. Aiken (personal communication, Fall of 2006) is an example of one who strategically plans her team's research to provide data for future policy issues.

In relation to the question "What characteristics of science and research make them most useful?" health policy influencers provided five general responses. These included the following:

- The research is credible
- Information is clearly presented in understandable lay terms
- Data are provided in quantitative mode
- Results give clear suggestions for actions to be considered
- Findings are framed in a policy context

Research credibility is a crucial characteristic for the results to be useable in policy decisions. Dickson and Flynn (2009), in their text *Nursing Policy Research: Turning Evidence Based Research Into Health Policy*, discuss the use of evidence-based decisions in organizational, health services, and patient safety health policy. As with other evidence-based practice texts, they discuss the characteristics and levels of evidence needed for policy decisions. They also address the second characteristic; information needs to be clearly presented in understandable lay terms, i.e., in terms that well-educated but nonhealth professionals are able to relate to and use. Gebbie, Wakefield, and Kerfoot (2000) interviewed leaders in nursing who are involved in health policy of the problems with leaders using research is the lack of its availability in common sources and in understandable language. Thus, it is important to present substantiated research for shaping health policy in understandable terms for both educated colleagues and policy makers.

Providing research data in a quantitative mode might seem initially problematic in nursing because of the discipline's strong support of qualitative, as well as quantitative, research. However, discussing this idea further with the national health policy influencers suggests that policy makers first value a "snapshot" of the information about the issue, then need to have stories and examples illustrating the policy issue and possible strategies. Thus, the quantitative data provide the initial snapshot, while the qualitative information is important for giving evidence-based stories and examples.

The last two valuable characteristics are related to and address the need for research to provide solutions or strategies for handling the policy issue. Furthermore, the solutions need to be framed in terms of a policy context that is relevant and valuable for society. Just providing strategies that are not interpretable for policy or policy makers is not helpful (M. Wakefield, personal communication, Spring of 2006). Dickson and Flynn (2009) address this research characteristic, suggesting that ongoing collaboration with policy makers is necessary to ensure that the research is relevant to specific policy issues, and results in recommendations that can be implemented in policy.

For the third question, "When are science and research *least* likely to be useful in policy making?" health policy influencers consistently provided four responses. Several of these responses were the negative counterpart to the answers given to Question 1:

- When information does not address critical public health issues
- When there is no window of opportunity for the information
- In times when policy makers hold strong values and beliefs
- When there are hidden agendas in the policy situation

For research to shape health policy, it must focus on critical public health issues. In the nursing profession, this is often the case, as nurse investigators ask many questions that focus on their clinical practice and the issues that their patients and families have to confront. As will be noted later, this is an important characteristic of the body of nursing research; the explicit targets are relevant clinical, societal problems. However, research can focus on an important public health issue, but not one that is of policy concern at the time, and thus, there is not a window of opportunity for the use of the findings. For example, patient safety issues are always important health issues but did not come to the attention of policy makers until the IOM (2000) published the report *To Err Is Human: Building a Safer Health System*. This report identified the critical nature of patient safety issues and the need to take a new systems perspective toward adverse events.

There are also times when research is more highly valued by policy makers in some organizations, administrations, and/or congresses than in others (Mecklin, 2009). When such groups hold strong values and beliefs, then research results may be of less value and use. In addition, in some situations, the policy maker(s) may hold a hidden agenda; that is, there is a particular outcome that is desired for the policy issue, e.g., a pet program. In these cases, research is less sought and is not valued unless it substantiates and supports the "hidden agenda."

In summary, discussions with the national health policy influencers were valuable in understanding when science and research are most and least valued for informing health policy. Surfacing a number of the characteristics that allow policy makers to relate to research as being useful and valuable helps to strategize how nursing research might more deliberately shape health policy.

Exploratory Study With Nurse Researchers

The purpose of this exploratory study was to consider more specifically how nursing research shapes health policy. The study used a qualitative approach with a randomly selected sample of nurse researchers with long-term, extramurally funded research programs. These were defined as nurse researchers holding a first or second competing continuation grant award from the NINR from 1986 to 2006. There were a total of 109 such investigators. A random sample of 32 such investigators was drawn. Ultimately, 23 nurse researchers participated in this exploratory study, for a response rate of 72%. The reasons for investigator nonparticipation were the following: an inability to contact the Nurse PI and/or an inability to set up a telephone interview within the time frame of the exploratory study. None of the nurse researchers who were able to be contacted directly within the study time frame declined to participate.

A semistructured questionnaire was used in eliciting the data. Content analysis (Neuendorf, 2002) was the qualitative method of choice. The content analysis was done by question; data responses were categorized with the frequency estimated for how often each type of response was recorded. Three to five of the nurse researchers had to provide a given type of response for the category to be reported. The categories are presented from the highest to the lowest in terms of frequency. The study was approved for human subject protection at the University of Michigan and the IOM.

To explore how nursing research was shaping health policy after two decades of stable, ever-increasing research financial support through the NINR, nurse investigators with long-term research programs were asked four questions. These included the following:

- What characteristics of their nursing research facilitated shaping health policy?
- What external factors assisted their nursing research in influencing health policy?
- What are the barriers that limit their nursing research in shaping health policy?
- What are the various ways that their nursing research has shaped health policy?

What Characteristics of Their Nursing Research Facilitated Shaping Health Policy?

Five categories of characteristics were identified from the nurse investigators' responses to Question 1: "What characteristics of their nursing research facilitated shaping health policy?" (Exhibit 1.1).

The PIs' responses varied from the importance of the public health issues studied to the value of the strong focus on clients, families, and communities in the research. The most frequently cited characteristic of nursing research shaping health policy was that the research addresses major public health issues. This category of responses is consistent with the information elicited from the national health policy influencers, as they also considered one of the most valuable characteristics of research for policy makers to be its relevance to public health issues. As Leavitt et al. (2006) suggest, policy and politics are consistently integrated; thus, research addressing the concerns of policy makers

---

EXHIBIT 1.1   *Characteristics of Nursing Research Shaping Health Policy, Ordered by Frequency of Response (N = 23)*

- Addresses major public health issues
- Research of interest to multiple disciplines and audiences
- Interdisciplinary team of investigators with multiple bodies of knowledge
- Research focused on clients/patients, families, and communities
- Research integrates complexity of health issues

and their constituents is a critical criteria. Nursing research that focuses on major public health issues will, by default, be targeting a number of voters' and society's concerns.

The involvement of interdisciplinary colleagues and ideas in nursing investigations is consistent and observable in the PIs' research programs. Two outcomes of this orientation are evident in the second and third characteristics categories of nursing research characteristic categories shaping health policy. The second category addresses the breath of interest in nursing research that results from the involvement of interdisciplinary colleagues; that is, multiple disciplines are vested in the results and their use. The science that flows from nursing research is also richer because of the several disciplinary perspectives that are involved with the investigations, which, in turn, enhances the science's ability to inform health policy.

The fourth category of responses suggests that an important characteristic of nursing research is the focus on the client, family, and community. This is one of the nursing research characteristics that caught the attention of the *New York Times* report in 1991. The IOM (2000, 2001, 2004) has recommended in a number of reports the need to focus healthcare on the patient and their context (family and community). A number of the nursing research programs were investigating patient safety outcomes and community, as well as school health promotion programs. For example, Gebbie et al. (2000) suggest that policy makers respond to the experiences and perspectives of nurses on health and illness, as well as their focus on clients and their families.

The final category focusing on nursing research characteristics that are valuable in shaping health policy is that the research integrates a complexity of health issues, e.g., a focus on the merger of biobehavioral concepts and indicators. As cited earlier, Gebbie et al. (2000) found in their study of nursing leaders in health policy that they were aware that policy makers appreciate and are attentive to the broad perspective that nursing brings to health and illness experiences. This category reinforces the richness of the evolving nursing research base.

What External Factors Assisted Their Nursing Research in Influencing Health Policy?

Four categories of external factors were cited as facilitating the nurse investigators' research programs to influence health policy (Exhibit 1.2).

A strong supportive research university environment was cited most frequently as assisting nurse investigators in being able to inform health policy with their long-term research programs. Many of the PIs who were interviewed were faculty in research-intensive universities. The presence of research infrastructures such as offices/research centers that assist with the identification of funding sources, grant submission, and grant management facilitated the investigators' success with their research programs. The fourth category of external factors, "Strong visibility by public and colleagues through

---

EXHIBIT 1.2 *External Factors That Facilitate Nursing Research Shaping Health Policy, Ordered by Frequency of Response (N = 23)*

- Based in strong supportive research university environments
- Partnered with multiple disciplines with visibility and access to diverse networks for dissemination
- Timeliness of research in informing major health issue or "window of opportunity"
- Strong visibility by public and colleagues through media attention and marketing of research

media attention, marketing, congressional testimony, and other examples," is also a factor of being in a strong research-intensive environment where resources are heavily invested in highlighting the faculty's research programs.

Being able to partner with multiple disciplines in their research programs was cited often by the nurse investigators as an important external factor to success in using their research to shape health policy. Linking with other disciplines brought access to diverse networks for research dissemination and use, thus increasing the visibility and communication opportunities for sharing their scientific findings. The PIs suggested that this led to opportunities to discuss their research with policy makers and to incorporate their work in organizational and national guidelines for healthcare.

The third most often cited external factor that helped nurse investigators use their research was when the findings from their research program coincided with a policy window of opportunity. Most of the investigators saw this happening by "luck" and were not involved in strategizing or planning for such an event. Just as nurse investigators have targeted their research programs to impact specific practice issues, they need to adopt the same approach to shaping health policy. Nurse investigators need to strategize their research programs to inform policy issues that will evolve from health and healthcare challenges for the next several decades. Such health challenges become policy and policy programs over time.

What Are the Barriers That Limit Their Nursing Research in Shaping Health Policy?

The nurse investigators of long-term research programs identified four categories of barriers that limited their ability to use their research in informing health policy (Exhibit 1.3).

The most frequently cited barrier was lack of congressional interest, which the nurse investigators interpreted as not having a window of opportunity. It could be theorized that although nursing research has matured dramatically in only two decades of stable funding, the field is just entering the stage of investigators planning for long-term research programs that can shape health policy. Another factor involved in being able to take advantage of policy windows of opportunity is to have a larger body of scientific knowledge that nursing leaders can access in providing information for numerous policy situations. This is a matter of the continuing evolution and maturation of the scientific body of nursing knowledge.

"Research not focused on major health concerns" was the next most frequently cited barrier. This finding contradicts the result reported under the nursing research characteristics that are most apt to assist in the use of the science to shape health policy. Several explanations may help to understand these findings. One, early in the establishment of the NCNR (now NINR), nursing research was scattered and focused on individual

---

EXHIBIT 1.3 *Barriers To Nursing Research Shaping Health Policy, Ordered By Frequency Of Response (N = 23)*

- Lack of congressional interest or no "window of opportunity"
- Research not focused on major health concerns
- Lack of economic outcomes
- Lack of research visibility to broader public and policy makers

practice issues that may or may not have reflected major public health issues. The development of the National Nursing Research Agenda and the subsequent NINR Strategic Plans and Areas of Emphasis facilitated the nursing scientific community in defining major public health issues that were also of concern to the nursing profession. Some nurse investigators focused their research programs around National Nursing Research Agenda priorities and the current Areas of Emphasis, whereas others used as criteria for forming their research programs the importance of selecting major public health concerns. A second explanation may be that this barrier seems to refer to not having the right research at the right time. It could relate more to the concept of a missed window of opportunity.

A number of the nurse investigators cited lack of economic outcomes as a barrier to being able to use their research in informing health policy. Many of their research programs provided data on quality outcomes in relation to nursing interventions being tested, but they could not speak to cost–benefit ratios or the cost of their interventions. In the judgment of the nurse investigators, policy makers required economic as well as quality outcomes in considering new health promotion or healthcare programs. The transitional care program of Naylor et al. (2004) for elderly patients and families provides information on the quality indicators for the clients and identifies the costs of transitional care.

The least frequently cited barrier was the lack of research visibility to the broader public and to policy makers. This was considered a major challenge for the future, how to enhance the visibility of nursing research and present it in a manner that it attracts the attention of health policy makers and those who influence such decision makers.

What Are the Various Ways That Their Nursing Research Has Shaped Health Policy?

The nurse investigators with long-term research programs suggested that their research had informed health policy in a number of ways. The manner in which nursing research shaped health policy was categorized in five areas, which are presented in order of the most to least frequent (Exhibit 1.4).

The five categories of ways nursing research informed health policy are indicative of the level of health policy that was influenced, except for one area, i.e., shaping health science policy. The most frequently cited way of informing health policy was informing organizational patient care policies. Often, these studies were also influential at a broader level. Metheny's chapter in this book, " From Bedside to Bench to Practice," changed a number of organizational patient policies on nasal-gastric tube placement while also being written into nursing and healthcare textbooks for several

---

EXHIBIT 1.4 *Ways of Shaping Health Policy Through Nursing Research, Ordered by Frequency of Response (N = 23)*

- Informed local practice in acute care organizations, such as hospitals
- Informed national health guidelines and standards
- Shaped health science policy
- Informed national health policy through federal agencies, congressional testimony, and Institute of Medicine citations
- Shaped state health policy

disciplines. Thus, the informing of health policy was at a local organizational level for hospitals across the country and at the national level through influencing educational processes.

A number of nurse investigators provided information on how they had been involved in developing different national health guidelines and standards. They were asked to be part of such processes based on their research expertise and programs of research. In addition, they were able to use their research findings in forming national guidelines. From a broad perspective, examples included shaping National Quality Forum documents, developing cancer pain guidelines, and generating national and international ambulatory guidelines for urinary incontinence (UI).

The third most frequently cited way for shaping health policy was different. This category refers to nursing research that influenced science policy. By definition, science policy refers to decisions and statements articulating the scientific directions and programs of institutions, associations, and/or local, state, national, and international governments. Such policy directs priorities for research programs and resource distribution. Examples from the interviewees generally related to aspects of an investigator's research that stimulated a Call for Proposals based on the importance of elaborating understanding of the scientific area. Another example was an institute intramural program of research that began in order to enhance one of the nurse investigators' program of study. In both of these examples, the nurse investigators had important programs of research that needed expansion in multiple directions and were involved in planning for the new science policy programs. Feetham's chapter in this text, "The Role of Science Policy on Programs of Research and Scholarship," provides multiple examples of how science policy is shaped and how, in turn, it informs health policy.

The fourth most frequently cited way for nursing research shaping health policy was to inform national health policy. The investigators cited multiple examples for this category, including consulting for federal agencies, providing congressional testimony on behalf of different professional associations, and having their research cited in IOM synthesis of research reports. In these cases, the investigators' involvement in consultation or testimony for congress or the IOM was based on their research expertise and sharing their research findings.

The least cited category of ways nursing research informed health policy was through shaping state health policy. The research program of Aiken et al. (2002) on the effect of organizational work environment on nurse and patient outcomes is an example of influencing state health policy. Several states, such as California, have passed legislation for patient–nurse ratios based on this scholarly work.

In summary, experienced nurse investigators provided a number of ways in which nursing research is shaping health policy at multiple levels. The ability to identify the nursing research characteristics that assist in informing health policy as well as the external factors and barriers that are part of nursing research's relationship to health policy are critical features in being able to explicitly plan and teach the processes for future generations.

General Themes Identified in Exploratory Study

Two broad themes were identified by the nurse investigators regarding nursing research and health policy. First was the need to educate nurse scientists about health policy. More specifically, they were concerned that as investigators, they did not have explicit knowledge of strategies and processes through which their research program findings could be used to inform health policy. Although doctoral programs in nursing do offer courses and content on health policy, models, strategies, and processes, understanding their relationship to individual research programs and planning for shaping health policy, as well as nursing practice, are rare. Only a limited number of the experienced nurse investigators interviewed stated that they consistently strategized and planned for how their research program findings could be influential over time. A number of nurse scholars have been concerned about this issue (e.g., Gebbie et al., 2000; Leavitt et al., 2006). This is an issue for both research and advanced practice doctoral graduates in nursing because the research-prepared doctoral individuals need to plan how the findings of their evolving research programs can inform health policy while the individuals with advanced practice doctorates will be teaming with them to translate research findings into health policy at multiple levels.

Second, the nurse investigators were concerned about needing a "Broker" system for moving research into health policy. Such a broker system could take multiple forms, e.g., organizational think tanks, professional associations, and doctorally prepared advanced practice nurses, who have an explicit objective for translating science to practice and health policy. An example of a formal organization that assumes this role is the IOM. The mandate of the IOM is as "Advisor to the Nation's Health." A great deal of their activity is directed at synthesizing multiple research studies from numerous disciplines to provide information for and elucidate what is known about specific policy issues and strategies as well as recommendations on how to handle them. The report *Keeping Patients Safe: Transforming the Work Environment of Nursing* (IOM, 2004) is an example of providing models, synthesized research, and recommendations on how the work environment and conditions of nurses influence patient safety. Sampselle's chapter in this text illustrates how a professional association was able to translate nursing research on UI into organizational patient care policies and into national guidelines on UI. In the future, as the cadre of Doctorate of Nursing Practice clinical scholars increases, these individuals, teamed with their research doctorally prepared colleagues, could also serve as brokers for moving the science of the discipline into both practice and health policy (Hinshaw, 2009).

Science shaping health policy is of concern to multiple disciplines and to society in order to be assured of health policies based on evidence from research. Whereas health policy reflects the influence of many factors, it is important in considering health decisions to have one of those factors be research. In addition, the research needs to bring multiple perspectives and reflect many disciplines. Nursing research, after almost 25 years of stable federal support, is clearly addressing important public health issues and providing information both to elucidate the health policy issues but also possible strategies for resolution.

Nursing research seems to have several of the major characteristics that national health policy influencers suggest make the information useable by policy decision makers. These characteristics include addressing major public health issues; focusing on the person, on his or her family, and on communities; and teaming with other disciplines to reflect a richness in the knowledge and perspective available to the policy process. The early promise of nursing research, as pointed out in the 1991 *New York Times* article "Beyond Tender Loving Care, Nurses Are a Force in Research" is being fulfilled. There is now evidence of the growth of the evolving knowledge base for the discipline and the ability of nursing research to shape both nursing practice (Hinshaw, Shaver, & Feetham, 1999) and health policy.

ACKNOWLEDGMENTS

The author thanks Drs. Suzanne L. Feetham and Patricia A. Grady for their systematic and thorough review of this chapter.

REFERENCES

Aiken, L. H., Clarke, S. P., Sloane, D. M., Sochalski, J., Silber, J. H. (2002). Hospital nurse staffing and patient mortality, nurse burnout and job dissatisfaction. *Journal of the American Medical Association, 288*, 1987–1993.

Birkland, T. A. (2005). *An introduction to the policy process: Theories, concepts and models of public policy making* (2nd ed.). Armonk, NY: M. E. Sharpe.

Block, L. E. (2004). Health policy: What it is and how it works. In C. Harrington & C. L. Estes (Eds.), *Health policy: Crisis and reform in the U. S. health care delivery system* (4th ed., pp. 4–14). Sudbury, MA: Jones and Bartlett Publishers.

Brody, J. (1991, August 13). Beyond tender loving care, nurses area force in research. *The New York Times.* Retrieved from http://www.nytimes.com

Dickson, G. L., & Flynn, L. (2009). *Nursing policy research: Turning evidence-based research into health policy.* New York: Springer Publishing Co.

Fawcett, J., & Russell, G. (2001). A conceptual model of nursing and health policy. *Policy, Politics & Nursing Practice, 2*(2), 108–116.

Feetham, S. L., & Meister, S. B. (1999). Nursing research of families: State of the science and correspondence with policy. In A. S. Hinshaw, S. L. Feetham, & J. L. F. Shaver (Eds.). *Handbook of clinical nursing research* (pp. 251–271). Thousand Oaks, CA: SAGE Publications.

Gebbie, K. M., Wakefield, M., & Kerfoot, K. (2000). Nursing and health policy. *Journal of Nursing Scholarship,* Third Quarter, 307–315.

Harrington, C., & Estes, C. L. (2004). *Health policy: Crisis and reform in the U. S. health care delivery system* (4th ed.). Sudbury, MA: Jones and Bartlett Publishers.

Hinshaw, A. S. (1988). Using research to shape health policy. *Nursing Outlook, 36*(1), 21–24.

Hinshaw, A. S. (1992). The impact of nursing science on health policy. *Communicating Nursing Research, 25*, 15–26.

Hinshaw, A. S. (2009, January). *Preparing doctoral students for health policy leadership.* Paper presented at the meeting of the American Association of Colleges of Nursing, 2009. Doctoral Education Conference. San Diego, CA.

Hinshaw, A. S., Shaver, J., & Feetham, S. L. (1999). *Handbook of clinical nursing research.* Thousand Oaks, CA: Sage Publishing Co.

Institute of Medicine. (2000). *To err is human: Building a safer health system.* Washington, DC: The National Academies Press.

Institute of Medicine. (2001). *Crossing the quality chasm: A new health system for the 21st century.* Washington, DC: The National Academies Press.

Institute of Medicine. (2004). *Keeping patients safe: Transforming the work environment of nurses.* Washington, DC: The National Academies Press.

Leavitt, J. K., Chaffee, M. W., & Mason, D. J. (2006). *Policy and politics in nursing and health care* (4th ed.). St. Louis: Saunders.

Longest, B. B. (1998). *Health policy making in the United States* (2nd ed.). Chicago: Health Administration Press.

Mecklin, J. (2009). The science of good government. *Miller-McCune,* July–August, 8–11.

Melynk, B., & Fineout-Overholt, E. (2005). *Evidence-based practice in nursing and healthcare.* Philadelphia: Lippincott Williams & Wilkins.

Milio, N. (1984). Nursing research and the study of health policy. *Annual Review of Nursing Research, 2,* 291–305.

Milio, N. (1989). Developing nursing leadership in health policy. *Journal of Professional Nursing, 5*(6), 315–321.

Milstead, J. A. (2004). *Health policy and politics: A nurse's guide* (2nd ed.). Sudbury, MA: Jones and Bartlett Publishers.

Naylor, M. D., Brooten D. A., Campbell, R. L., Maislin, G., McCauley, K. M., & Schwartz, J. S. (2004). Transitional care of older adults hospitalized with heart failure: A randomized clinical trial. *Journal of the American Geriatrics Society, 52*(5), 675–684.

Neuendorf, K. A. (2002). *The content analysis guidebook.* Thousand Oaks, CA: Sage Publications, Inc.

Richmond, J., & Kotelchuck, M. (1983). Political influences: Rethinking national health policy. In C. H. McGuire, R. P. Foley, A. Gorr, R. W. Richards, & Associates (Eds.). *Handbook of health professions education* (pp. 386–404). San Francisco: Jossey-Bass.

Shamain, J., Skelton-Green, J., & Villeneuve, M. (2003). Policy is the lever for effecting change. In M. McIntyres & E. Thomlison (Eds.). *Realities of Canadian nursing: Professional and practice's power issues* (pp. 83–104). Philadelphia: Lippincott, Williams and Wilkin.

2

Research: A Foundation for Health Policy

Patricia A. Grady

INTRODUCTION

Policies help to guide our behavior and priorities within society. Policy can be considered from many perspectives, and different types of policies permeate our lives in a variety of ways: public policy, social policy, health policy, institutional policy, and organizational policy (Mason, Leavitt, & Chaffee, 2007; Dickson & Flynn, 2009). Those in health science disciplines are in the unique position to influence most or all of these policy types within their professional and personal spheres. Nurses can and should be involved in health-related public policy (International Council of Nurses, 2000).

Within the healthcare delivery system, policies assume a primary role related to human safety and well-being. The circumstances accompanying policy change or creation can vary markedly. Policies can be formulated by design or by convention, by political or situational influences, or by hard core data or compelling anecdotes. In an ideal world, policy is formulated by evidence or data that inform or point the way toward best solutions or strategies. There is a recognition that, over the past several decades, research has had a modest influence on policy making (Chelimsky, 1991; Weiss, 1977, 1988) but that current circumstances favor the value of research in policy making (McCall, 2009). With the coming of age of nursing research, we have a new opportunity and a new imperative to generate and implement the results of well-designed studies to provide the foundation for evidence-based practice and policies.

GENERAL CONTRIBUTIONS OF NURSING RESEARCH

Our healthcare system will encounter new and significant challenges as we face the future. With the advent of the 21st century, a dramatic change in our demographics is becoming apparent. Our population continues to grow, to age, and to become more culturally and ethnically diverse. Many diseases that were once acute and life-threatening, such as heart disease, diabetes, and HIV, are now treated as long-term and chronic conditions. In addition, the long-term effects of endemic problems such as poverty and poor nutrition are evident. New global health threats continue to emerge along with reemerging threats that were thought to have been conquered, such as tuberculosis and malaria.

Nursing research gained a significant place in our nation's science and healthcare enterprise with the founding of the National Center for Nursing Research on the campus of the National Institutes of Health (NIH) in 1986. The National Center for Nursing Research began to address the pressing research needs for nursing at that time, and by 1994, it became the National Institute of Nursing Research (NINR). The research done by the pioneering nursing scientists has begun to establish the foundation for evidence-based practice and evidence-based policy. The year 2010 will mark the institute's 25th anniversary at the NIH.

Research carried out by scientists and primarily supported by the federal government and private organizations continues to be vital in addressing the wide-ranging and ongoing health needs of our nation. Nurses, as the largest group of health professionals at 2.9 million in the United States alone, have a particular opportunity to identify health issues in greatest need of attention by clinical and basic researchers. In part, this relates to the unique importance of the nursing profession in identifying the needs of patients and their families. Nurses can communicate effectively with the various members of the health team and patients, the former in the technical language of science and medicine and the latter in terms understood by the general public. It is our sincerest hope that the foundation of solid science that these scientists have built over the past several decades and that they continue to generate as we go forward will contribute heavily in meeting the local, national, and global healthcare challenges the years to come.

Creating a healthier America—improving the public health and the delivery of healthcare—is not easy, but our nation has put this goal at the forefront of our national agenda. Over the years, it has become clear that the health of an individual is closely linked to the broader health of the community—the health of the community where individuals live, work, and play (Healthy People, 1990; World Health Organization, 2008; Oregon Health Fund Board). Health promotion and prevention are hallmarks of nursing research and its application to clinical practice.

By the same token, community health is profoundly affected by the collective beliefs, attitudes, and behaviors of everyone who resides in the community. To reemphasize, individual health is inseparable from the health of the larger community, and the health of every community in every state and territory determines the overall health status of our nation. And the health of nations, both resource rich and resource poor, determines the global health.

In 1990, for the Healthy People initiative, we came together to articulate a national vision—a vision that has helped to stimulate the creation of subsequent national frameworks that have guided our efforts in improving the health of our nation. This vision is carried through in Healthy People 2010, and we carry it with us in our current efforts to advance the health of our nation. This vision is reflected from the corridors of the Congress to the corridors of schools and community centers. Community-based and school-based approaches that are widely used by nurse clinicians and researchers in testing out and implementing health improvement interventions can be viewed as resulting from such frameworks (Gross et al., 2009; Gross, Sambrook, & Fogg, 1999; Hill et al., 2003; Harrell et al., 1996).

We know that much remains to be done, that while we make advances on certain fronts, new challenges arise and other challenges persist or recur, such as the continuing disparities in healthcare in our society and the escalating costs at all levels. Every generation has faced comparable challenges, and the health and welfare of our nation and the health of our citizens and communities are some of the most critical challenges of our generation. How we meet these challenges will determine the health and well-being of generations to come. Our hope is that evidence-based practice and evidence-based policy will be available to meet these challenges. It is up to the members of the healthcare cadre to make this happen (McClellan et al., 2007). The nursing profession has a vital role to play in meeting these challenges.

Today, stakeholders are demonstrating an increasing interest in the policies that influence their daily lives. Reflective of evolutions in social interactions and technologies, our framework for advancing the nation's health in the next decade and beyond will incorporate an ever-expansive public dialogue, as health forums are held across the nation, as interactive technologies allow us to share our ideas and ingenuity on unprecedented scales, and as we strive, as a nation, to develop a healthcare system that successfully promotes the health of all members of our society. Activities such as these provide unprecedented opportunities to participate in policy making.

WAYS IN WHICH NURSING RESEARCH IS USEFUL IN HEALTH POLICY PROCESSES

Health policy can emerge from a variety of sources. Research studies, practice guidelines, community preferences, and information from practice-based settings may all play a role in the process. Thus, being able to think broadly and then generalize from research results is a key step in paving the way for change. Nursing research, with its emphases on behavior as a predicate for good health, symptom management in chronic illness, health promotion, health disparities, and caregiving, is ideally suited for the policy issues facing us today and for centuries to come.

Although we focus primarily on national policy as the first step, many of the same factors operate also on a global level. As our society becomes increasingly diverse and multicultural, our ability to understand and accommodate the needs of ethnically and culturally diverse groups must be enhanced. In regard to this, Madon et al. urged investigators to develop quantitative, scientific frameworks to guide healthcare "scale-up" in developing countries (Madon et al., 2007, p. 1728). This scaling up is best informed by evidence-based knowledge generated from well-designed clinical studies.

Unlike traditional research paradigms, which identify and address barriers related to the performance of specific projects, Madon et al. stress "implementation science" that creates generalizable knowledge that can be applied across settings and contexts and addresses those questions that will translate research into local communities of practice. But despite formidable gaps between innovations in healthcare and the delivery of findings to the communities in the world, "action-based," "community-based," "participatory" research lies at the very core of nursing science (Ledogar, Acosta, & Penchaszadeh, 1999). Rosenkoetter and Nardi (2006, 2007), in an American Academy of Nursing Brief, eloquently reiterate this point, stating, "International researchers need to demonstrate how their products increase the research capacity so desperately needed in developing countries, and develop models to facilitate international research participation and exchanges (Rosenkoetter and Nardi 2006, p. 114)." It is clear that as we look to build international communities of research, we must go beyond traditional methods of the conduct of science and become advocates for participatory, action-oriented initiatives that link neighborhoods with effective, evidence-based healthcare research. These efforts will bring science into transcultural, evidence-based programs that will engage the participation and acceptance of practice communities.

Nursing research can be helpful in health policy processes at virtually every juncture, from changing practice at the bedside to changing policy in the halls of the Congress. From the health practices that are taught to parents of small children to faculty who are teaching the next generations of health professionals, from assisted living to hospice, from adult housing communities to community centers, nurses have the broadest reach of all professionals, and those who are scientists have the opportunity to rewrite the future.

UNDERSTANDING HOW TO INFLUENCE POLICY

Policy making is a complex process, and health policy can be even more complicated. There are many players and influences to understand in order to access the system. The system itself is composed of checks and balances, which provide for differing strategies. There are many points of access, and each of these points can be associated with success. Primarily, the institutions include federal, state, and local governments in the public sector and healthcare providers, purchasers, industries, and consumers in the private sector. Professional societies and health advocacy groups are also major players in facilitating policy change. Any of these groups mentioned can be involved throughout the process, and collectively, they may all be involved depending on the scope and interest of the policy change being contemplated. However, depending on the magnitude of the change under consideration, it is likely that only a smaller number of parties may be involved at any one time. Although this may seem unnecessarily complicated, the system is designed to provide for checks and balances. Despite what may seem like deterrents to change, the system is designed to provide for thoughtful deliberation and interactive analysis. It is important to have an understanding of the structure and process of the organization, national, regional, or local, to best be able to influence changes in policy.

When America was founded, it was informed by a system of separation of powers and of checks and balances. This has the advantage of providing many points of access for making change, and it also prevents change from occurring too rapidly during a time when passions shed more heat than light on critical problems of the day. The latter sometimes proves frustrating for those who call for urgent change, but it also provides time for deliberation and exposition of differing points of view. In the United States, there are the legislative, executive, and judicial branches of the government. This was intended to create a separation of powers that govern. The Congress is the primary legislative or policy-making branch, whereas the executive branch is primarily responsible for implementing policies. The judicial branch is principally dedicated to resolving constitutional and legal conflicts. Interestingly, according to the Constitution, both the president and the executive branches of government are charged with implementing policies approved by the Congress (Patel & Rushefsky, 2006).

A familiar example of how this operates is that of the NINR. The NINR is part of the NIH, which is a component of the Department of Health and Human Services (DHHS). The secretary of the DHHS is a political appointee and reports directly to the president of the United States. The DHHS is a part of the executive branch of the government. As such, the director of the NINR works for and ultimately reports to the president of the

United States as well. Scientists who interface with the NINR are not always aware that when budget testimony is presented to the Congress, the director is actually testifying on behalf of the president's budget for the institute. Any other position on the budget could be viewed as lobbying and is in fact illegal. In a typical scenario, the NINR director testifies yearly before both the House and Senate Appropriations committees, who then each craft their own version of the budget bill. The two branches of the Congress then meet to try to reconcile their respective versions and produce a Conference bill, which is usually a compromise or composite stemming from their two bills. The conference bill is then presented to the president, who either signs or vetoes the bill. When the final bill is signed by the president, it then becomes law, and we have a budget for the coming fiscal year. Halfway through each fiscal year, the process begins again for the following fiscal year.

In actual fact, the budget for the NINR, as for the other NIH institutes, is a line item in the budget bill. In effect, the NINR and other NIH institutes receive their budget from the Congress (with the approval of the president), not from the NIH director, as is commonly (and understandably) believed. The NIH director can influence the budget with the Congress and also has a discretionary budget available for special programs that he or she wishes to stimulate, which generally span the missions of the institutes and centers across the NIH. Examples of this have included the Shannon Awards, Areas of Emphasis, and Roadmap programs (Garnett, 2004).

Private citizens have the right and are, in fact, encouraged to make their wishes known to their Congressional representatives in both the House and the Senate. Elected representatives are very sensitive to the needs of their constituents, who have placed them in their respective positions through the elective process and whom they wish to serve in those positions. Congressional offices are established in home districts and states, and members of the Congress spend time in these offices meeting with constituents and traveling throughout their states and districts in order to keep their fingers on the pulse of the people they represent. This time spent at home provides many opportunities for constituents, including scientists, to relate their messages to elected officials. Since nurse scientists have a major role in improving the health of the American people, elected officials are typically very receptive to hearing what these researchers have to say.

The idea of communicating to the Congress is an important one and can be facilitated in many ways. Knowing how to craft messages to reach Congressional members is an acquired skill. Since Congressional time is limited, it is important to consider the type of message that will best communicate the issue you wish to bring forward. This message should be concise, bulleted, and memorable. The time available is often about 15 minutes, and it is important to make the most of it. A number of organizations have detailed reference guidelines for visiting your members of the Congress and tend to be very helpful. Examples of such guidelines include those provided by the American Association of Colleges of Nursing, American Association of Medical Colleges, and Society for Neuroscience. Many universities and colleges also have staff liaisons to the Congress. Many of the larger universities even have a Washington office to facilitate Congressional interface. All these avenues are useful to explore before setting off on a mission. One other consideration is that, even if you meet with a Congressman, the person you may really be talking to is the congressional staff. Staffers are usually assigned to offices for short terms, extremely energetic, incredibly hardworking, well-informed, and committed to carrying out the goals of the congressional representative they work for. They can be helpful to constituents, and they should be treated well.

Local Versus National Politics

It is a well-known truism that "all politics is local," and it is a useful guide when considering effecting a policy change. Identify pressing issues on a national level, but consider how one might create change in a familiar environment. Many of the same constraints and operative issues are likely to be similar. Moreover, the key players will be familiar, and what factors they are likely to respond to or want will be more apparent to you. Making local change in a hospital, community, or organization can often serve as a useful pilot for taking your ideas or models to a larger scale or audience.

CONSIDERATIONS FOR INFLUENCING HEALTH POLICY

Health policy has grown to encompass prevention and wellness as well as care delivery. Contemporary health promotion requires more than simply educating individuals about healthy practices. It includes efforts to change organizational behavior, as well as the physical and social environment of communities. It is also about developing and advocating for policies that support health, such as economic incentives (U.S. DHHS, 2005).

Influencing policy is facilitated when approached early in the planning process. When thinking about doing research that will change policy or practice, it is important to consider the following points.

What Is the Need? Where Is the Gap?

This is an area where the clinician–researcher partnership is crucial. Clinical nurses see researchable problems on a daily basis, and together, researchers and clinicians can quickly establish which of these areas is most important, feasible for study, and likely to be implemented.

Who Is the Patient Population? Who Will Benefit From This Change and How Wide Will the Effect Be?

The larger the potential patient population, the greater is the potential impact and, often, the potential for implementation. The potential impact is also increased when working with special populations, such as women, children, underserved minority, and rural populations, because their health needs have been historically understudied, so the need for information is greater in many areas.

What Level of Evidence Is Required?

The level of evidence required may depend on a variety of influencing factors, ranging from the best evidence to the most readily available evidence. Time frames during which issues are thought to have a life span may also be a major influencing factor.

There are many good references and texts that have considered this issue in detail (LoBiondo-Wood & Haber, 2010; Melnyk & Fineout-Overholt, 2005; Polit & Beck, 2008). In general, it is accepted that the seven levels (level I being the best) in an evidence hierarchy include the following: Level VII, opinions of authorities and expert communities; Level VI, single descriptive or qualitative study; Level V, systematic review of descriptive and qualitative studies; Level IV, single correlational observational study; Level III, systematic review of correlational/observational studies; Level IIa, single randomized controlled trial (RCT); Level IIb, single nonrandomized trial; Level Ia, systematic review of RCTs; and Level Ib, systematic review of nonrandomized RCTs.

In addition to levels of quality of evidence, other perspectives encompass components of robustness, which include credibility, generalizability, reliability, objectivity, and rootedness (Shaxson, 2005) or standards for efficacy, effectiveness, and dissemination (Flay et al., 2005). Since nothing is ever proven beyond a shadow of a doubt or with absolute certainty, it is important to select reasonable criteria within an appropriate context and to make known both the context and the criteria that are used.

What Level of Evidence Is Already Available From the Literature and Evidence-Based Studies?

Two issues are of importance here: first, knowledge of what has already been done and, second, consideration of how the proposed project will fit into the larger body of knowledge. With regard to the first, most are familiar with Medline, CINAHL, The Cochrane Library, and other major resources for conducting literature searches. It is also useful to determine whether any major reports or consensus conferences have been done in your area of interest from the NIH in Bethesda, Maryland, or the Institute of Medicine of the National Academy of Sciences in Washington, DC. The Brookings Institute, the Rand Corporation, and other large think tanks often have publications of interest related to health and health policy. These sources are helpful in assessing what has been done and often include recommendations for future needs. Information sources such as these are helpful with regard to the second consideration mentioned, the assessment of how any potential effort will fit into and contribute to the available body of knowledge. Identifying a need or gap is important, but in order to maximize the full impact of a planned study or the results of one, it is important to be able to place it in a broader context. An example of this is seen in studies using the Transitional Care Model (Naylor et al., 2004), which has been successful in several patient populations. Using those early successes, subsequent studies are now moving it closer to policy and practice. This is explicated in detail in a later chapter, but a key point was matching the design with a significant health system need. In a representative study, the patient population selected was the elderly with "common medical and surgical conditions," which was coincidental with those conditions that represented the top 10 in Medicare reimbursement. This information generated from the study would potentially be of interest to third-party payers. Thus, from the outset, it could be expected that if results were positive, they had the potential to improve the quality of life for a large segment of our elderly citizens as well as the potential for substantial cost savings to our health-care system.

Who Needs to Know About the Results and How Do I Reach Them?

Defining the population of interest is critical in each step of the process to change health practice and policy. It is important in refining the question being asked, in identifying and recruiting subjects to participate, in enlisting effective advocates, and in disseminating the results. Increasingly, new technologies, databases, and communication modalities exist to facilitate this process. Examples are seen in health promotion programs that seek to address health problems across this spectrum employing a range of strategies and operating on multiple levels (U.S. DHHS, 2005). With the advent of communication technologies including the Internet, PDAs such as the Blackberry and the iPhone, and social marketing approaches, there are a range of innovative possibilities to assist with this challenge.

Who Are My Allies in This Endeavor? Who Will Be Able to Help Accomplish This Change? Who Are the Interested Parties and What Is Their Specific Interest?

Interdisciplinary, experienced people who have successes and lessons learned and who have an interest in the outcome are on this list. This will often include private–public partnerships and academic ones. Community leaders are important in these endeavors and can become part of the team in creative ways.

What Can Be Done to Facilitate Translation? Is It Possible to Design a Study With Translation in Mind?

When designing a study, it is useful to consider these questions. In addition to designing the study according to sound research principles, it is important to consider what might facilitate the translation of the results. For example, if you are testing ways to check for accurate feeding tube placement as described in detail later, the easier to administer and more portable the test, the more widespread positive impact the results are likely to have. In other words, a complicated test would, at best, be used in critical care settings and, possibly, step-down units but would be less likely to be used at home or by family members. Likewise, if a strategy is successful in a research study but is difficult to implement, its likelihood of getting into practice is limited. Factors that influence this include, but are not limited to, unreasonable limitations on lifestyle; decrease in quality of life; uncomfortable, painful, or unpleasant side effects; or unacceptable costs. An interesting analogy to consider is a lesson taken from our basic science colleagues, who often do their studies in animal models. They have learned that when using model systems, the closer the model is to the human condition, the greater is the likelihood of translating their successes into the clinical setting.

What Role Does Timing Play?

Clearly, an important part of the process of identifying an area for study is looking at areas of need, but timeliness influences the receptivity for most ideas. Any area is more likely to garner interest or attention if it affects a large segment of the population or a specialized segment, such as the underserved. Timing is an aspect that should be considered when trying to maximize the potential for change. This can mean anticipating an impending change or being opportunistic when a change occurs unexpectedly. Most major changes seem to be influenced by fortunate or unfortunate timing. Timing favors the impact that a study can have if it addresses an emerging problem such as HIV/AIDS in the late 1980s and 1990s or end of life during the emergence of assisted suicide, because the interest is heightened during these periods. A current example of this includes the enhanced interest in chronic illness and end-of-life issues that have emerged with the aging of our population.

Certain practical matters are important as well. The Congressional schedule of when the Congress is in session, the budget cycle, and the election cycle are all contributors to the receptivity levels.

Networks and Influence Groups

Another important aspect of creating policy change is the effective utilization of networks and influence groups, including professional societies, community, and advocacy groups. Aspects to consider are briefly reviewed in the following paragraphs.

Professional Societies

There may be a tendency to endow governmental bodies with the primary responsibility for change. Surely, the government has a critical role. Yet professional societies can be very powerful agents for change because they have a central mission in which members are invested, and these groups often have memberships of considerable size. Professional societies frequently have well-developed and highly skilled components that address ways to monitor and influence policy in areas of interest to their constituents. Grassroots efforts in legislative activities are informed and encouraged. Membership training seminars and information are available to assist members with regard to legislative processes and ways to access public policy systems. Excellent examples of such member guides include *A Guide to Grassroots Activism* (American Association of Colleges of Nursing, 1998) and *Guide to Public Advocacy* (Society for Neuroscience; www.sfn.org).

Community Groups

It is important to consider that every citizen has a role in formulating policy. Whether it is exercised through active involvement or ceded to others by noninvolvement, the potential for creating remarkable change does exist. Often, the potential is realized only when the occasion arises, such as seen in the potential of building toxic waste dumps or building superhighways through prized neighborhoods. Recalling the dictum "all politics is local," nurses, as an important part of the fabrics of the communities in which they live, have an almost unmatched opportunity to tap into the grassroots network to help bring about change. In fact, nurses, who typically top public opinion polls (Gallup Polls; Harris Polls) as the most trusted healthcare professionals, occupy a unique position of trust and respect in communities and are often consulted with regard to health issues.

Increasingly, the public is becoming more involved in issues they care about. In efforts to reform healthcare, Health Care Community Discussions were held across all 50 states and the District of Columbia, in which there were more than 9,000 participants. Friends, families, neighbors, and coworkers came together in homes, offices, coffee shops, fire houses, universities, and community centers with a common purpose: to discuss reforming the healthcare system. The DHHS collected and analyzed the data from these initial discussions and published the results in March 2009 in *Americans Speak on Health Reform: Report on Health Care Community Discussions*. The input from participants in the Health Care Community Discussions and similar forums is increasingly being used to frame our national policy needs. Public input continues to be needed to inform the Congressional and executive initiatives that support and achieve healthcare reform.

Another example of a national forum for civic participation is HealthReform.gov, where citizens can provide input and comments on health reform online or in "face-to-face meetings." However, a third ongoing policy initiative is Healthy People 2020. As part of this initiative, public participation is being gathered through meetings and online venues to engage citizens and to integrate their ideas and innovations into the Healthy People 2020 strategic plan.

Translation and Communication

One of the major challenges in the translation of research into practice and policy is developing effective strategies. This is where considering the target audience and avoiding putting up barriers before the onset of the research are important. Having considered this in the design of the study gives the researcher an advantage, but there are still challenges to face. Communication of the information is critical. Simply stated, what to say and where to say it are the key. One of the first challenges is to publish the results where they will reach the largest proportion of the audience who will be interested in and/or impacted by the results. This may mean publishing in what were traditionally referred to as "nonnursing" journals, or clinical journals. Another strategy, rather than choosing the either/or approach, is to consider that most robust studies have several strong components and look for the portions of the study that are most appropriate to different audiences and different journals. However, another complementary approach is to publish a plain-language version for association newsletters, general publications, and community-oriented publications. For example, the most highly cited publication list has often been headed by the recently retired *Reader's Digest*. Although *Reader's Digest* is not a scientific journal, it has been a widely read journal, by virtue of the fact that it was created to reach a broad, general audience. Therefore, any items that appear in a publication of this type will be viewed by a large cross-section of the populace and are likely to have high visibility with less time and effort required than with many other strategies.

Successful Application of Strategies[1]

The following research studies that have been successful in influencing policy have considered and incorporated important strategic principles previously mentioned. Later chapters of this book examine in detail some illustrative case studies of linking research to policy. The following are brief examples that provide a basis for the later stories and case studies. These mini-examples highlight the importance of asking strategic research

---

[1] Adapted from *Changing Practice, Changing Lives* (2005).

questions that address barriers to optimal care or prevention. They also show how researchers strategically link their research management with the policy process.

Identifying a Significant Clinical Problem

In applying these principles, Drs. Nancy Bergstom and Barbara Braden identified a *major health problem*, that of pressure ulcers, and moved from the clinical setting to policy setting in a remarkably short period of time.

Pressure sores, also known as pressure ulcers or bed sores, represent a serious health problem in hospitals, nursing homes, and other healthcare settings. These sores develop when a bedridden or otherwise immobilized patient remains in one position for too long. More than 4 million people develop pressure sores each year, primarily the elderly and persons suffering a major injury or disease, adding roughly $9 billion in annual healthcare costs. Pressure sores also complicate patient care and delay recovery. The best treatment for pressure sores is prevention, and improved methods of assessment can help identify individuals at risk for pressure sores before they develop.

These investigators developed and tested the Braden Scale for Predicting Pressure Sore Risk.

This instrument is designed to help healthcare providers determine a patient's risk for pressure sores by assessing six parameters: ability to change positions, physical activity capability, nutrition and hydration status, exposure of the skin to moisture, exposure of the skin to friction or shearing during movement, and the ability to sense and respond to pressure-related discomfort. Findings supported the predictive value of the Braden scale to identify those patients at high risk for pressure sores.

The Braden scale is now widely used in nursing homes and hospitals all over the world due to a series of strategic activities. Dr. Bergstrom has chaired two panels of the Agency for Health Care Policy and Research, now the Agency for Healthcare Research and Quality, to determine best practice on pressure sore prevention. Her research and knowledge was instrumental in writing *Pressure Ulcers in Adults: Prediction and Prevention* and *Pressure Ulcer Treatment*, from which the current Agency for Healthcare Research and Quality clinical guidelines for prevention and treatment of pressure sores were developed (Bergstrom, Braden, Kemp, Champagne, & Ruby, 1996).

Building Upon and Enhancing Seminal Work

Another example of strategic planning is the work of Dr. Margaret Grey, who identified a *significant clinical problem*, adapted the study design for a *specialized population* (teenagers), and built upon and *enhanced previous work* of other disciplines.

It is significant that Type 1 diabetes, a disease that affects how the body uses sugar for energy, is one of the most prevalent chronic conditions among the young, affecting over 200,000 children and adolescents in the United States. However, diabetes management, which involves frequent testing of blood sugar levels and injections of insulin, often proves very difficult among adolescents. Uncontrolled, diabetes can lead to problems such as poor circulation, high blood pressure (HBP), kidney damage, and blindness. Research on teenagers with diabetes has shown that they have difficulties in diabetes management, often in association with social situations involving peer pressure and fear of being seen as different.

Dr. Margaret Grey developed and tested an intervention called Coping Skills Training (CST) to improve diabetic teenagers' coping and communication skills, healthy behaviors, and conflict resolution, in conjunction with routine diabetes management. This program was designed to increase teenagers' sense of competence and mastery by redirecting inappropriate or nonconstructive coping styles into more positive behavior patterns.

CST's effectiveness was tested in an RCT in teenagers with Type 1 diabetes. Both the control and study groups received usual care. The teenagers in the intervention group also received CST in small class sessions, using role playing to explore common, difficult situations that they might face with friends. These included issues such as managing food choices, making decisions about drugs and alcohol, and facing interpersonal conflicts.

Both groups were followed for a year to assess their diabetes control and quality of life. Compared with teenagers in the control group, the teenagers who received CST maintained better metabolic control and showed a significant improvement in long-term blood sugar levels and reported a better quality of life (Grey, Davidson, Boland, & Tamborlane, 2001).

Using Clinical Expertise to Translate

Relying on her background as a nurse practitioner, Dr. Grey has facilitated the translation of these results into practice. So far, over 100 practices that manage the care for teenage diabetics have requested the CST manual developed by Dr. Grey and her team to incorporate this training into their routine care. Furthermore, current clinical guidelines on child and adolescent diabetes care emphasize the need for comprehensive behavioral care, not just disease management. This work is even timelier now, as it is being extended to teenagers with Type 2 diabetes, a disorder on the increase in the young.

This example shows a progression toward "personalized" healthcare and builds on a successful study, the Diabetes Complications and Control Trial, funded by the National Institute of Diabetes, Digestive and Kidney Diseases, NIH. In fact, it enhances the reach of the Diabetes Complications and Control Trial, which was thought to be successful in teenagers during the trial, an effect that did not persist when initially translated into general practice, a good example of identifying a gap.

Selecting the Best Setting

It is also important to identify the best settings in which to accomplish research goals. Dr. Joanne Harrell's work has focused on disease and risk factor prevention and used novel strategies to help incorporate her findings more broadly. Dr. Harrell's work is described in more detail elsewhere; a quick look at the strategies is described here.

While cardiovascular disease (CVD) usually strikes adults over 40 years of age, lifestyle behaviors that contribute to its development often begin in childhood. Childhood overweight and obesity rates are rising, often due to inactivity and poor nutrition. Children are increasingly found to have hypertension and elevated cholesterol levels. Smoking also tends to start during adolescence. Nurses working with children and teenagers can foster healthy lifestyle patterns to prevent the early development of CVD.

Dr. Harrell was the principal investigator for the NINR-funded Cardiovascular Health in Children and Youth (CHIC) studies. As a result of her work, Dr. Harrell has developed education and exercise programs that focus on improving physical activity and reducing long-term cardiovascular risks for use in schools across North Carolina, which has one of the highest rates of death from CVD and stroke in the United States.

The CHIC study involved elementary school students. In the program, the students received classes on the importance of exercise, selecting "heart-healthy" foods, and the dangers of smoking. In addition, they participated in a physical activity class that involved fun, noncompetitive aerobic activities including jumping rope and dancing. Compared with children in a control group who continued in their standard physical education classes, children in the CHIC program had significantly greater knowledge about healthy habits and reported more physical activity. They also had lowered their cholesterol level and body fat, increased their aerobic power, and had a smaller rise in their diastolic blood pressure (BP) than did the controls (Harrell et al., 1996).

During her studies, Dr. Harrell developed the novel approach of sending "report cards" to the Congressional representatives of the state, informing them as to how well their respective districts were faring in health outcomes. This was a rapid and efficient way of getting their interest in the research she was doing, because it was in their home territory.

Incorporating Stakeholders in Planning and Implementation

Community involvement is a strategy that has been successful in reaching difficult-to-reach populations with significant, persistent health problems. Community involvement of this type can be an important upfront step toward translating and incorporating the research into everyday lifestyles. An excellent illustration of these principles is focusing on urban African American men, an underserved population prone to high blood pressure (HBP) (Hill et al., 2003). This is also a good example of the effective use of interdisciplinary approaches.

High BP, also known as hypertension, is the most common chronic disease among Blacks in the United States and a major cause of disability and death, contributing to the mortality gap between Blacks and Whites. HBP management often involves behavioral changes and dietary modifications, along with a regimen of antihypertensive medications that require close follow-up from a healthcare provider. Black men living in urban or impoverished communities have a high incidence of HBP, and they generally have poor access to health services and often do not seek care or remain in treatment.

This research group developed a program using a multidisciplinary healthcare team, led by a nurse, to work with Black men with HBP. To evaluate the program, they recruited Black men diagnosed with HBP and living in inner-city Baltimore. Although many of the men reported taking some form of antihypertensive medication, half had no health insurance or regular doctor, and fewer than one in five had achieved adequate BP control. Roughly one quarter showed evidence of heart and/or kidney damage. This was especially significant given the relatively young age of the men (Hill et al., 2003). The healthcare team tested a program that taught all of the study participants about the benefits of HBP control and monitored health outcomes. Half of the men, serving as the control group, received referrals to community healthcare sources for usual HBP care. The rest were enrolled in the HBP team intervention. The healthcare team consisted of a nurse practitioner, a community health worker, and a physician consultant. The team intervention included follow-up care, ongoing assessments, home visits, and referrals to social services and job training as part of the study. At the conclusion of the study, men in both the control and the intervention groups showed decreases in smoking and consumption of salty foods. However, the men in the HBP team intervention showed a significant decrease in their systolic and diastolic BPs, with 44% lowering their BP to within the normal range, and fewer signs of heart and kidney damage. They also reported more regular use of healthcare services and antihypertensive medications than did the control group.

According to Dr. Hill, no previous hypertension studies have focused on high-risk, young urban Black men, who are frequently underserved by the healthcare system. She used a comprehensive, community-based, healthcare team approach with these men. The team approach was key to achieving control of hypertension over 3 years' time. As past president of the American Heart Association, Dr. Hill has worked closely with the American Heart Association to incorporate these principles in their guidelines. This is a good example of translational and community research, and interacting with one's professional society to facilitate policy guideline formulation.

Using Impact Measures That Translate

With the aging of the U.S. population, a greater number of older adults are living longer with chronic health conditions. Our current healthcare system tends to focus on acute care provided in hospitals. Less emphasis has been placed on home care after patients leave the hospital, where recovery and rehabilitation continue.

The following program provides good examples of interdisciplinary research approaches to address problems associated with the increasing prevalence of chronic illness in our society and also addresses the issue of providing an evidence base for care that is clinically effective and cost-effective (Naylor et al., 2004).

This research group has worked with an interdisciplinary research team testing ways to improve the outcomes and reduce the costs of care for elders living in the community. They have developed and tested a transitional care model to provide hospital discharge planning and transitional care for a variety of vulnerable patient populations.

In RCTs in the elderly with chronic illness, patients who had received the intervention had fewer total rehospitalizations, hospital days, and deaths than did the control group that continued in standard care. Improvements were also noted in patient satisfaction and quality of life. Total healthcare costs were lower for those in the intervention group. Details of efforts to translate this work into policy are detailed in a subsequent chapter.

Using Interdisciplinary Approaches

As we face the 21st century and our population becomes increasingly multicultural, our research strategies must address these issues in order to be meaningful. In addition, there is an increasing appreciation that health disparities disproportionately affect certain segments of our society, and we must address these issues as well. This example of Dr. Kate Lorig's work incorporates these principles using interdisciplinary teams (Lorig, Gonzalez, & Ritter, 1999).

Chronic conditions such as arthritis, CVD, and diabetes are the principal causes of disability in the United States, and they account for a large percentage of all healthcare costs. Treatment plans often depend on patient self-management, which may involve strict medication schedules, diets, and exercise regimens, along with education programs that teach healthy behaviors, recognition of adverse symptoms, and coping with discomfort and disability.

More than one in eight people in the United States are of Hispanic origin. Roughly one fifth of Hispanics lack proficiency in English, which tends to isolate them from accessing or using community health resources, whereas nearly one third lack any form of health insurance. Many older Hispanics do not have access to healthcare or to useful health information about chronic diseases, especially health materials written in Spanish.

Dr. Kate Lorig and her research team have designed programs aimed at improving health status, delaying deterioration, and reducing the need for healthcare visits related to chronic health conditions. Much of their initial research was devoted to arthritis. Successful outcomes resulted in the 6-week Arthritis Self-management Program, which helped to reduce pain and the need for physician visits while increasing the activity levels for arthritis sufferers.

Using Novel Strategies to Translate

Despite successful outcomes, the Arthritis Self-management Program was not reaching the Hispanic population across the United States, where arthritis is a leading cause of disability. In order to make the courses available to all Spanish-speaking persons, Dr. Lorig developed a new program, based on her previous work, that included a 6-week series of classes along with a book, *Como Convivir con su Artritis* (*How to Live With Your Arthritis*). In an effort to be culturally sensitive, healthcare class leaders were recruited from the Hispanic community and received training to teach the course. The classes were held at local community sites. The book and the class materials contained detailed information in Spanish about self-management of arthritis, along with audiotapes to promote exercise and relaxation. Each class also included additional family members who wanted to learn about the disease. One year after the program, a follow-up evaluation found that the study participants reported increased self-efficacy in managing their arthritis; improved activity levels and general health; decreased pain, disability, and depression levels; and fewer visits to a physician, compared with a control group that received standard care.

Dr. Lorig expanded her research on arthritis self-management to develop a new program, *Tomando Control de su Salud* (Taking Control of Your Health), designed to address a variety of chronic conditions, including heart disease, hypertension, diabetes, and lung disease. Several organizations in the United States are now offering this model of chronic disease self-management. In addition, the National Health Service of England has adopted it as a nationwide program and is presently implementing it in primary healthcare sites. Organizations and communities in Canada, Europe, Australia, China, Taiwan, Japan, Korea, and South Africa are using her work. This self-management model is making a difference in the lives of chronically ill adults throughout the world. Dr. Lorig's research continues to develop and evaluate community-based self-management programs.

SUMMARY

I am confident that nurse scientists will continue to be leaders in the overall research community and that, in the days ahead, they will pioneer ever more effective ways to translate research into effective, broad-based practice and to help shape and implement the policies essential to transform and advance healthcare for today and tomorrow. We must remind ourselves that we, as individuals, ultimately control our own health and critically influence the health of our families, the health of our communities, and the health of our nation. It is crucial that we, as health professionals, proactively engage our interdisciplinary professional communities, and we must find the time for civic participation—to be fully active as citizen scientists in the shaping of healthcare policies and in the planning and funding decisions that will determine the quality and effectiveness of our healthcare system.

ACKNOWLEDGMENTS

The author is grateful for the helpful reviews and suggestions of Drs. Robert Hamill, Ada Sue Hinshaw, and Dushanka Kleinman in the preparation of this chapter.

REFERENCES

Bergstrom, N., Braden, B., Kemp, M., Champagne, M., & Ruby E. (1996). Multi-site study of incidence of pressure ulcers and the relationship between risk level, demographic characteristics, diagnoses, and prescription of preventive interventions. *Journal of the American Geriatrics Society, 44*(1), 22–30.

Chelimsky, E. (1991). On the social science contribution to governmental decision making. *Science, 254,* 226–230.

Dickson, G. L., & Flynn, L. (2009). *Nursing policy research.* New York: Springer Publishing Company.

Flay, B. R., Biglan, A., Borouch, R. F., Castro, F. G., Gottfriedson, D., Kellan, S., et al. (2005). Standards of evidence: Criteria for efficacy, effectiveness, and dissemination. *Prevention Science, 6*(3), 151–175.

Gallup Poll. Polls accessed via: http://www.gallup.com

Garnett, C. (2004). Director's discretionary fund to mark 15 years. *NIH Record.* Retrieved June 8, 2004, from http://nihrecord.od.nih.gov

Grey, M., Davidson, M., Boland, E. A., & Tamborlane, W. V. (2001). Clinical and psychosocial factors associated with achievement of treatment goals in adolescents with diabetes mellitus. *Journal of Adolescent Health, 28*(5), 377–385.

Gross, D., Garvey, C., Julion, W., Fogg, L, Tucker, S., & Mokros, H. (2009). Efficacy of the Chicago Parent Program with low-income African American and Latino parents of young children. *Prevention Science, 10,* 54–65.

Gross, D., Sambrook, A., & Fogg, L. (1999). Behavior problems among young children in low-income urban day care centers. *Research in Nursing & Health, 22,* 15–25.

Harrell, J. S., McMurray, R. G., Bangdiwala, S. I., Frauman, A. C., Gansky, S. A., & Bradley, C. B. (1996). Effects of a school-based intervention improve to reduce cardiovascular disease risk factors in elementary-school children: The Cardiovascular Health in Children (CHIC) Study. *The Journal of Pediatrics, 128,* 797–805.

Harris Interactive. The Harris poll. Available at www.harrisinteractive.com

Healthy People 1990, 2000 (National Health Promotion and Disease Prevention Objectives, [1990]); Healthy People 2010 (Pt 1, 2, 3, [1999]), and Healthy People 2020 (Phase 1 [2008]). U.S. Department of Health and Human Services. Washington, DC.

Hill, M. N., Han, H., Dennison, C. R., Kim, M. T., Roary, M. C., Blumenthal, R. S., . . . Post, W. S. (2003). Hypertension care and control in underserved urban African American men: Behavioral and physiologic outcomes at 36 months. *American Journal of Hypertension, 16,* 906–913.

International Council of Nurses. (2000). *Participation of nurses in health services decision making and policy development: Position statement.* Geneva.

Ledogar, R. J., Acosta, L. G., & Penchaszadeh, A. (1999). Building international public health vision through local community research: The El Puente-CIET partnership (Editorial). *American Journal of Public Health, 89*(12), 1795–1797.

LoBiondo-Wood, G., & Haber, J. (2010). *Nursing research: Methods and critical appraisal for evidence-based practice.* St. Louis: Mosby Elsevier.

Lorig, K., Gonzalez, V. M., & Ritter, P. (1999). Community-based Spanish language arthritis education program: A randomized trial. *Medical Care, 37,* 957–963.

Madon, T., Hofman, K. J., Kupfer, L., & Glass, R. I. (2007). Implementation science. *Science, 318,* 1728–1729.

Mason, D. J., Leavitt, J. K., & Chaffee, M. W. (2007). *Policy and politics in nursing and health care.* St. Louis: Elsevier.

McCall, R. B. (2009). Evidence-based programming in the context of practice and policy. *Social Policy Report, XVIII* (III), 1–20.

McClellan, M. B., McGinnis, M., Nable, E. G., & Olsen, L. M. (2007). *Evidence-based medicine and the changing nature of health care.* Washington, DC: The National Academies Press.

Melnyk, B. M., & Fineout-Overholt, E. (2005). *Evidence-based practice in nursing and healthcare. A guide to best practice* (1st Ed.). Philadelphia: Lippincott, Williams & Williams.

Naylor, M. D., Brooten, D. A., Campbell, R. L., Maislin, G., McCauley, K. M., & Schwartz, J. S. (2004). Transitional care of older adults hospitalized with heart failure: A randomized, controlled trial. *Journal of the American Geriatrics Society, 52*, 675–684.

Patel, K., & Rushefsky, M. (2006). *Health care politics and policy in America*. London: M.E. Sharpe.

Polit, D. F., & Beck, C. T. (2008). *Nursing research: Generating and assessing evidence for nursing practice.* Philadelphia: Lippincott, Williams & Wilkins.

Rosenkoetter, M. M., & Nardi, D. A. (2006) American Academy of Nursing. White paper on global nursing and health: a brief. Nursing Outlook., Mar-Apr; *54*(2):113–115.

Rosenkoetter, M. M., & Nardi, D. A. (2007). American Academy of Nursing Expert Panel on Global Nursing and Health: White paper on global nursing and health. *Journal of Transcultural Nursing, 18*(4), 305–315.

Shaxson, L. (2005). Is your evidence robust enough? Questions for policy makers and practitioners. *Evidence and Policy, 1*, 101–111.

U.S. Department of Health and Human Services. (2005). *Changing practice, changing lives: 10 landmark nursing research studies*. Bethesda, MD: Office of Science Policy and Public Liaison, National Institute of Nursing Research, National Institutes of Health.

Weiss, C. H. (1977). Introduction. In C. H. Weiss (Ed.), *Using social research in public policy making* (pp. 1–22). Lexington: Lexington Books.

Weiss, C. H. (1988). Evaluation for decisions: Is anybody there: Does anybody care? *Evaluation Practice, 9*(1), 5–19.

World Health Organization. (2008). *2008–2013 action plan for the global strategy for the prevention and control of noncommunicable diseases.* Retrieved from http://www.who.int/nmh/publications/9789241597418/en/index.html

3

Shaping Health Policy: The Role of Nursing Research—Three Frameworks and Their Application to Policy Development

Judith Shamian and Moriah Shamian-Ellen

INTRODUCTION

One of the key responsibilities of a government is to develop policies for the better management of societies and for the protection of their citizens' well-being. Public policy, health policy, environmental policy, and financial policy are all tools that are used to shape governments' actions to govern. We often find that on the same issue, different countries have different policies. Some countries will have a national healthcare system that is financed by governments through different taxation systems; other countries have healthcare systems that are a mix of private and public funding. Immunization and maternal child policies are examples where different countries have different policies regarding who to immunize while the international scientific evidence is the same. In the area of human resources, we will find the same phenomena; different countries fund and prepare healthcare providers using different skill mixes, different number of years of education, and different standards. The question to be asked is why are all these, and many other policies, so different from each other and how do government and policy makers make their decision?

Policy making is complex, and many factors play into it. Factors like political ideology, political will, public opinion, stakeholder engagement, media coverage, and others, influence the policy-development process. In recent years, evidenced-based policy has received increased attention (Campbell et al., 2009; de Bont, Stoevelaar, & Bal, 2007; Griffin et al., 2006; Hennink & Stephenson, 2005; Madden, King, & Shiell, 2009; Shamian & El-Jardali, 2007; Shamian & Griffin, 2003; Shamian, Skelton-Green, & Villeneuve, 2002; Wilfond & Thomson, 2000). While there is a growing awareness that research evidence should shape, contribute, and influence policy, the factors affecting the development of policy also influence whether evidence is used, resulting in limited examples of evidence-based policy. For example, governments all over the world make policies and decisions regarding who will receive and should receive seasonal flu shots. While the evidence worldwide for the benefits of seasonal flu shots are the same; different governments make different decisions. Some governments offer the flu shots to all citizens over 65 years of age, others offer it to all their citizens, and yet there are many other combinations. Policy decisions of governments are so different despite the fact that there is only one set of evidence. This chapter will help readers understand the factors that contribute to final decision making.

While the notion of evidenced-based policy is used in most policy development, there is growing science to help advance and strengthen this practice. Over the last couple of decades, both scientists and policy makers realized that it is beneficial to work together to inform policy development at all levels. Furthermore, there is a growing number of commissioned targeted research to answer questions that require public or health policies. As the demand for evidence for policy making grew, the need for models to guide the evidence contribution expanded. The frameworks described in this chapter are examples of such models that help to conceptualize and follow a systematic process so effective evidenced-based policy can be accomplished.

The purpose of this chapter is to describe three such models that integrate evidence in the policy-making process, where research can be used to inform policy. Examples are provided on the applications of these models at the institutional, national, and international levels. This chapter makes recommendations for researchers to apply the models and examples to frame their research programs and scholarship to inform policy.

In order to execute evidenced-based policy development, there is a need for international, national, and local data that can assist to determine recommended policy. Such data sets usually will be large data sets that can be used for secondary data analysis. For example, to make policy recommendations regarding the number of nursing education seats in universities and colleges required for the country to provide appropriate levels of care and to implement "Needs Based Health Human Resources Planning (HHR) Planning" (O'Brien-Pallas & Tomblin Murphy, 2007), there is a need for data on current health professions, healthcare requirements, scope of practice, and many other factors. National data sets can be used to provide evidence for policy, and they are available only in a handful of countries and a few international agencies (Canadian Institute for Health Information and Organisation for Economic Co-operation and Development).

Some of the critical questions facing researchers, policy makers, politicians, stakeholders, and others are how to advance evidence-based policy development. Models and frameworks for policy development offer a systematic approach that guides and informs the process.

MODELS

While there are several models that describe the processes of using evidence to inform policy, this chapter will describe three of these models. Numerous models have been developed over the last few decades (Dobbins, Ciliska, Cockerill, Barnsley, & DiCenso 2002; Green & Bennett, 2007; Lavis et al., 2003; Lavis et al., 2002; Lomas, 2000b; Shamian et al., 2002; Weinick & Shin, 2003). The models discussed below were selected because they were developed to serve a broad agenda in different countries, are most applicable to nursing, and focus specifically on healthcare policy. They are widely generalizable and have applicability to both developing and developed countries. The models described in this chapter place a major emphasis on the use of evidence in the policy-making process.

While research is not always included in the policy-making process, it is critical that the use of evidence in the policy setting continuously be discussed and brought to the forefront. The models can also serve as diagnostic tools to assist in determining how to advance the policy-development process and why, frequently, the process comes to a halt or falls off the government agenda all together.

The three models described below are the following:

1. Data-Driven Policymaking (Weinick & Shin, 2003)
2. Evidence-Informed Health Policy (Green & Bennett, 2007)
3. The Policy Cycle: Moving From Issue to Policy (Shamian et al., 2002)

Framework 1: Data-Driven Policymaking (Weinick & Shin, 2003)

In 2003, the Agency for Healthcare Research and Quality (AHRQ), a U.S.-based government-funded agency, published three data books containing over 118 measures, as well as tools, to help analysts, decision makers, policy makers, and planners in the policy-setting process. In addition to these extensive data projects, the AHRQ (2004) disseminated a data-driven

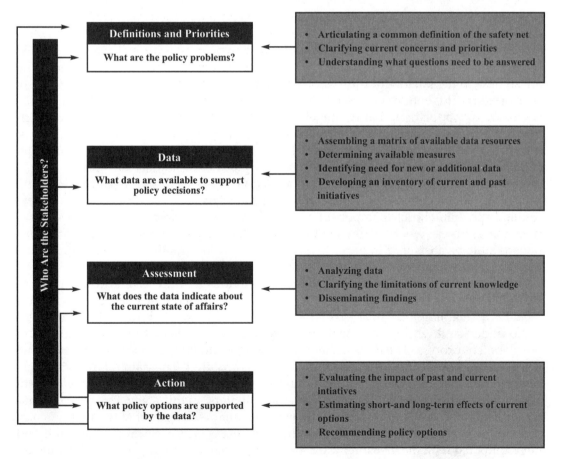

FIGURE 3.1 Data-driven policymaking (Weinick & Shin, 2003).

policy framework that includes "a four-stage process for developing data-driven capabilities to support policy decision making" (Figure 3.1). This model was chosen as one of the frameworks utilized in this chapter since it was developed by a U.S. government agency and incorporated as a baseline component in the integration of stakeholders. The framework provides suggestions for identifying the necessary data and using these data to create buy-in with different stakeholder groups.Furthermore, as will be described below, the framework includes four basic stages that encompass the major steps in ensuring that research, if available, is utilized in policy formulation.

An underlying component of the model is "who are the stakeholders," that is, who should be sitting at the table at different points throughout the process. Having the right stakeholders around the table will ensure buy-in and is likely to influence the process. The stakeholders can range from government officials to hospital representatives to community activists. The important aspect here is that all potential stakeholders be considered and included at each stage of the process: this will facilitate a broader scope of alternatives, ideas, and insight. The four-stage process includes the following:

1. Definition and priorities
2. Data
3. Assessment
4. Action

The first stage, *definition and priorities*, includes three main activities that ultimately assist in identifying the policy issues/problems. The first activity includes developing a *common definition*, as this is necessary to ensure that the different stakeholders, who are coming to the table with different backgrounds, are working under the same set of assumptions. This model discusses three aspects of developing a common definition, which are by population, that is, homeless or persons with special needs; by providers, that is, hospitals, clinics, or school-based health centers; and by funding stream, that is, Medicaid, Medicare, or State funding. The definition process naturally leads into *understanding other members' concerns and priorities*. Each stakeholder, and the group it is representing, has their key issues and concerns, and understanding what concerns and priorities other members have and other organizations have can shape the overall policy-setting approach. The last component of this stage includes *understanding the questions to be answered*, that is, what the key issues are that the group will discuss and what questions need to be answered in order to have the proper information to make appropriate policy recommendations.

The second stage, *data*, includes four main activities that are geared toward identifying the appropriate data to support the policy recommendations and decisions. This includes assembling a *data matrix* that serves as a reference tool for all the stakeholders to understand what data sources and resources are available to support the policy-development process. The data matrix should address the importance of the data, what it represents, how helpful it is, and how it can be acquired. The data matrix will likely identify data that are available from a number of different sources, that is, government agencies, local hospitals, and community health centers. In this stage, the group should also identify and *determine available data measures*, that is, length of stay, readmissions, and turnover rates; once these are identified, baseline measures can be captured and then compared with the measures after the policy implementation, and thus, the policy's impact can be determined. Based on the data, policy decisions can be made at various levels. If the data show a shortage of nurses, then the appropriate decision maker might invest in additional educational seats. On the other hand, if turnover is a major issue related to workload or workplace issues, governments and employers might introduce different policies that will deal with reduction of turnover, which will lead to both more cost-effective operation and better clinical outcomes (O'Brien-Pallas, Tomblin Murphy, & Shamian, 2008). It will be essential to have baseline data before policies are introduced and implemented and an evaluation plan so the policy impact can be evaluated. In the process of developing the data matrix and determining available data measures, the *need for new or additional data* will be identified (O'Brien-Pallas et al., 2006). The last component in the data section is to record all *previous initiatives* that have been undertaken with respect to this policy and their impact. Through this analysis, it will be possible to determine which policies had the most impact. Those policies that had minimal or no impact might be recommended for elimination. If this is national policy, it would have to go to the legislature/ governing body for change. For example, at the institutional level, there might be policies and funding in place for child care for hospital staff. However, if most of the staff have no young children and, therefore, no need for these services, such a service, while costly, will also have little value to improve the retention strategies. Appropriate data usage can lead to the optimal use of resources, optimal staff satisfaction, and patient outcome.

The third stage, *assessment*, basically entails taking all the information generated in the previous two stages, that is, defining priorities and questions, collecting the data, and assessing the current situation. This stage includes *analyzing the data*, which can be done using a number of policy analysis frameworks. *Limitations of current knowledge* should be understood in this stage as well. Very rarely is all the information readily available and easily understood, and it is important for the stakeholders to be inclusive in this process and understand the current situation, including what information is missing in this decision-making process. The final component in the assessment phase, and one of the most crucial, is *disseminating the findings* of the process. The stakeholders can view the findings, mull over options, and use the findings to determine what is feasible to accomplish and how to proceed to the policy adoption phase. Furthermore, the findings can form the baseline to monitor the policy process and evaluate its impact.

The final stage in this framework is *action*, which entails assessing and selecting policy options. In this stage, it is recommended to *estimate the impact* of previous and current initiatives in conjunction with the potential impact of current options to mitigate the negative outcome of previous initiatives. Determining ways to evaluate the policy and to identify its failures and successes also occurs in this stage. The recommendations, the final component of this framework, should be presented to the stakeholders and their respective organizations. The recommendations should be presented with the data analysis and evidence supporting the ultimate recommendation. Often, policy development is incremental and might take years of development until a comprehensive policy is in place. Therefore, policy recommendations should be revised and adjusted based on both new emerging data and policy impact evaluation.

Summary

This framework provides an overview of how data can and should influence the policy-development process. One weakness of this model, as opposed to the following two models, is that this one does not represent a cyclical approach to policy development, but rather a linear approach to ensuring the incorporation of data in the policy-development process. This model emphasizes the importance of having clarity of the issue/problem that the policy will deal with. Based on this model, when the various stakeholders achieve an understanding of the issue/problem then the data gathering process can be initiated. The tools in this model and the data matrix are useful in demonstrating how data can be utilized at the policy-development process.

Framework 2: Evidence-Informed Health Policy (Green & Bennett, 2007)

In 2007, the World Health Organization (WHO) developed an extensive review on enhancing capacity for developing appropriate health policy. This model has international significance and was developed through the collaboration of scientists from many countries. This model can be used with, in, and among countries providing a consistent framework and language. Within this review, a framework for evidence-informed policy was developed and explained. For a broader description of the WHO's initiative, please see the electronic document at http://www.who.int/alliance-hpsr/resources/Alliance_BR.pdf (Green & Bennett, 2007). While the WHO developed this framework to

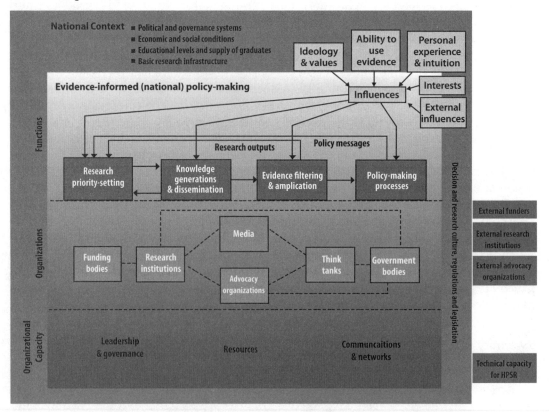

FIGURE 3.2   Evidence-Informed Health Policy-Making (Green & Bennett, 2007).

assist developing countries, this framework is built on the most advanced knowledge on policy development and relevant to all settings. The review emphasizes the need for not only evaluative research but also research that is also "descriptive, analytical, diagnostic, theoretical and prescriptive" (Green & Bennett, 2007). This is a goal that is sometimes difficult to obtain in both developing and developed countries, including most of the Organization of Economic Cooperation and Development countries. While evidence is essential, the overall framework highlights the necessary functions, actors, and organizational capacity requirements in order to enable evidence-informed policy, in any environment.

The WHO framework in Figure 3.2 is composed of three main levels. The first level consists of the four main functions that occur between research and policy setting. The second level focuses on the organizations that execute the four main functions, and the third level highlights the necessary organizational capacities required to carry out the functions. Each of these levels will be discussed, but initially, the underlying basis of the framework is described.

The WHO framework utilizes the term *evidence-informed* health policy making as opposed to *evidence based*. This is because policy setting is highly political, and many factors come into play, not just the role of research. While data should play a key role, to date, data and research have not been highly utilized in the policy-setting arena (Green & Bennett, 2007). Research is not the only factor that should be considered when developing policy, and this is demonstrated by the underlying influences that affect the four main functions in Figure 3.2. Policy makers' ideologies, values, and interests, which either they hold themselves or various interest groups have presented to them, play a key role in the policy decision-making process. In addition, the external influences exerted by interest groups, organizations, and networks influence the policy-making process. Policy makers' personal experiences and intuitions will undoubtedly come into play in the policy-making process. These components are justifiable and acceptable influences into the policy-making process, and these components may or may not align with the research and evidence (Wilfond & Thomson, 2000).

Another major influence of the increased usage of knowledge translation initiatives is the ability of policy makers, their staff, and their organizations to obtain and appropriately interpret the evidence. All of these influences need to be taken into consideration before one can begin to understand the four main functions. Policy makers come to the table with their own beliefs and ideologies, and sometimes, the evidence supports this and it is aligned and easily interpreted. Other times, there may not even be evidence to inform the process, and then there is an identifiable void.

Another underlying aspect of this framework is to recognize that these influences and levels are occurring in a broader arena, that is, a national and international context. At the international level, there are political and economic factors that influence policy setting, which can, and do, override the influence of research. At the national level, these issues exist as well, but another factor comes into play. Even when research is sought to inform policy, at times, the necessary data are not available, and even if these are available, there is a lack of experts who can interpret the data and make these useful for policy makers. In some countries, these issues are stronger than others, but in any case, they need to be considered as underlying factors in the broader policy-making process.

These influences affect the four components of the functional level. The first component is priority setting for research. These decisions are made by different organizations, that is, the funding bodies, the research organizations, universities, and the policy-making bodies (which can overlap and be the funders as well). In recent years, the priority-setting component has become more formal, and funders have started grappling with where the funds would be most appropriately used. Increased and continued collaboration between researchers, funders, and decision makers is needed in deciding what priority areas should be focused on, not only in the policy realm but also in the research arena. In some instances, this can take on the role of specifically commissioned research to address a priority area, whereas in other instances, research findings can bring new priority areas to light.

The second component is the generation and dissemination of knowledge. In the past, new knowledge was usually generated at the university level and dissemination consisted of publications. Researchers and decision makers have worked in silos, each not necessarily understanding each other's needs and focusing on their own interests (Lomas, 2000a). Over time, this evolved in two ways. First, many organizational bodies, not just universities, produce knowledge, and secondly, dissemination is much broader and requires much more effort than just publications. Recent studies have demonstrated an increase in communication and collaboration between researchers and decision makers (Campbell et al., 2009; Tourangeau, Coghlan, Shamian, & Evans, 2005).

This is manifested by the third component, evidence filtering and amplification. Various organizations filter through the vast amount of research findings and amplify the ones that they feel are relevant and can strongly influence the beliefs, values, and mindsets of policy makers. The final component, the policy-making process, is meant to include all the factors of the policy-development process, that is, agenda setting, policy development, implementation, and evaluation. These four components are all linked together, as demonstrated in Figure 3.2, which demonstrates a connection between all different components and different stages through the various organizations that play a part in the policy-making process.

The four functions described above are carried out by different organizations, as reflected by the organizational level in the WHO framework. No specific connections are made between specific organizations and the functions, since some of these organizational types can carry out multiple components in the functional realms, at different times and stages. The organizations are placed under the functions that would most obviously be related to their organizational type; however, that may not be their only role. For example, advocacy organizations may generate knowledge and disseminate it, but they may also fund certain types of knowledge generation. The dotted lines between the organizations demonstrate that they all work in informal or formal networks, and through these networks, they develop and influence the four components of the functional realm. However, they can do this only if they have certain aspects of organizational capacity.

Organizational capacity, as pictured in the third level of the framework, highlights three main organizational behavior variables necessary in organizations in order to facilitate the four functional components. The first organizational capacity variable is "leadership and governance." This variable addresses the need for not only individual leadership but also organizational leadership and appropriate governance within policy setting. Having strong leadership and the appropriate governance structures can influence the extent to which the capacity in the organization is developed. The reason the term *appropriate governance* structures was utilized is that different organizations require different governance structures, and therefore, there is no ideal setting, but rather, organizations need to evaluate and determine what is most beneficial to their institution. The second variable that is essential in building an organization's capacity is "resources": Having a sufficient amount of resources can ensure the necessary success. Human resources, that is, staff, financial resources, funds, physical resources, and computers, are necessary for an organization to appropriately accomplish its task. Lastly, "communication and networks" are essential since organizations need to be able to communicate their work and also create and foster the relationships that they create with other groups in their network. Bringing all of the elements in the model will enable evidence-informed policy making.

Summary

This model offers a comprehensive approach to scientists, decision makers, and stakeholders. Its use of all types of evidence, not just the pure quantitative science, broadens the availability of data to support policy considerations. Furthermore, the model recognized the complexity and the various levels of organizations, individuals, and resources required in the policy-development process.

This model reminds the readers that we are dealing with evidenced-informed processes rather than evidenced-based policy development. The nuance of the language is very important, and it is important to be clear that, at best, data will inform policy decisions. Furthermore, this model is uniquely suited to both developed and developing countries. The model can also be useful for international policy engagement as different countries can benefit from using similar models for policy setting and decision makers can have a common framework and language that can guide their negotiations and agreements. This model also recognizes the importance of all data levels: descriptive, qualitative, and others, in addition to the traditional quantitative data sets. Finally, this model suggests that countries consider linking funding priorities to policy issues and reminds funders and others that the proper conditions (funding, human resources, etc.) need to be in place in order to develop and make data available for policy-development purposes.

Framework 3: The Policy Cycle: Moving From Issue to Policy (Shamian, Skelton-Green, & Villeneuve, 2002)

This policy framework was developed to support the work of the Office of Nursing Policy (ONP) at Health Canada, at the Federal Government of Canada. The ONP was established in 1999 to provide input and advice to Health Canada and the Canadian healthcare system on a wide range of issues. One of the authors of this chapter was the inaugural executive director of the ONP.

In order to provide systematic, high-quality, evidenced-based policy advice, the ONP needed a framework to guide its work and its partnerships inside and outside of governments and other stakeholders. After careful review of the available models at the time this policy cycle was developed, it was determined that existing models did not meet the needs of the ONP, and therefore, this model was adopted based on the previous work by Kingdon (1955), Milstead (1999), and Tarlov (1999). These previous models were not as comprehensive and do not encompass all of the four stages, dealing with only some aspects of the issues at hand. The integration of various components of these previous models leads to a modified model that could address policy formulation without the need of using multiple frameworks for the same purpose.

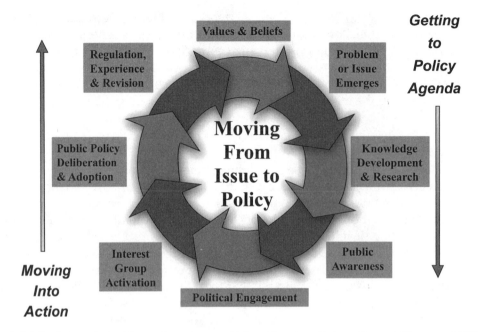

FIGURE 3.3   Policy Cycle: Moving from Issue to Policy (Shamian, Skelton-Green, Villeneuve, 2002).

The policy-development framework has four distinct stages:

1. Setting the policy agenda
2. Moving into action/legislation
3. Policy implementation
4. Policy evaluation

The policy cycle (Figure 3.3) deals mostly with Stages 1 and 2, but the complete framework requires Stages 3 and 4 to be exercised.

Parts 1 and 2 of the framework and what is described in the policy cycle consist of eight steps, which are (1) values and cultural beliefs, (2) emergence of problems or issues, (3) knowledge and development of research, (4) public awareness, (5) political engagement, (6) interest group activation, (7) public policy deliberation and adoption, and (8) regulation. The first four steps of the policy cycle lead to "getting to the policy agenda." These four steps are essential building blocks to get the issue on the policy agenda and on the radar screen of decision makers that can move it into policy. If citizens, communities, interest groups, organizations, and politicians do not value and believe in the issues that are highlighted in the policy arena, the issues will not be addressed and the policy-development process will come to a halt, for this specific issue.

The second phase in the cycle that is composed of Steps 5 to 8 leads to "moving into action." It is anchored by political engagement as a required building block. For a problem to press forward into the policy setting and action realms, political engagement is essential. If policy makers are not engaged and involved, then policy issues can be discussed, debated, and acknowledged by numerous stakeholders, but they will not result in policy change. This model initially developed and used to develop a case and promote policy development related to nurses' health and healthy work environments. The model guided the problem definition, the evidence identification and evidence building, and the engagement of stakeholders and opinion leaders and resulted in ongoing significant policy work in this area in Canada at the Federal, provincial and local levels (Kerr, Laschinger, Severin, Almost, & Shamian, 2005; McIntyre, Thomlinson, & McDonald, 2003; Registered Nurses of Ontario; Shamian & El-Jardali, 2007).

The third stage of the framework, "policy implementation," can take place only once the policy development has been accomplished. The journey from policy adoption to implementation is equally complicated and requires numerous steps. While the policy implementation requires the engagements of governments, decision makers, and/or funders, the focus shifts from decision makers to implementers. At this stage, it is important to have very clear processes and expectations so what is gained through the policy adoption is not lost through implementation.

Finally, the fourth stage of the framework, the "policy evaluation," provides all stakeholders with the analysis if the right policy was adopted, implemented, and if it achieved the desired impact. This stage requires systematic data gathering and analysis, which is based on the data used at the "setting the policy agenda" stage.

The Policy Cycle, which constitutes the first two stages of policy development (Figure 3.3), has eight elements, which are described below:

Values and Cultural Beliefs

This element anchors the first phase of the policy-development process. The various stakeholders in the policy-setting process share some of the values and beliefs related to the issue at hand in order to move forward. The stakeholders involved in a certain policy-setting process identify their beliefs on the issue so open dialogue and discussion can occur. Some policy makers will have the same values and beliefs, yet the importance they place on them may differ. For example, a group of stakeholders may value home care for the elderly, preventative healthcare, and early childhood vaccinations, and they may think that these are all valuable and important initiatives. However, if there were resources available only for certain initiatives, the stakeholders may differ on which initiative they think is most important, based on their past experiences, values, beliefs, and interests. Furthermore, some political groups would believe that the government's role is to establish the standards to which the citizens might choose or choose not to comply other political ideologies will support the findings and reinforcement of such policies. Thus, it is essential to know what the political ideology in place is and frame the policy recommendations accordingly. Identifying stakeholders' values and articulating them to those involved are essential not only in the beginning of the policy-setting process but also throughout the process, to ground the various stakeholders and to continuously obtain and reinforce buy-in.

Emergence of Problem or Issue

The second element, "problems and issues," can come from any source and at any time (Kingdon, 1995). Some problems can be in existence for years and no policy development can occur from it. Some interest groups can work for many years to bring an issue to the forefront, for example, the role of nurse practitioners or the necessity of primary healthcare to build healthy nations, whereas other issues spring to the limelight due to some unforeseen episode, for example, SARS (Severe Acute Respiratory Syndrome). It is not sufficient for an issue just to exist, but rather, it needs to have a sense of urgency that results in political will for the policy. In order for policy makers to focus on a problem, the problem needs to scream "look at me." It needs to be brought to policy makers' attention. There are a number of ways to do so, such as through interest group activities, lobbying, media coverage, and/or research findings. Workplace health was one of such areas in which the data, stakeholders lobbying activities, interest group involvement, and media attention all helped to put it on the national and international agenda.

Furthermore, if data supporting an issue are not acted upon when brought to the forefront, then interest in the issue might fade, and the opportunity to act on that initiative again may not occur for some time. It is important to note that policy makers can deal at any given time with only a few of the many issues that are put in front of them. Each policy development takes a long time, and it requires engagement of multiple levels and branches of government, that is, legislative arm, regulatory, finance, and others.

Knowledge and Development of Research

The third element of research and evidence should be used to provide solid support to the issue. Research can propel an issue into the spotlight, but at the same time, it can be used as factual evidence to anecdotal perceptions. For example, nurses have the highest absenteeism rate among all employee categories (Canadian Nurses Association, 2006). This data point, coupled with other evidence that emerged from works of Aiken et al. (2001), Bruce, Sale, Shamian, O'Brien-Pallas, and Thomson (2002), Shamian, Kerr, Laschinger, and Thomson (2002), and others, propelled this agenda forward, and over the last decade, ongoing research and findings helped to further strengthen the policy direction in the area of workplace health.

Public Awareness

The fourth element and the last step of the first phase in the policy cycle is the development of public awareness of the problem, as well as the potential solutions. All potential stakeholder groups should be addressed, and ideally, the message should be customized for the different groups. In order to do this, one needs to research the values and interests of the different groups and then appropriately customize the message.

For example, if trying to implement evidence-based nursing practice, then when speaking to the funders, the message of improved efficiency should be portrayed; when speaking to patient advocacy groups, the message of higher quality care should be emphasized; and when speaking to nursing groups, the messages of higher quality care, as well as more manageable workload, should be demonstrated. Creating buy-in is one of the main goals of this stage. Furthermore, different means of communication should be utilized, for example, Web sites, local newspapers, radio interviews, and conference presentations. While research should influence policy, it is wrong to imply that research should be the only driving force, since other factors drive the policy-making process as well, such as the media, different interest groups, and political engagement, as discussed in the next few steps (Orosz, 1994).

Political Engagement

The fifth element is political engagement, where politically engaging key figures are the anchor of the start of the second phase of the policy-setting cycle of "moving into action/legislation." To propel an issue from "just being an issue" to policy makers' agenda political engagement is a required step. In order for an issue to be on the political agenda, it should have research backing, but it also needs to be "softened up"; that is, policy makers and stakeholders need to become accustomed to the issue and potential solution so that buy-in can occur (Kingdon, 1995). While evidence should be used, it is important to "humanize" the issues and make them real-life concerns, which can be accomplished through personal stories or individual's anecdotes (Milstead, 1999). Buy-in will need to be built up, and for this to occur, the government structures and interest groups must be well understood and targeted, carefully consider each contact and the best way to approach them, customize the messages, and keep the stakeholders and contacts regularly updated as to the progress (Shamian, Skelton-Green, & Villeneuve, 2002). Canada is a Federated model where the Federal Government and the provinces have to work together to achieve national policy. The ministers of health meet annually, and in 2000, a National Nursing Strategy was approved. It had 11 recommendations, one of which was to establish a national forum to develop recommendations to the ministers of health on how to deal with issues related to workplace health and the health of nurses. This recommendation led to the Canadian Nursing Advisory Committee (CNAC) report called *Our Health, Our Future: Creating Quality Workplaces for Canadian Nurses*, which outlined 51 recommendations to ministers, employers, unions, educators, and others. This watershed document, which was accepted by the ministers, has been guiding the policy development and implementation in this area in Canada and has also been picked up by other countries and organizations like the WHO.

Interest Group Activation

The sixth element is interest group activation. Interest groups should be involved throughout the process, but it is important to highlight their engagement. For example, during the work of CNAC, all stakeholders participated: unions, healthcare executives, nurse executives, scholars, and others. This supported early adoption and buy-in to the proposed recommendations to the ministers. Some of the groups issue ongoing report cards that assess their government's success in delivering their commitments (Canadian Federation of Nurses Unions, 2003). Interest groups are some of the key stakeholders in the process. They provide the opportunity for the issue and potential policy solution to be repeated over and over again, through every medium, that is, direct mail, e-mail, speeches, publications, networking, and radio, in addition to meeting and pressuring politicians and others.

Public Policy Deliberation and Adoption

The seventh element is public policy deliberation and adoption. Once buy-in is obtained at an acceptable level, and there is enough support and interest in the issue, the policy deliberation should be brought to the agenda by government officials. At this point, the potential solution and policy formulation should be deliberated. If the policy is not able to reach this point, then the success of the previous steps should be evaluated and assessed. Once it has reached this point, in order for it to be sustainable, it must meet the following five criteria: technical feasibility, value acceptability within the policy community, tolerable cost, anticipated public agreement, and a reasonable chance for elected officials to be receptive to the policy ideas (Kingdon, 1995). For example, when the minister of health approved the National Nursing Strategy in 2000, it was acknowledged that nurses' health and workplace issues were of concern to the nation. Later on, when the CNAC report was released in 2002, the ministers of health felt compelled to act on it, as it was both commissioned by the ministers and was an evidence-based multistakeholder report.

Regulation

The last step, and the eighth element of the policy cycle, includes the proposed policy becoming a law, including regulations and other directives associated with the policy adoption. The recommendations from CNAC and other research led to various policy and regulation changes in provinces. For example, the Government of the Province of Ontario, which is the largest province in Canada, issued a standard of 70% full-time and 30% part-time or casual employment. Institutions that are funded by the government need to submit annually their data including the full-time/part-time ratio and what is the action plan to achieve the required 70/30 policy. Other provinces put in regulations regarding the use of lifts to reduce back injury. All provinces increased the production of nurses and expected educational institutions to meet new targets. The magnitude of action is tremendous and further described in *Healthy Workplaces for Health Workers in Canada: Knowledge Transfer and Uptake in Policy and Practice* (Shamian & El-Jardali, 2007).

Following the completion of Stages 1 and 2, Stages 3 and 4 (policy implementation and policy evaluation) have to take place. Research and data play a very significant role in both of these stages. While Stage 3 requires the implementers to do the bulk of the work, scientists can gather data on how policy is implemented. The policies that are implemented are meant to deal with the problem that led to the policy development in the first place. Ongoing research and evaluation will help decision makers to determine if the problem has been resolved, if the policy instruments used are the correct ones to resolve the problems, and if further work is needed to resolve the problem.

At the fourth stage, "policy evaluation," data will be gathered to demonstrate the impact of policy implementation. To have an optimal policy evaluation, the data elements to be assessed should be decided during Stages 1 and 2 to the policy process. In the event of nurses' health and workplace health, a national study was carried out by Statistics Canada to determine the progress (Statistics Canada, 2006). Scientists, stakeholders, and governments are also conducting their own evaluations.

Summary

This model provides a systematic approach for a comprehensive policy development, from determining the social/political values present that will impact whether there will be an interest and willingness to deal with some societal problems to the evaluation of policies. The model recognizes that there can be back-and-forth movements in the process, and some policy issues might get stuck in one of the steps for lengthy periods of time or fall off the cycle altogether based on internal and/or external factors.

The model also offers a very good diagnostic tool in determining how one should proceed, what the next logical steps are, or why some policy development runs into roadblocks. This model has been used and is well tested in both nursing and health policy.

CONCLUSION

This chapter described three models of evidence-based policy development. The examples presented are meant to reinforce the importance of data and research in building evidence-based policy development, implementation, and evaluation. It is essential to keep building evidenced-based policies, and furthermore, it is essential for decision makers and researchers to keep an ongoing exchange of information so both can benefit from the expertise they bring to the table.

During the last few decades, we have developed numerous large data sets that provide better evidence than do single studies. These large data sets galvanized the ability to advance evidence-based policy development. It also allows ongoing review of progress without requiring major financial investments. For example, census data in most countries can shed light on overall health of populations.

All of the models presented emphasize the importance of having good data and using the available information in defining the issue/problem for which there is a need for a new or revised policy. Decision makers, stakeholders, and researchers can all benefit from understanding the various models described in this chapter and how these models can be used to resolve problems in a manner where policies are developed based on existing data. It is important to note that the evidence to guide policy development, while essential on its own, will not achieve policy development and implementation. The various other aspects of policy development, like stakeholder involvement, public engagement, and others, are all relevant to achieve policy development and implementation.

The role of advocacy and stakeholders in policy influence has been recognized for decades and centuries, but the role of evidence is a more recent development and is still in the process of integration into the policy-development strategies. In order to enhance the use of evidence into policy, researchers, funders, decision makers, and stakeholders need to understand both the importance of evidence and how it can be integrated in the process. The models described in this chapter help to integrate the data in the process of policy making and offer mechanism for all relevant players to see what their role can be in this process. The models accept implicitly and explicitly that, often, there are missing data, and policies may be made with less than optimal data. The challenge is to make sure that the existing research, data, and opinions get examined and used in a manner that provides as much evidence as available to frame both the issue and proposed policy solutions.

While all three models show some systematic stepwise process, the models of Green and Bennett (2007) and Shamian et al. (2002) emphasize how to navigate the complexity of the policy process. The policy process can take decades. With complex issues like anti-smoking policies or use of cellular phones while driving, it can take decades to build the evidence and to have decision makers and politicians put in place the necessary policies. Often, the progress is incremental in small steps, and at times, it takes years from point one to point two. In nursing, one just needs to look at how many decades we have had the evidence to support the role of nurse practitioners. Despite this evidence, most countries do not have the policies, educational programs, and funding in place, regardless of the ongoing pressure to advance primary healthcare. One look at how long it takes to put in place policies for the practice of nurse practitioners, one can understand the meaning of "messiness," "politics," and "time," regardless of the availability of the best research.

Furthermore, policy can start at any place, might skip steps, stay on one step forever, or fall off the policy agenda altogether. Working through this process, it is also important to know how to compromise, as some policy improvement is better than none. Incremental policies take more time but could lead to the desired outcome over time. The evaluation process becomes very important in moving to the next stage of policy development. The healthcare and nursing community can benefit significantly by adapting the tools for evidence-informed policy development. One of the fundamental requirements is to learn how to work with various stakeholder groups within nursing, healthcare community, public, media, governments, and others that are relevant for the process. Using the models offered here and others, coupled with a growing body of data, we can offer leadership in building policies that will lead to improved health systems, healthy populations, and healthy providers.

REFERENCES

Aiken, L. H., Clarke, S. P., Sloane, D. M., Sochalski, J. A., Busse, R., Clarke, H., . . . Shamian, J. (2001). Nurses' reports of hospital quality of care and working conditions in five countries. *Health Affairs, 20*, 43–53.

Agency for Healthcare Research and Quality (AHRC) (2004). U.S. Department of Health and Human Services Public Health Service. *Monitoring the health care safety net—developing data-driven capabilities to support policymaking.* AHRQ Pub. No. 04-0037. http://www.ahrq.gov/data/safetynet/weinick.pdf

Bruce, S., Sale, J., Shamian, J., O'Brien-Pallas, L., & Thomson, D. (2002). Musculoskeletal injuries, stress and absenteeism among Ontario nurses: Interviews with nurses, hospital administration and occupational health and safety. *Canadian Nurse, 98*(9), 12–17.

Campbell, D., Redman, S., Jorm, L., Cooke, M., Zwi, A. B., & Rychetnik, L. (2009). Increasing the use of evidence in health policy: Practice and views of policy makers and researchers. *Australia and New Zealand Health Policy, 6*, 21.

Canadian Institute for Health Information (CIHI). http://secure.cihi.ca/cihiweb/dispPage.jsp?cw_page=home_e

Canadian Nurses Association. (2006). *Towards 2020: Visions for nursing.* Ottawa, ON: Author. The statistics found in the *Vision 2020* document were based on data from the 1987, 1992, 1997, 2001, 2002 and 2005 Statistics Canada Labour Force Survey.

Canadian Federation of Nurses Unions (CFNU) (2003). *Action to stem the nursing shortage/implement CNAC—report card.*

Canadian Nursing Advisory Committee (CNAC) (2002). *Our health, our future: Creating quality workplaces for Canadian nurses.* http://www.hc-sc.gc.ca

de Bont, A., Stoevelaar, H., & Bal, R. (2007). Databases as policy instruments. About extending networks as evidence-based policy. *BMC Health Services Research, 7*, 200.

Dobbins, M., Ciliska, D., Cockerill, R., Barnsley, J., & DiCenso, A. (2002). A framework for the dissemination and utilization of research for health-care policy and practice. *The Online Journal of Knowledge Synthesis for Nursing, 9*(7).

Green, A., & Bennett, S. (Ed.). (2007). *Sound choices enhancing capacity for evidence-informed health policy.* Geneva: Switzerland.

Griffin, P., Grinspun, D., Bajnok I., Tucker, D., El-Jardali, F., & Shamian, J. (2006). What's the fuss about? Why do we need healthy work environments for nurses anyway? Longwoods eLetter, February 28, 2006. Longwoods Publishing Corporation.

Hennink, M., & Stephenson, R. (2005). Using research to inform health policy: Barriers and strategies in developing countries. *Journal of Health Communication, 10*, 163–180.

Kerr, M. S., Laschinger, H. K., Severin, C. N., Almost, J. M., & Shamian, J. (2005). New strategies for monitoring the health of Canadian nurses: Results of collaborations with key stakeholders. *Canadian Journal of Nursing Leadership, 18*(1), 67–81.

Kingdon, J. W. (1995). *Agendas, alternatives, and public policies.* New York: Harper Collins College Publishers.

Lavis, J. N., Robertson, D., Woodside, J. M., McLeod, C. B., Abelson, J., & The Knowledge Transfer Study Group. (2003). How can research organizations more effectively transfer knowledge to decision makers? *The Milbank Quarterly, 81*(2), 221–248.

Lavis, J. N., Ross, S. E., Hurley, J. E., Hohenadel, J. M., Stoddart, G. L., Woodward, C. A., & Abelson, J. (2002). Examining the role of health services research in public policymaking. *The Milbank Quarterly, 80*(1), 125–154.

Lomas, J. (2000a). Using 'linkage and exchange' to move research introduction policy at a Canadian foundation. *Health Affairs, 19*(3), 236–240.

Lomas, J. (2000b). Connecting research and policy. *Isuma: Canadian Journal of Policy Research,* 140–144.

Madden, L., King, L., & Shiell, A. (2009). How do government health departments in Australia access health economics advice to inform decisions for health? *A survey. Australia and New Zealand Health Policy, 6*(6).

Milstead, J. A. (1999). *Health policy and politics: A nurse's guide*. Gaithersburg, Maryland: Aspen Publication Inc.

McIntyre, M., Thomlinson, E., & McDonald, C. (2003). *Realities of Canadian nursing: Professional, practice, and power issues*. Philadelphia, PA: Lippincott Williams & Wilkins.

O'Brien-Pallas, L., Griffin, P., Shamian, J., Buchan, J., Duffield, C., Hughes, F., Lashinger, H., North, N., Stone, P., & Hayes, L. (2006). The impact of nursing turnover on patient, nurse and system outcomes: A pilot study and focus for a multi-center study. *Policy, Politics and Nursing Practice, 7*(3), 169–179.

O'Brien Pallas, L., &, Tomblin Murphy, G. (2007). *Health human resources modelling: Challenging the past, creating the future*. Canadian Health Services Research Foundation.

O'Brien-Pallas, L., Tomblin Murphy, G., & Shamian, J. (2008). *Understanding the costs and outcomes of nurses' turnover in Canadian hospitals*. TOS Final Report. FRN# 66350. http://www.hhrchair.ca/images/CMSImages/TOS_Final%20Report.pdf

Organisation for Economic Co-operation and Development (OECD), http://www.oecd.org/statsportal/0,3352,en_2825_293564_1_1_1_1_1,00.html

Orosz, E. (1994). The impact of social science research on health policy. *Social Science and Medicine, 39*, 1287–1293.

Registered Nurses of Ontario (RNAO). (Ongoing). Healthy work environments best practice guidelines. Accessed November 2, 2009 from http://www.rnao.org/Page.asp?PageID=861&SiteNodeID=241

Shamian, J., & Griffin, P. (2003). Translating research into health policy. *Canadian Journal of Nursing Research, 35*(3), 45.

Shamian, J., Kerr, M. S., Laschinger, H. K. S., & Thomson, D. (2002). A hospital-level analysis of the work environment and workforce health indicators for registered nurses in Ontario's acute care hospitals. *Human Resource Planning Focus Issue of the Canadian Journal of Nursing Research, 33*(4), 35–50.

Shamian, J., & El-Jardali, F. (2007). Healthy workplaces for health workers in Canada: Knowledge transfer and uptake in policy and practice. *Healthcare Papers, 7*, 6–25.

Shamian, J., Skelton-Green, J., & Villeneuve, M. (2002). Policy: The essential link in successful transformations. In M. McIntyre, E. Thomlinson, & C. McDonald (Eds.), *Realities of Canadian nursing professional, practice, and power issues* (2nd ed., 6, 94–111). Philadelphia: Lippincott Williams, & Wilkins.

Statistics Canada. (2006) *National Survey of the Work and Health of Nurses (NSWHN)*. Record number:5080. http://www.statcan.gc.ca/cgi-bin/imdb/p2SV.pl?Function=getSurvey&SDDS=5080&lang=en&db=imdb&adm=8&dis=2

Tarlov, A. (1999). *Public policy frameworks for improving population health* (Vol. 896, pp. 281–293). The New York Academy of Sciences.

Tourangeau, A. E., Coghlan, A. L., Shamian, J., & Evans, S. (2005). Registered nurse and registered practical nurse evaluations of their hospital practice environments and their responses to these environments. *Canadian Journal of Nursing Leadership, 18*(4) 54–69.

Weinick, R. M., & Shin, P. W. (2003). *Developing data-driven capabilities to support policymaking*. George Washington University: The Agency for Healthcare Research and Quality's (AHRQ).

Wilfond, B. S., & Thomson, E. J. (2000). Models of public health genetic policy development. In M. J. Khoury, W. Burke, & E. J. Thomson (Eds.), *Genetics and public health in the 21st century* (pp. 61–81). New York: Oxford University Press.

4

The Role of Science Policy in Programs of Research and Scholarship

Suzanne L. Feetham

As nursing research and nursing science have progressed over the last decades, observation and engagement with active scientists and doctoral students demonstrate that few deliberately address the role of science policy in their programs of research and scholarship. The purpose of this chapter is to describe science policy, provide exemplars of recent science policy and their influence on research, and provide some direction to scientists to address and inform science policy.

SCIENCE POLICY

Science policy defines what is recognized as science and therefore guides research direction, development, and funding as well as determining the focus of and resources for research education and training. Science policy is at the intersection between public policy and research and acts to justify, manage, or prioritize support of scientific research and development. It can be seen as a mechanism for advancing a field/area of science by alerting scientists to gaps in science (Feetham & Meister, 1999). Science policy may establish the standards for science and for academic research programs. It consists of decisions that, formally or informally, shape the allocation of scarce resources to support scientist training and to support scientific work. Science policy is influenced by its perceived social utility and the potential for solving problems (Huston, 2008). The allocation of the National Institutes of Health (NIH) budget to the 27 institutes and centers within NIH is a reflection of both science policy and political will[1] and determines the resources of the NIH and each institute to implement science policy (Feetham & Meister, 1999; Richmond & Kotelchuck, 1993; The AIP Bulletin of

[1] Political will is one component required to affect change in policy. Political will is governments (policy makers) and the public giving priority to issues to enact legislation. Political will requires understanding and support and is influenced by public opinion, the intensity of interest in the topic, and the degree to which the topic is considered relevant. Feasible solutions are needed to inform political will (Lezine & Reed, 2007; Richmond & Kotelchuck, 1993).

Science Policy News; http://www.aip.org/fyi/2009/016.html). An example of science policy familiar to most nurse researchers is the strategic plan of the National Institute of Nursing Research, 1 of the 17 NIH institutes (http://www.ninr.nih.gov/AboutNINR/NINRMissionandStrategicPlan/).

PUBLIC POLICY TO SCIENCE POLICY

Understanding the association of public policy to science policy and science policy to programs of research and scholarship should be an expectation of active scientists and for scientist education. When this context is lacking in scientific education, scientists are not prepared for the environment in which they will compete for funding and conduct and disseminate their research.

A primary tenet for scientists is that with finite resources, all science is political. Almost all people agree that "science should be supported." Beyond that, consensus quickly breaks down (The AIP Bulletin of Science Policy News; http://www.aip.org/fyi). Public policy is made in the name of the "public" and is generally made or initiated by government conveying what the government intends to do and what it chooses not to do. Most political issues in the United States have a scientific component, such as stem cell research, energy conservation, health equity, and climate change. What scientists sometimes forget or negate is that policy is interpreted and implemented not only by the public policy makers, but also by individuals in the private sector and individuals and groups outside of the public realm, such as nonprofit organizations and universities. Scientists and the public may expect that policy development is rational and based on evidence, but unfortunately, this is not the usual case (Birkland, 2005; Wilfond & Thomson, 2000). For example, in recent years, policy development at the federal level in the United States is perceived by many as more grounded in partisanship rather than the needs of the public (Mecklin, 2009).

Most developed countries have a specific national body overseeing national science (including technology and innovation) policy. This national body may be the conduit for the application of public policy to science policy. The processes to implement science policy are reflective of political will, relevant knowledge, and information related to the issue and social strategy (Huston, 2008; Richmond & Kotelchuck, 1993). Policy implementation is also the result of legislation and regulation. The process for scientists to inform policy must be deliberative and continue over time using established relationships with policy makers so that there is an increased potential that cumulative scientific evidence will inform policy. Scientists can contribute to better science policy by improving the scientific quality of the evidence from their research and then communicating the research knowledge more effectively to policy makers.

Embryonic Stem Cell Research as an Example of Public Policy to Science Policy

It is important that scientists understand the interdependence between public and science policy. Policies for embryonic stem cell research are one example of the influence of public policy to science policy and the effect of political and social will on science policy. In August 2001, President G. W. Bush signed a directive that limited federal research funds to embryonic stem cell lines created before August 9, 2001. At that time, the understanding of scientific advisors was that the existing cell lines were sufficient to meet the research needs. Further examination revealed that the actual number of cell lines was much smaller than initially reported and insufficient to meet scientists' needs. This public policy directive immediately affected science policy as federal funding for embryonic stem cell research was discontinued.

The outcomes of this science policy can be interpreted as both limiting and advancing embryonic stem cell science (D. M. Burke, personal communication, September 10, 2007; *Fumento, 2009; National Research Council, 2007*). The scientists conducting research using embryonic stem cells reported that the loss of funding resulted in scientists leaving the United States to conduct their research in other countries and that there were fewer applications by students to work in the laboratories of scientists conducting embryonic stem cell research. The 2001 directive can also be interpreted as resulting in the more rapid advancement of stem cell science as alternative sources of stem cells and scientists identified alternative funding sources for their research.

Although President Obama signed Executive Order 13505[2] to remove barriers to responsible scientific research involving human stem cells, other policy actions accompanied this order. After the executive order, the NIH published draft guidelines for embryonic stem cell research and sought public comments on the guidelines. The NIH then posted a Web site for approval of embryonic stem cell lines (stemcells.nih.gov/policy/ 2009guidelines.htm) and appointed a nine-member advisory working group that included scientists, a law professor, and a medical ethicist (stemcells.nih.gov/policy/taskforce/ workinggroups/resourceaccess/). This is but one example of the interdependence of science and policy and reinforces the need for scientists to understand this relationship.

MODELS FOR PUBLIC POLICY AND SCIENCE POLICY

Wilfond and colleagues (Wilfond & Nolan, 1993; Wilfond & Thomson, 2000) distinguish policy development as extemporaneous and evidentiary. They describe the history of policy development for genetic screening and use the policy development for cystic fibrosis newborn screening as an exemplar of the models for policy development. They report that many policies are based on limited or no data, with excessive credence being placed on one or a small number of studies. In some instances, data not supportive of the policy being developed are disregarded, resulting in the loss of scientific integrity in the process. Both public and science policy can be developed extemporaneously, meaning they can be based on high political and public will due to current circumstances and, with rapid implementation, may lack scientific evidence. In extemporaneous policy development, forces affecting the use of the information can be consumer and commercial interests. Actual implementation "establishes" the policy test, and costs drive the resulting care and practice.

In contrast, the evidentiary policy model applies data from multiple sources such as epidemiological and clinical studies and works for public and professional consensus. Scientific evidence is used in its entirety to formulate policy and is given equal if not greater weight than other elements in the policy process. In contrast to extemporaneous policy development, the evidence-based standards of care and practice resulting

---

[2] Executive order 13505, March 9, 2009 (http://edocket.access.gpo.gov/2009/pdf/E9-5441.pdf).

from evidentiary policy drives utilization and costs (Wilfond & Nolan, 1993; Wilfond & Thomson, 2000). In evidentiary policy, whereas scientific evidence is the foundation of the policy, political will from public opinion is integral to the process, and the policy is analyzed in terms of costs and benefits. Researchers are better positioned to be able to inform policy when they understand the expectations of policy makers and include the expectation to inform policy through the continuum of their program of research and scholarship (Berkowitz & Gebbie, 2009; Feetham & Meister, 1999).

In 2009, there is some evidence of a stronger political will to use scientific data for evidence-based policy and decision making. Building on a speech by President Obama in September 2009, the National Academy of Sciences conducted a symposium on the dissemination and use of scientific data to inform government policy. At the same time, the National Research Council, through the Division of Behavioral and Social Sciences and Education, established an ad hoc committee to conduct a study to develop an agenda for research on the public policy uses of knowledge from social science research (The National Academies, 2009; http://www8.nationalacademies.org/cp/CommitteeView. aspx?key=49136). The committee is charged with improving the use of social science evidence in the policy process. Supporting the need for this committee, Mecklin (2009) reports that we lack the science to know what types of research best informs what types of policy and what are the most efficient and effective ways to disseminate research findings to decision makers.

In addition to understanding evidentiary and extemporaneous models of policy development, it is critical that researchers appreciate the gaps that exist in the application

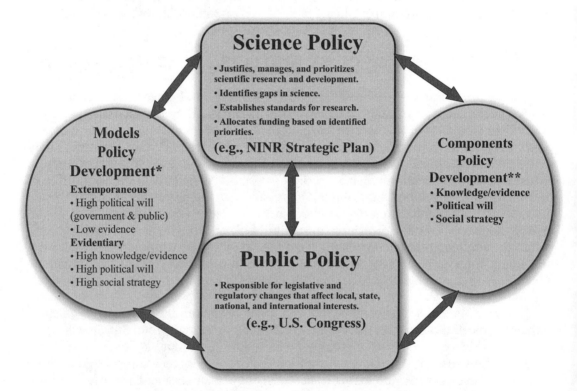

FIGURE 4.1 Integration model of science policy and public policy framed from models of policy development* and components of policy**. Copyright 2009 by S. Feetham and J. Moore. *Wilfond & Thomson, 2000. **Richmond & Kotelchuck, 1993.

of science to policy development. For example, scholars (Mecklin, 2009; Orosz, 1994) report that it is not known why some research is used and other research is not used in policy development. Although advancing the best science is a priority for researchers, understanding the processes and relationships of public policies, science policies, and the influence of politics is essential to fully advance science.

Another example of the efforts to advance evidentiary policy development is the work of the American Association for the Advancement of Science (AAAS). The AAAS, an international nonprofit organization dedicated to advancing science around the world, established the Center for Science, Technology, and Congress in 1994. The center's purpose is to provide objective information to the Congress on relevant science and technology issues to assist the scientific community in their understanding of the issues and to work with Congressional policy makers. The Center conducts targeted initiatives to bridge the gap between public policy and science policy (http://cstsp.aaas.org/). In 2009, the center briefed the Congress on "Climate Change: Health & Policy Implications," published an issue of *Science* on *Science and Technology in Congress,* and provided public comment to the Department of Health and Human Services on Objectivity in Research, the NIH Stem Cell Guidelines, and the Presidential Memo on Scientific Integrity (http://www.aaas.org/spp/cstc/, accessed November 20, 2009). Attention to the work of the AAAS can inform scientists on useful processes to monitor public and science policy. In addition, the AAAS provides examples of testimony and responses for public comment to scientific areas of interest to investigators.

SCIENTISTS' ROLES IN GOVERNMENT AND SCIENCE POLICY

Scientists are needed in the government at local, state, and national levels to inform and guide policy development and decisions related to science. The complexity of policy issues confronting the nation, including environmental concerns and the health of individuals, families, and communities, requires that there be scientists within the government who understand and can interpret science to the policy makers and to the public. When scientists transition from the conduct of their programs of research to government policy development, there is a shift from one's personal scientific knowledge and contributions to a focus on the larger public and national interests. As with one's program of research, informing policy requires recognizing that the evidence from the research to policy changes may take years as the changes diffuse from the national level to affect the public's health at the local level.

The potential to inform policy at the point of development can be seen as an opportunity. Chubin and Maienschein (2000) note that scientists who engage in policy development should not be seen as digressing from "real science" but as facilitating the expanding reach of science (p. 1501) and are a necessary part of the scientific enterprise.

Exemplars of Science Policy

Although scientists may recognize the following exemplars, they may not view these examples in the context of science policy. For nurse scientists, a central source of science policy that informs and affects research resources is the NIH. This section will describe several examples of science policy to demonstrate their processes and outcomes. Exemplars include the NIH, the largest federal funder for health research, and the Health

Resources and Services Administration (HRSA). These exemplars demonstrate the federal role of identifying gaps in the science and serving as a catalyst to bridge the gaps.

NIH Roadmap

In 2002, the Director of the NIH led a process with the nation's scientific community to develop a Roadmap to guide health research in the 21st century. The process included meetings with more than 300 leaders in academia, industry, government, and the public (http://nihroadmap.nih.gov/). The purpose of the Roadmap was to identify opportunities and gaps in biomedical research that were believed best addressed by the NIH as a whole. The Roadmap's purposes include new pathways to discovery, describing the research teams of the future, and reengineering the clinical research enterprise while sustaining the cutting-edge contributions of NIH-funded scientists. Among the outcomes of the Roadmap were changes in the structures and priorities for the review and funding of research and policies affecting investigators as individuals and research teams. The end goal of the Roadmap is the promotion of science to extend the quality of healthy life for people in this country and around the world (http://nihroadmap.nih.gov/).

Multidisciplinary to Transdisciplinary Research Teams

As part of the Roadmap initiative, multiple approaches have been taken by the NIH to change the structure and education of research teams. For example, there are changes in the expectations of research teams, with emphasis on the diversity of team members to combine the skills and disciplines of the physical, biological, and social sciences. The changes resulted from the recognition of the complexity of today's research problems, a complexity that requires scientists to collaborate across disciplines, rather than the more siloed traditional research and organizational models. To conduct complex health research, teams are required that include the biological, medical, behavioral, nursing, quantitative, informatics, engineering and computer sciences. Although each discipline brings its own strengths, perspectives, language, and methods, the intent of the Roadmap science policy is to provide incentives for multiple disciplines to develop transdisciplinary research. Transdisciplinary extends interdisciplinary and multidisciplinary research. It is an integrative process in which researchers work jointly to develop and use a shared conceptual framework that synthesizes and extends discipline-specific theories, concepts, methods, or all three, to create new models and language to address a common research problem (Kessel & Rosenfield, 2008; Rosenfield, 1992).

Multiple approaches have been supported by the NIH, the National Science Foundation, and the Agency for Healthcare Quality and Research to advance from interdisciplinary to transdisciplinary research (National Science Foundation; http://www.nsf.gov/funding/pgm_summ.jsp?pims_id=5261). For example, in 2003, the NIH implemented the Curriculum Development Award in Interdisciplinary Research that supports the development of innovative courses, curricula, and educational approaches designed to train interdisciplinary scientists in emerging areas of biomedical, behavioral, and quantitative sciences. Also, as part of the NIH Roadmap, a program to support Exploratory Centers for Interdisciplinary Research was initiated in fiscal year 2004 (RFA-RM-04-004; http://

grants1.nih.gov/grants/guide/rfa-files/RFA-RM-04-004.html), with the goal of creating full interdisciplinary research consortia.

Another key initiative of the Roadmap affecting research team composition was the transition of the longstanding General Clinical Research Centers (GCRC) to the model of Clinical Translation Science Awards (CTSA). These awards were a significant departure from the GCRC focus, with new emphasis on transdisciplinary research and research training and the development of new research partnerships with organized patient communities, community-based healthcare providers, and academic researchers. In the process of developing competitive CTSA applications, nurse scientists from nursing schools were often engaged as leaders or coleaders of components of the infrastructure such as community-based centers. With the science policy incentive of the CTSA initiative, scientists have demonstrated the contributions of nursing science and the skills of nurse scientists as leaders in research collaboration.

To further advance the goal of research team diversity, in 2006, the National Cancer Institute sponsored a meeting on the "Science of Team Science" (http://cancercontrol. cancer.gov/brp/scienceteam/index.html). (The findings from this meeting are also available as a supplement to the *American Journal of Preventive Medicine, 35*(2s) August 2008, ajpm-online.net.)

Team science is recognized as a rapidly emerging field concerned with understanding and managing circumstances that facilitate or hinder the effectiveness of large-scale research, training, and translational initiatives (National Science Foundation Profiles in Team Science; http://depts.washington.edu/teamsci/pdfs/_TeamScienceComplete_ sm.pdf). The characteristics of team science include teams where independent researchers bring their disciplinary science to provide interdisciplinary expertise. All members of the team work toward a specific scientific goal that would not be realized by any single component or discipline of the team. The results may be a new science building from the scientific language and methods across the science of the team members. Team science initiatives are designed to promote collaborative cross-disciplinary methods to examine research questions about complex phenomena such as the interdependence of genes, with the physical and social environments, and human behavior to health (Hiatt & Breen, 2008).

It has required more than the initiatives described above to change the structure and composition of research teams. Another significant policy change enables more than one principal investigator on grants and with the possibility of the principal investigators being from more than one institution (http://grants.nih.gov/grants/guide/notice-files/ NOT-OD-07-017.html). This policy change is another incentive for scientists to move toward transdisciplinary research (Stokols, Hall, Taylor, & Moser, 2008).

Summary

The multiple approaches of the NIH and other federal agencies to advance the diversity of research teams demonstrate their commitment to inform the research community and support the transition to diverse research teams (http://nihroadmap.nih.gov/). These approaches are strong examples of science policy resulting in changes in the education of researchers, the structure of research teams, and the engagement of the scientific communities. Such changes would not have occurred without these science policy incentives. It is important for scientists to monitor the reports and Web sites of funding agencies and foundations to identify changes in science policy and to use this information to inform their programs of research and scholarship.

The New Expectations of Conducting Research: Sharing Data and Common Measures

Issues regarding sharing data have been reported from before the time of Galileo (Brandt-Rauf, 2003). However, in the United States, large amounts of scientific and technical data and information are available to the public. These data sources are often supported by the government, nonprofits, and universities through public archives, libraries, data centers, and, more recently, through open Web sites. In this section, some history and context for the issues and importance of data sharing, the rationale, challenges, and expectations of researchers are described. Data containing genetic information are used as an exemplar of both the public and science policy as databases and repositories with genetic information are integral to the future for supporting bio-behavioral research. It is important that researchers know the language and issues of such databases and repositories.

The availability of data is reported to strengthen the economic and intellectual capacity in the United States. It is also noted that the same forces (academia and corporate) that benefit from public access to scientific information are also known to challenge the system to delay or have more control over public access to data (Esanu & Uhlir, 2003). Not surprisingly, the scientific advances in digital technologies have also resulted in concerns regarding public access to data (Brandt-Rauf, 2003; Hilgartner, 1997; Hilgartner & Brandt-Rauf, 1994). For research involving human subjects, there are strong regulations protecting privacy. Although this protection is essential, it can also delay or appropriately prevent access to some data.

When data are not available to other scientists, there can be redundancy of effort, resulting in wasted resources, and the trajectory to discovery can be delayed as scientists do not have data and information to build on. Froese and Reyes (2003) report that, over time, the retention of data by individuals or institutions results in a cumulative loss of knowledge because data are not archived and made accessible to scientists and the public. In addition, without open data, collaboration among scientists can be diminished.

In the United States, the intensity of public challenges for access to data supporting policy and regulation has varied over recent decades. For example, in the 1990s, the private sector requested public access to federally funded scientific data because of the perceived lack of government transparency for data used to support regulations by the Environmental Protection Agency. Differing congressional actions were taken in response to these demands, without resolution that was acceptable to both the public and governmental agencies' stakeholders. The challenges to congressional actions increased with the Data Quality Act of 2001 and continue today. The Data Quality Act required federal agencies to report the sources of their scientific data and information. These data are expected to be useful and open to independent analysis by scientists and policy makers (http://www.whitehouse.gov/omb/fedreg_reproducible/; http://www.ftc.gov/ogc/sec515/).

Despite the resistance and challenges, there is an increasing expectation for scientists to openly share their data from federally funded research. Researchers need to understand the context of the public policy and science policy behind these expectations.

Changing Culture of Sharing Data: Science Policy and the NIH

For decades, the NIH has funded individual researchers and teams of researchers to study selected disorders continually funding the collection of biological samples for research involving similar or the same disorders. In addition, the NIH has funded studies that attempt to answer similar or the same questions regarding individuals' and families' responses to health and illness, sometimes using the same and sometimes using quite disparate psychosocial and behavioral measures. These samples and data were rarely shared beyond the individual researcher or his or her research team. Although the findings from these research projects were disseminated in individual scientific publications, the findings were not often examined across studies except through periodic publications of meta-analyses. Disparate research findings and conclusions often went unnoticed, and similar discoveries across studies were not treated as accumulating evidence. This pattern of retaining samples and data by individual researchers or their institutions is reported to have resulted in a loss of knowledge and great redundancy in funding of like studies and research efforts (Froese & Reyes, 2003). This lack of access to samples and data also limited the researchers' ability to understand that with appropriate informed consent on the part of the participant, they might have used the samples for multiple purposes or even shared them more widely with other interested researchers.

In recent years, the NIH has dramatically changed its policies related to shared access for both samples and data collected as a part of NIH (federally funded) studies. This process of widespread data sharing began in the early 1990s, during the time of the *Human Genome Project (HGP)*. During the HGP, all genomic data generated as a part of the HGP were placed in a public database every evening and made freely and rapidly available on the Internet so that they would become immediately accessible to the worldwide research community. This served to accelerate the pace of scientific and medical discovery around the globe.

As a result of the widespread data sharing that occurred with the HGP, the benefits of sharing data widely and openly became clear, leading the NIH to reexamine the tradition of single research teams holding their own data. As a result, since 2003, the NIH has determined that investigators funded by them (the U.S. tax payers) should be required to share their data if their project is funded at the level of more than $500,000 per year in direct costs (http://grants.nih.gov/grants/policy/data_sharing/). Like the HGP, these data are expected to be widely shared and are considered community resources.

Although important research findings are widely shared by publishing them in scientific journals, it began to become clear that many individuals and groups did not have access to these publications because they were not members of the associations that published the journals that contained the findings. Furthermore, many people had no access because they could not afford to buy subscriptions or purchase individual journal articles over the Internet. In the early 2000s, the issue of public access to research findings that resulted from studies funded by the tax payers began to draw much attention. There were meetings and Congressional hearings to explore how these findings could become more widely accessible without negatively affecting the publishing world and infringing on U.S. copyright laws.

These deliberations resulted in the passage of a law, The NIH Public Access Policy implements Division G, Title II, Section 218 of PL 110-161 (Consolidated Appropriations Act, 2008), which states:

SEC. 218. The Director of the National Institutes of Health shall require that all investigators funded by the NIH submit or have submitted for them to the National Library of Medicine's PubMed Central an electronic version of their final peer-reviewed manuscripts upon acceptance for publication, to be made publicly available no later than 12 months after the official date of publication: Provided, That the NIH shall implement the public access policy in a manner consistent with copyright law. (http://publicaccess.nih.gov/policy.htm)

This Public Access Policy ensures that the public has access to the published results of NIH-funded research. It requires scientists to submit final peer-reviewed journal manuscripts that arise from NIH funds to the digital archive PubMed Central (http://www.pubmedcentral.nih.gov/). The policy requires that these final peer-reviewed manuscripts be accessible to the public on PubMed Central to help advance science and improve human health.

It is expected that science will be advanced through these policies. As noted, the impetus of more data sharing comes from the experiences with the HGP and also from the NIH Roadmap—New Pathways of Discovery. The intent is to advance the understanding of complex biological systems and health research through wide access to databases, technologies, and other resources (http://nihroadmap.nih.gov/).

Databases and Repositories Including Both Genotypic and Phenotypic Information

The NIH has developed a comprehensive database of genotypes and phenotypes, which is called "dbGaP." dbGaP was developed to collect, organize, and distribute data from numerous studies that have explored the associations between specific genotypic information (genetic and genomic) and phenotypic traits (e.g., blood pressure, weight, and presence or absence of a disease). Increased understanding of these associations (and, eventually, contributions and even causation) can be important for learning more about both human health and illness; the nature, biological processes, and prognoses of a particular illnesses; prediction of disease; and new preventive, diagnostic, and treatment modalities, with resulting improved healthcare outcomes. The dbGaP Web site is located at http://www.ncbi.nlm.nih.gov/entrez/query.fcgi?db=gap and is managed by the NIH Center for Biotechnology Information of the National Library of Medicine.

The dbGaP has become the repository for many other studies, resulting in extremely large amounts of genomic and phenotypic data becoming available, including those resulting from the Cancer Genome Atlas, 1000 genomes project, medical sequencing projects, the Framingham SHARe Project, the Framingham SHARe Social Network Project, and many more. The advances in genomic technologies and increasing amounts of health data (especially in electronic health records) allow for more rapid collection, storage, and distribution of these data so that they can be analyzed by researchers from around the world.

Relatively limited amount of study data (e.g., summaries including variables measured, but not individual-level data) can be directly accessed by anyone through the National Center for Biotechnology Information's Web site. To be given access to the vast majority of the data (which are not publicly available), researchers from around the world must apply to gain access to the individual-level data through an NIH Data Access Committee. The individual-level data can be examined and analyzed only by approved users, who agree to adhere to all of the participant protection policies (http://edocket.access. gpo.gov/2007/pdf/E7-17030.pdf). The researchers' agreements must also be agreed to by the researchers' institutional officials.

At this time and for the foreseeable future, it is imperative that nurse researchers learn how to access and utilize this and the numerous other databases to which they already have access. To see some of the existing databases in addition to dbGaP, visit www.ncbi. nlm.nih.gov/guide/genetics-medicine/.

Challenges and Issues to Data Repositories

The establishment of the NIH-sponsored central repository is another example of science policy. From a scientific standpoint, a central repository such as dbGaP offers a number of important advantages as individual investigators and many institutions may lack the infrastructure to develop and sustain the repository. Leaders of the NIH make the case that through a central repository, there can be stricter and more coherent control over the quality and standards of the genotype and phenotype data. They note the ability to up-date terminology and format as technologies and methodologies change. Furthermore, they argue that there can be consistent, defined, and transparent security and standards for access to the data; a long-term commitment to data maintenance after studies have been completed; a common point of entry for all investigators who use the data; a consistent and defined approach to data removal in the event of withdrawal of participant consent; facilitation of meta-analyses and analyses that use data from multiple studies; and the ability to implement consistent participant protections at the level of data submission and data access (http://ohsr.od.nih.gov/guidelines/45cfr46.html#46.101; https://gwas. lifesciencedb.jp/cgi-bin/gwasdb/gwas_top.cg; www.genome.gov/gwastudies/).

One of the potential disadvantages is that there may be some data that should not be retrievable through a single or central repository, particularly those residing at the NIH (an entity of the federal government). There are those individuals who express concerns about the federal government having access to private information about individuals. Furthermore, data stored through the NIH may be accessible through the Federal Freedom of Information Act. For data where there are legitimate reasons, they should not be accessed, such as drug use or sexual behavior of adolescents; there is an exemption that may be claimed, "Personal Information Affecting an Individual's Privacy." This exemption permits the government to withhold all information about individuals in "personnel and medical files and similar files" when the disclosure of such information "would constitute a clearly unwarranted invasion of personal privacy" (http://www. corporateservices.noaa.gov/foia/foiaex.html).

The NIH developed guidance and policies that would ensure security for participants and also allow access to the data by approved users to promote efficient and effective scientific discoveries (Policy for sharing of data obtained in NIH supported or conducted Genome-Wide Association Studies (GWAS), 2007). At the beginning of these activities, there were lengthy discussions among the scientists and ethics consultants about how much data (particularly genomic and genetic data) could be included in the open-access (publically available) database. The remainder of the data was placed in the controlled access component of the database.

In studies over the past decade, scientists have reported that by examining smaller and smaller amounts of genetic or genomic data, they can determine if an individual is a member of a larger group by matching genomic data from that individual. Jacobs (2009) and Jacobs et al. (2009) reported that they could identify both case and control individuals when they had access to the individual's genetic data and aggregate Genome-Wide Association Studies (GWAS) data. Other studies (Craig et al., 2005; Homer, 2008; Homer et al., 2008) have demonstrated that it is possible to identify that certain individuals are included in a GWAS sample even when an extremely small amount of genomic information is made available. In addition to the current DNA matching, researchers agree that in the near future, there will be sufficient knowledge, experience, and data to conduct DNA profiling using physical traits that predict hair color, eye color, stature, and others. Further privacy concerns are raised as information can be inferred from data that become available when data across data sets are combined (Greenbaum, Du & Gerstein, 2008; P³G Consortium et al., 2009).

In response to these findings, the NIH has changed its policies regarding the amount of data placed in the open-access component of dbGaP. Although consideration of these studies resulted in less information being made available in the open-access component of the database, it demonstrated the value of a national repository, where new data can be carefully and rapidly considered by experts and new safeguards can be quickly put in place to protect the privacy of human subjects (Kaye, Heeney, Hawkins, de Vries, & Boddington, 2009). Scientists anticipate that in the future, other methods for identification of individuals will be developed and that policies and practices for genomic data sharing will likely need to be continuously updated to protect and ensure participant privacy. Despite the privacy risks that may come with central data repositories, they are seen as effective, efficient, economical, and essential in promoting high-quality science and reducing duplication of expensive research efforts (Foster & Sharp, 2007; Jacobs, 2009; Wang, Barratt, Clayton, & Todd, 2005). Ethical concerns about the development and maintenance of such databases must always be kept in the foreground as this type of research moves forward.

Summary

As nurse scientists integrate genomic science advances into their research programs, it is important that they are fully informed of the public policy and science policy that affect their science. It is essential to understand the trajectory for the development of the dbGaP, the GWAS databases, and the public policy and science policy affecting access to and sharing of data, including the requirements for the protection of human subjects. Nurse scientists funded for a project where data sharing is required need to inform the study participants of this expectation. The responsibility of investigators to inform and protect their research subjects is imperative and requires understanding the advances in genomics and the resulting issues of anonymity and privacy (Clayton et al., 1995; Wallace & Clayton, 2006).

Patient-Reported Outcomes Measurement Information System

In a further effort to advance science and related to the expectations of data sharing is the NIH-initiated multicenter cooperative group Patient-Reported Outcomes Measurement Information System (PROMIS). The intent of PROMIS is to build and validate common, accessible item banks to measure key symptoms and health concepts applicable to a range of chronic conditions. Access to data banks of valid items will result in comparable data across studies of different chronic conditions. Rolland (1984, 1987; Rolland & Williams, 2005) and Gallo et al. (2009) have demonstrated that although there may be some condition-related responses, individual and family responses are related to the characteristics of the illness/condition, which supported this focus on the PROMIS initiative. This "noncategorical," non-disease-specific approach should encourage scientists to apply research findings across conditions.

This multisite initiative is a major shift from the traditional investigator-developed or selected measures used in NIH-funded research. Although such measures have evidence of reliability and validity, because the findings have not been examined across multiple studies, the potential to advance science and knowledge of health and illness is more limited. Criteria for the development of the core set of PROMIS measures include that they will be drawn primarily from existing items for the most common dimensions of patient-reported outcomes that are relevant to a wide range of chronic diseases. The items will have been used in large diverse samples. In the early phases of PROMIS, there was a focus on pain and fatigue (Chen, Revicki, Lai, Cook, & Amtmann, 2009; Christodoulou, Junghaenel, DeWalt, Rothrock, & Stone 2008). State-of-the-science measurement theory is used to develop common metrics for the measures (Hays, Bjorner, Revicki, Spritzer, & Cella, 2009; Irwin, Varni, Yeatts, & DeWalt, 2009).

The measures developed through the PROMIS initiative could provide an opportunity for research teams focusing on disease-/condition-specific research to realize the potential of advancing science as they demonstrate that their data are comparable with data from individuals and families across other diseases/conditions. Recognizing that data are comparable across studies could result in increased dialogue and collaboration across clinical investigators from diverse areas of specialization, such as one chronic illness to another. For example, using common measures, scientists studying diabetes could conduct research in collaboration with those who study the same concepts such as fatigue, pain, and/or family decision making in individuals with cancer. The findings from such collaboration could result in discoveries with relevance to practice across conditions and diseases that would not result from the traditional disease-focused research.

To encourage the use of the PROMIS repository feasibility studies, a plan to maximize acceptance and a plan for public private partnership to sustain the repository are in process. An anticipated outcome is the development of common measures of patient-reported outcomes for use in clinical trial research and clinical practice application. The PROMIS measures repository will be publicly available on a Web-based system. The PROMIS initiative as an example of science policy demonstrates the infrastructure required to support change in the scientific community (http://www.nihpromis.org/WebPages/PositiononRoadmap.aspx).

A potential limitation of the PROMIS is that the frequently used measures of individual and family responses to health and illness tend to be measures of negative outcomes, such as depression, and studies are conducted with the assumption that quality of life is diminished. Researchers do not tend to measure resiliency and processes for positive or neutral health outcomes. To date, family measures are not included in most health research (Feetham & Thomson, 2006; Grzywacz & Ganong, 2009). Unless scientists engaged in the PROMIS initiative recognize these gaps, this initiative will not reach its potential to advance the science and our knowledge of responses to health and illness. Scientists can inform the PROMIS process by monitoring the PROMIS Web site and studying the research of scientists engaged in this initiative.

Health Resources and Services Administration Core Clinical Measures

Another example of public policy influencing science policy and the federal role in addressing science gaps is the Department of Health and Human Services Health Resources and Services Administration (HRSA) initiative for core clinical measures for HRSA grantees providing health services (http://www.hrsa.gov/quality/coremeasures.htm accessed 11/22/09). Public attention to safety and quality has increased since the Institute of Medicine (1999) report *To Err Is Human: Building a Safer Health System* and the subsequent report *Crossing the Quality Chasm: A New Health System for the 21st Century* (Institute of Medicine, 2001). Public accountability was one reason for the core clinical measures initiative, as HRSA grantees providing health services to the public receive reimbursement from multiple funding sources including federal and state funds. A characteristic of HRSA-supported health centers is that they meet performance and accountability requirements regarding administrative, clinical, quality, and financial operations (Institute of Medicine, 2002).

The HRSA Federally Qualified Health Centers are the agency's largest clinical services program. In 2008, health centers cared for more than 17 million patients, employed more than 113,000 people in underserved communities, and leveraged more than $8 billion in other health resources. For more than 40 years, HRSA-supported health centers have provided comprehensive, culturally competent, quality primary healthcare services to medically underserved communities and vulnerable populations. Health centers serve people of all ages, races, and ethnicities; those without and with health insurance; and special populations including migrant and seasonal farm workers and their families. Health centers also serve the homeless and residents of public housing and outpatient health programs/facilities operated by tribal organizations (http://bphc.hrsa.gov/).

Traditionally, except for descriptive data in the Uniform Data System, when the health centers and other HRSA clinical service grantees reported their clinical outcomes, each grantee selected its own outcome measures. This resulted in data that were not comparable across HRSA grantees and, in most instances, not comparable to nationally recognized standards. Therefore, the Health Center Program was not able to communicate to the Congress and other stakeholders clinical outcome data across all grantees. In 2005, through a HRSA-wide initiative implemented by the agency's scientists and clinicians, existing reports were reviewed, as well as national measures reported by the National Quality Forum, the National Committee on Quality Assessment, and the former Ambulatory Care Quality Alliance, now known as the AQA alliance. The National Committee on Quality Assessment is the national leader for the Healthcare Effectiveness Data and Information Set, a tool used by more than 90% of America's health plans to measure performance on important dimensions of care and service. From this review of reports from HRSA-service-providing grantees and standard measures, HRSA scientists and clinicians identified potential core measures.

Additional evidence of the alignment of public policy to science policy is that the core measures address priority health conditions of HRSA populations and that they are of complex conditions of high cost and morbidity in the United States. These measures cover the age continuum and include screening for colon, breast, and cervical cancer. These are cancers that disproportionately affect HRSA populations and for which early detection and care can significantly decrease mortality and improve 5-year survival. In addition, the HRSA core measures set includes measures for prenatal HIV screening, access to prenatal care, and appropriate immunizations by life cycle. Chronic disease management performance measures are included for diabetes and hypertension. Another criterion for the measures is that they are amenable for quality improvement. These core measures are presented to all HRSA grantees providing health services in a standard format that includes the science and evidence for each measure (www.hrsa.gov/quality/coremeasures.htm).

To reflect HRSA's important role in population and community health, additional Core Clinical measures are planned in the areas of mental health, oral health, asthma, obesity, and smoking. Quality measures for patient safety, patient satisfaction, and health literacy/communication are also being considered. This initiative demonstrates HRSA's commitment to quality improvement and begins to measure and demonstrate the quality of care across the agency as a whole (http://www.hrsa.gov/quality/coremeasures.htm, accessed November 22, 2009). As these data are reported beginning in 2010 and are made available to researchers, they will inform community-based health services and clinical research. Being able to report on clinical performance measures that align with major national quality improvement organizations to make evidence-based statements about the impact of their grantees providing health services on improving access to cost-effective care for the nation's underserved populations. In addition, HRSA grantees will have the ability to measure the quality of care delivered to their patient populations.

This exemplar on HRSA core measures is important in several ways; it demonstrates the role of science and scientists in informing federal programs (Chubin & Maienschein, 2000) and the federal role in identifying gaps in policy and bridging those gaps. A nurse scientist was the initial lead on this project, and federal nurses were a significant part of the HRSA-wide team. This initiative also demonstrates the cycle of public policy development, the application of science policy, and the eventual effect on health policy.

ROLE OF SCIENTISTS IN SCIENCE POLICY

There are repeated calls for scientists worldwide to become involved in guiding government decisions concerning science. In the United States, science policy-making positions range from political appointees (advisory panels, review groups, and professional associations) to consultants, to career scientists in federal, state, and local governments. In these roles, scientists may provide leadership on programs, science and technology issues, and budgets. What is needed is knowledgeable "civic scientists" as staff in public service to provide informed science policy making (Chubin & Maienschein, 2000).

RESPONSIBILITIES OF SCIENTISTS TO INFORM AND MONITOR SCIENCE POLICY

Changes in science policy from federal agencies come primarily as a result of processes evident to the public and with opportunities for public input. It is therefore imperative that scientists monitor the Web sites of funders and those of the federal agencies and the

Federal Register (http://www.gpoaccess.gov/fr/) for opportunities for public comment on new policies and requests for information (RFI). An example is the 2007 RFI regarding the peer review process at the NIH (RFI: "NIH System to Support Biomedical and Behavioral Research and Peer"), where the NIH sought comments regarding the NIH's support of biomedical and behavioral research, including peer review. The goal of the RFI was to examine the current system to optimize its efficiency and effectiveness. In this RFI, the NIH stated that it was interested in creative suggestions, even if they involve radical changes to the current approach (http://grants.nih.gov/grants/guide/notice-files/NOT-OD-07-074.html). Scientists had the opportunity to provide information regarding proposal page limits, composition of study sections, and the processes for peer review, including the presence of the principal investigator during reviews. It appears that few nurse scientists responded to this opportunity. Although the majority of responses appeared to come from biological scientists, the resulting changes in the peer review process affected the scientists across all disciplines.

To be better informed scientists, researchers need to first understand what science policy is and its impact on programs of research and then focus on health, public, and science policy relevant to their programs of research. Scientists need to serve on advisory committees and study sections, monitor and respond to RFIs, participate in policy fellowships, and design their programs of research to inform policy. An example of a policy fellowship is the interdisciplinary Robert Wood Johnson Foundation Health Policy Fellowship (www.healthpolicyfellows.org/).

To improve the development of programs of research that have the potential to effectively inform and influence policy, nurse scientists should answer the following questions:

- Will the research improve health outcomes?
- What is the effect on healthcare service, including costs?
- Which institutions or agencies of government may be interested in the findings?
- Will the research findings be able to be translated into current practice? Are the interventions practical for larger scale application?
- Will the research findings have the capacity to potentially affect a large group of people that are identified as national priority areas?
- How can the results be made a permanent part of healthcare?
- Does the current political climate possess the political will to change current practices based on the research findings?
  - In what ways can the intended research be adjusted to accommodate this reality?
  - Is there flexibility as the political climate changes?

(Feetham & Meister, 1999; Richmond & Kotelchuck, 1993; J. Moore, personal communication, December 5, 2009).

SUMMARY

Science policy influences the context, resources, and parameters for the conduct and dissemination of science. It is an iterative and interdependent process among public policy, science policy, and researchers. Scientists need to assume a more focused role in monitoring and informing science policy by responding to RFIs, providing congressional testimony, and serving on advisory committees and study sections (www.csr.nih.gov/

Committees/rosterindex.asp; cms.csr.nih.gov, resources for Applicants; www.ninr.nih. gov/NR/rdonlyres/1E4D1CA0-FA23-4819-8A6C-4B9C59FA4B46/5109/Febmin01.pdf 11-09-2009). More academic and corporate scientists need to pursue roles as staff in public service to provide informed science policy making. The trajectory from public policy to science policy does not occur in isolation. With limited resources for science, passivity by researchers is not an option.

ACKNOWLEDGMENTS

The author thanks Barbara Barth Frink, PhD, RN, FAAN, Pam S. Hinds, PhD, RN, FAAN, Jennifer Moore, BSN, MS, RN, and Elizabeth Thomson, DNSc, MS, RN, CGC, FAAN, for their reviews and critique of the chapter.

REFERENCES

American Association for the Advancement of Science. (2009). *Policy Brief May 2009*. Retrieved from http://www.aaas.org/spp/cstc/briefs/stemcells/index.shtml

American Association for the Advancement of Science. Center for Science, Technology and Congress. Retrieved November 20, 2009, from http://www.aaas.org/spp/cstc/

Berkowitz B., & Gebbie K. M. (2009). Nurses and policy: What more is there to say? *Nursing Outlook, 57*(2), 69.

Birkland, T. A. (2005). Models of the policy process. *An introduction to the policy process: Theories, concepts, and models of public policy* (pp. 200–232). New York: M.E. Sharpe Inc.

Brandt-Rauf, S. (2003). The role, value, and limits of S&T data and information in the public domain for biomedical research. In J. M. Esanu & P. F. Uhlir (Eds.), *The role of scientific and technical data and information in the public domain: Proceedings of a symposium*. Washington, DC: National Academies Press.

Chen, W. H., Revicki, D. A., Lai, J. S., Cook, K. F., & Amtmann, D. (2009). Linking pain items from two studies onto a common scale using item response theory. *Journal of Pain and Symptom Management, 38*(4), 615–628.

Christodoulou, C., Junghaenel, D. U., DeWalt, D. A., Rothrock, N., & Stone, A. A. (2008). Cognitive interviewing in the evaluation of fatigue items: Results from the patient-reported outcomes measurement information system (PROMIS). *Quality of Life Research, 17*(10), 1239–1246.

Chubin, D., & Maienschein, J. (2000, November 24). Staffing science policy-making. *Science, 290*, 1501.

Clayton, E. W., Steinberg, K. K., Khoury, M. J., Thomson, E., Andrews, L., Kahn, M. J., Kopelman, L. M., & Weiss, J. O. (1995). Informed consent for genetic research on stored tissue samples. *Journal of the American Medical Association, 274*(22), 1786–1792.

Craig, D. W., Huentelman, M. J., Hu-Lince, D., Zismann, V. L., Kruer, M. C., Lee, A. M., . . . Stephan, D. A. (2005). Identification of disease causing loci using an array-based genotyping approach on pooled DNA. *BMC Genomics 6*, 138.

Data Quality Act. (2001). Retrieved November 20, 2009, from http://www.whitehouse.gov/omb/fedreg_reproducible/; http://www.ftc.gov/ogc/sec515/dbGaP Database Genotype and Phenotype. Retrieved October 20, 2009, from http://www.ncbi.nlm.nih.gov/gap

Esanu, J. M., & Uhlir, P. F. (Eds.) *The role of scientific and technical data and information in the public domain: Proceedings of a symposium*. Washington, DC: National Academies Press.

Feetham, S. L., & Meister, S. B. (1999). Nursing research of families: State of the science and correspondence with policy. In A. S. Hinshaw, S. Feetham, & J. Shaver (Eds.), *Handbook of clinical nursing research* (pp. 251–272). Thousand Oaks, CA: SAGE Publications.

Feetham, S. L., & Thomson, E. J. (2006) Keeping the individual and family in focus. In S. M. Miller, S. H. McDaniel, J. S. Rolland, & S. L. Feetham (Eds.). *Individuals, families, and the new era of genetics—Biopsychosocial perspectives*. New York, NY: WW Norton & Company.

Foster, M. S. & Sharp, R. R. (2007). Share and share alike: Deciding how to distribute the scientific and social benefits of genomic data. *Nature Reviews Genetics, 8,* 633–639.

Froese, R., & Reyes, Jr., R. (2003). Use them or lose them: The need to make collection databases publicly available. In A. Legakis, S. Sfenthourakis, R. Polymeri, & M. Thessalou-Legaki (Eds.). *Proceedings of the 18th International Congress of Zoology* (pp. 585–591).

Fumento, M. (2009). The dirty secret of embryonic stem cell research—Science, funding and stem cell research. Retrieved from Forbes.com

Gallo, A. M., Knafl, K. A., & Angst, D. B. (2009). Information management in families who have a child with a genetic condition. *Journal of Pediatric Nursing, 24*(3), 194–204.

Greenbaum, D., Du, J., & Gerstein, M. (2008). Genomic anonymity: Have we already lost it? *American Journal of Bioethics, 8,* 71–74.

Grzywacz, J. G., & Ganong, L. (2009). Special issue: Families and health. *Family Relations, 58*(4), 373–379.

GWAS Genome Wide Association Studies data base. https://gwas.lifesciencedb.jp/cgi-bin/gwasdb/gwas_top.cgi

Hays, R. D., Bjorner, J., Revicki, R. A., Spritzer, K. L., & Cella, D. (2009). Development of physical and mental health summary scores from the Patient Reported Outcomes Measurement Information System (PROMIS) global items. *Quality of Life Research, 18*(7), 873–880. (PMCID: Pending)

Health Resources and Services Administration core measures. Retrieved November 22, 2009, from http://www.hrsa.gov/quality/coremeasures.htm

Health Resources and Services Administration Federally Qualified Health Centers. Retrieved November 10, 2009, from http://bphc.hrsa.gov/

Hiatt, R. A., & Breen, N. (2008). The social determinants of cancer: A challenge for transdisciplinary science. *American Journal of Preventive Medicine, 35*(2S), S141–S149.

Hilgartner, S., & Brandt-Rauf, S. I. (1994). Data access, ownership, and control: Toward empirical studies of access practices. *Knowledge: Creation, Diffusion, Utilization 15*(4), 355–372.

Hilgartner, S. (1997). Access to data and intellectual property: Scientific exchange in genome research. In National Research Council, *Intellectual property rights and research tools in molecular biology* (pp. 28–39), Washington, DC: National Academy Press.

Homer, N. (2008). Resolving individuals contributing trace amounts of DNA to highly complex mixtures using high-density SNP genotyping microarrays. *PLoS Genet, 4*(8), e1000167.

Homer, N., Szelinger, S., Redman, M., Duggan, D., Tembe, W., Muehling, J., . . . Craig, D. W. (2008). Resolving individuals contributing trace amounts of DNA to highly complex mixtures using high-density SNP genotyping microarrays. *PLoS Genet, 4*(8), e1000167.

Huston, A. C. (2008). From research to policy and back. *Child Development, 79*(1), 1–12.

Irwin, D. E., Varni, J. M., Yeatts, K., & DeWalt, D. A. (2009). Cognitive interviewing methodology in the development of a pediatric item bank: A Patient Reported Outcomes Measurement Information System (PROMIS) study. *Health and Quality of Life Outcomes, 7,* 3. (PMCID: PMC2642767)

Institute of Medicine. (1999). *To err is human: Building a safer health system.* Washington, DC: National Academy Press.

Institute of Medicine. Committee on Quality of Health Care in America. (2001). *Crossing the quality chasm: A new health system for the 21st century.* Retrieved August 17, 2006, from http://www.nap.edu/books/0309072808/html/

Institute of Medicine. (2002). *National priorities for action: Transforming health care quality.* Washington, DC: National Academy Press.

Jacobs, K. (2009, October 05). NIH-led study confirms ability to identify individuals from GWAS data. *GenomeWeb Daily News.* Retrieved from http://www.genomeweb.com

Jacobs, K. B., Yeager, M., Wacholder, S., Craig, D., Kraft, P., Hunter, D. J., . . . Chatterjee, N. (2009). A new statistic and its power to infer membership in a genome-wide association study using genotype frequencies. *Nature Genetics, 41*(11), 1253–1257. Epub 2009 Oct 4.

Kaye, J., Heeney, C., Hawkins, N., de Vries, J., & Boddington, P. (2009). Data sharing in genomics—re-shaping scientific practice. *Nature Reviews Genetic, 10*(5), 331–335.

Kessel, F. S., & Rosenfield, P. L. (2008). Toward transdisciplinary research: Historical and contemporary perspectives. *American Journal of Preventive Medicine, 35*(2S), S225–S234.

Lezine, D. A., & Reed, G. A. (2007). Political will: A bridge between public health knowledge and action. *American Journal of Public Health, 97*(11), 2010–2013.

Mecklin, J. (2009). The science of good government. *Miller-McCune, 2*(4), 8–10.

National Institutes of Health (2009). *Guidelines on stem cell research.* Retrieved November 20, 2009, from http://stemcells.nih.gov/policy/2009guidelines.htm

National Institutes of Health Roadmap. Retrieved October, 2009 http://nihroadmap.nih.gov/

National Institutes of Health Roadmap. Exploratory Centers for Interdisciplinary Research. Retrieved October 2009 RFA-RM-04-004 http://grants1.nih.gov/grants/guide/rfa-files/RFA-RM-04-004.html

National Institutes of Health, National Cancer Institute *Science of Team Science* Meeting October 2007; http://cancercontrol.cancer.gov/brp/scienceteam/index.html

National Institute of Nursing Research Mission and Strategic Plan. Retrieved June, 2009, from http://www.ninr.nih.gov/AboutNINR/NINRMissionandStrategicPlan/

National Research Council (U.S.). (2007). *The National Academies' 2007 amendments guidelines for human embryonic stem cell research.* Washington, DC: National Academies Press.

National Science Foundation. *Profiles in Team Science.* Retrieved from http://depts.washington.edu/teamsci/pdfs/_TeamScienceComplete_sm.pdf

National Quality Forum. (2004). *National voluntary consensus standards for nursing-sensitive care: An initial performance measure set. A consensus report.* Retrieved August 17, 2006, from http://www.qualityforum.org/txNCFINALpublic.pdf

Orosz, E. (1994). The impact of social science research on health policy. *Social Science and Medicine, 39*(9), 1287–1293.

P³G Consortium, Church, G., Heeney, C., Hawkins, N., de Vries, J., Boddington, P., . . . Weir, B. (2009). Public access to genome-wide data: Five views on balancing research with privacy and protection. *PLoS Genet, 5*(10), e1000665. doi:10.1371/journal.pgen.1000665.

Policy for sharing of data obtained in NIH supported or conducted Genome-Wide Association Studies (GWAS). (2007). National Institutes of Health, HHS. *Federal Register.* 72:166 Tuesday, August 28, 2007 49290. Retrieved from http://edocket.access.gpo.gov/2007/pdf/E7-17030.pdf

Patient Reported Outcomes Measurement Information System. (2009). Retrieved October 10, 2009, from http://www.nihpromis.org/WebPages/PositiononRoadmap.aspx

Richmond, J. B., & Kotelchuck, M. (1993) Political influences: Rethinking national health policy. In C. Mcquire, R. Foley, A. Gorr, & R. Richards (Eds.), *Handbook of health professions education* (pp. 386–404). San Francisco, CA: Jossey-Bass Publishers.

Rolland, J. S. (1984). Toward a psychosocial typology of chronic and life-threatening illness. *Family Systems Medicine, 2*, 245–263.

Rolland, J. S. (1987). Chronic illness and the life cycle: a conceptual framework. *Family Process Journal, 26*, 203–221.

Rolland, J. S., & Williams, J. K. (2005). Toward a biopsychosocial model for 21st century genetics. *Family Process Journal, 44*, 3–24.

Rosenfield, P. L. (1992). The potential of transdisciplinary research for sustaining and extending linkages between the health and social sciences. *Social Science & Medicine, 35*, 1343–1357.

Rossi, P. H., & Freeman, H. E. (1993). *Evaluation: A systematic approach* (5th ed.). Newbury Park: Sage.

Stokols, D., Hall, K. L., Taylor, B. K., & Moser, R. P. (2008). The science of team science overview of the field and introduction to the supplement. *American Journal of Preventive Medicine, 35*(2S), S77–S89. Retrieved from http://cancercontrol.cancer.gov/brp/scienceteam/ajpm/ScienceTeamScienceOverviewFieldIntroductionSupplement.pdf

The AIP Bulletin of Science Policy News. Accessed February, 2009, from http://www.aip.org/fyi/2009/016.html

The National Academies (2009). *A research agenda for the use of social science evidence in public policy.* DBASSE-CFE-09-09. Accessed October 2009, from http://www8.nationalacademies.org/cp/CommitteeView.aspx?key=49136

Wallace, C., & Clayton, D. G. (2006). Appropriate use of information on family history of disease in recruitment for linkage analysis studies. *Annals of Human Genetics, 70*(Pt 3), 360–371.

Wang, W. Y., Barratt, B. J., Clayton, D. G., & Todd, J. A. (2005). Genome-wide association studies: Theoretical and practical concerns. *Nature Reviews Genetics, 6*(2), 109–118.

Wilfond, B.S., & Nolan, K. (1993). National policy development for the clinical application of genetic diagnostic technologies. *Journal of the American Medical Association, 270*(24), 2948–2954.

Wilfond, B. S., & Thomson, E. J. (2000). Models of public health genetic policy development. In M. J. Khoury, W. Burke, & E. J. Thomson (Eds.), *Genetics and public health in the 21st century.* New York: Oxford.

5

Changing Health Science Policy: The Establishment of the National Institute of Nursing Research at the National Institutes of Health

Ada Sue Hinshaw and Janet Heinrich

INTRODUCTION

Although the history of nursing research goes back to the systematic care studies in hospitals that Nightingale conducted during the Crimean War (1853–1856), nursing research was not a recognized part of mainstream biomedical research in the United States until the establishment of the National Center for Nursing Research (NCNR) (1986), later redesignated the National Institute of Nursing Research (NINR) (1986), at the National Institutes of Health (NIH).

The establishment of the NINR, within the NIH, informed and influenced science policy. Science policy is defined as documents and statements articulating the scientific interests, directions, and programs of institutions, associations, and/or governmental agencies. Such policies direct research resources distribution.

The NIH mission focuses on biomedical and behavioral research that, in 1986, was heavily centered on the etiology of diseases, mechanisms of spread and injury, and appropriate therapies. The NINR brought a new perspective that was complementary to the biomedical approach. The integration of such a new disciplinary approach at the NIH brought new values, language, and focus to the agency.

Nursing research reflects the profession's commitment to patient-centered care within the family, community, and health systems context. The focus is on health promotion/risk reduction, even within illnesses. There is an emphasis on individuals or families and their illness experience and, in particular, a concern with symptom management of the consequences of illnesses and the side effects of medical therapies. Preserving the dignity of individuals and families during health, illness, and end of life is a special consideration of the profession and discipline (Cabinet on Nursing Research, 1985). These premises guide nursing research programs. However, such a different perspective could not help but reshape health science through new priorities, calls for applications and proposals, and grant award funding with a strong interdisciplinary, collaborative component.

What were the political and policy context and processes that supported the successful legislation creating a place for nursing research within "the mainstream of scientific investigation?" This chapter will examine the context and processes surrounding the establishment of the NINR at the NIH.

LEGISLATIVE PROCESS TO ESTABLISH THE NCNR/NINR

The legislative process to establish the NCNR/NINR began in the Fall of 1983 and extended through to April of 1986, when the center was created under the Health Research Extension Act of 1985. Since this chapter will refer repeatedly to this successful legislative process in telling the story of the NCNR/NINR, the key events and dates for the political process will be outlined.

The two-year process was as follows:

- Fall of 1983: Congressman Edward Madigan (R-Illinois) introduced legislation to amend the NIH reauthorization to create a National Institute of Nursing (NIN), among other changes.
- November of 1983: The above amendment was passed by the House of Representatives.
- Early 1984: Senator Orrin Hatch (R-Utah) introduced legislation to create a Center for Nursing Research in The Bureau of Nursing, Health Resources and Services Administration (HRSA).
- Fall of 1984: Two bills, House and Senate, were resolved in the conference but vetoed by President Reagan as he awaited the 1984 NIH Structure Report from the Institute of Medicine (IOM).
- Early Fall of 1985: New legislation for the creation of the NIN was introduced in the House and Senate.
- October of 1985: Two bills were reconciled in conference committee. Negotiations with the White House led to the NCNR.
- November of 1985: President Reagan vetoed the legislation, calling it micromanagement of the NIH.
- November of 1985: The House of Representatives and Senate overrode the Presidential veto by overwhelming majorities.
- April 16, 1986: The NCNR was established under the Health Research Extension Act of 1985.

THEORETICAL CONTEXT FOR CREATION OF THE NCNR/NINR

The Shamian, Skelton-Green, and Villeneuve (2003) model, entitled "From Talk to Action" is utilized to understand the political legislative process and the professional context surrounding the NCNR/NINR's creation. The model's stages and steps are created to lead to health policy change.

The Shamian et al. (2003) model for moving a public health issue into policy consists of two stages: getting to the policy agenda and moving into action. The initial stage, getting to the policy agenda, includes five steps: (1) values and cultural beliefs, (2) emergence of problems or issues, (3) knowledge and research development, (4) public awareness, and (5) political engagement.

The second stage consists of three steps, including (1) interest group activation, (2) public policy deliberation and adoption, and (3) regulation, experience, and revision. Establishing the NINR within the "mainstream of health science" encompassed all of these steps.

Values and Cultural Beliefs

The importance of nursing research for improving patient care and the general public health was evolving over a period of 30 years. Nursing research grants and fellowship programs of the Public Health Service (PHS) were established in 1955 (Gortner & Nahm, 1977, p. 27). At this time, there was $500,000 for research grants and $125,000 for fellowships allocated for nursing research, operated out of the Institute of General Medical Sciences of the NIH. From this small beginning, the number of nurse scientists grew, as did the number of universities offering doctoral programs in nursing and related biomedical and behavioral fields. By the mid-1970s, nursing research was funded in the areas of cancer, aging, mental health, and maternal and child health, with the major focus of nursing research centered in the Division of Nursing, a component of the Bureau of Health Manpower in the Health Resources Administration. The research programs were administered by the Division of Nursing as of 1967, where they were closely linked with nursing education and nursing practice. Funding for nursing research was steady at approximately $5 million per year, although yearly appropriations were a constant battle to be won (Gortner & Nahm, 1977, p. 28).

In 1956, Virginia Henderson wrote a guest editorial in *Nursing Research*, noting that nurse studies outnumbered nursing practice studies 10 to 1 and that more than half of doctoral theses focused on nursing education (Gortner & Nahm, 1977, p. 20). There was a growing concern that more research should address practice and patient care issues. Gortner, Bloch, and Phillips (1976) proposed the following framework for nursing research on patient care:

> Nursing research has been less concerned with physical and mental diseases than with the general and specific impairments of man such as pain, anxiety, suffering and hospitalization and attendant stress. Instead, the term patient care research has become synonymous with much of the recent activities in nursing research: the growth of clinically relevant studies over the past four years has been remarkable. . . . While our knowledge in many areas remains insufficient, there is neither the dearth of information nor the apparent lack of interest in practice-related research that was evident just five years ago. . . . [Moreover] the growth in practice-related research has been accompanied by increasing rigor and sophistication, both in the choice of problems and the design of the studies (Gortner & Nahm, 1977, p. 24).

The evolving research could be understood with a set of classification categories that the above authors proposed. The classification categories included building a science of practice or identification of individual and group health needs, the artistry of practice or clinical therapeutics and procedures, experimental studies of the physical and social environments in which nurses and clients interact, the development of methodologies or measurement tools such as indicators of care quality, and the application of research findings to improve care in controlled studies (Gortner & Nahm, 1977, p. 24).

In the mid to late 1970s, a small group of nursing research leaders were concerned about the lack of visibility and limited resources for nursing research, both at the NIH and on Capitol Hill. Two or three investigators were making visits to elected officials to talk about the potential nursing research contributions. Ada Jacox and Barbara Hansen, nursing research pioneers, visited their elected officials and members of the Appropriations Committees in both the House and the Senate. Others, including JoAnne Stevenson and, later, Nola Pender and Nancy Woods, were talking to officials at the NIH to explore funding opportunities from organizations other than the Division of Nursing, without much success.

A nursing research network was formed in the late 1970s, initiated by Carolyn Williams and implemented by Ada Sue Hinshaw, as a component of the American Nurses Association (ANA), Cabinet on Nursing Research, to develop examples of nursing research that could inform the Congress on the need for funding. Participants in this legislative network were encouraged to contact their elected officials to explain their research findings. Early examples of study topics included low-birth-weight infants care, pain management, and quality of patient care. At this time, some of the prominent nursing research leaders were beginning to talk about the need for nursing research to be a part of the biomedical and behavioral research mainstream, in other words, a part of the NIH.

Many nursing leaders believed strongly that any talk of moving nursing research into the mainstream of biomedical and behavioral research at the NIH was dangerous and naïve. They considered nursing research to be in an early and formative stage that benefited from linkages with nursing education and practice.

Emergence of a Problem or Issue

In 1983, the IOM issued a report on the future of nursing, *Nursing and Nursing Education: Public Policy and Private Actions*, that recommended that nursing research be part of the biomedical and behavioral research mainstream, which nursing assumed was the NIH (IOM, 1983). The report specifically recommended, "establish an entity for nursing research in the mainstream of scientific investigation" (IOM, 1983, p. 19). The report recommendations became an issue of discussion at major nursing organization meetings. A group of organizations, called the Tri-Council, including the ANA, National League for Nursing, American Association of Critical-Care Nurses, and, later, the American Organization of Nurse Executives, was formed to consider concerns about moving nursing research to the NIH. Many nursing leaders voiced strong opposition to the idea and concerns that the Division of Nursing and all other nursing programs would be harmed by such a move. The Division of Nursing was seen by some as the one and only base for all of nursing in the Federal government. Leadership within the Cabinet on Nursing Research (chair, Nola Pender), a component of the ANA, was very enthusiastic about moving nursing research to the NIH, as were some of the leaders in the other organizations.

At the same time, the legislation for the reauthorization of the NIH was being considered in Committee in the House of Representatives. Congressman Madigan (R-Illinois) introduced an amendment to the reauthorization creating a NIN within the NIH, thus implementing the recommendation from the IOM report. Although not all nursing leaders were supportive of the idea at the time, they did not speak publically against the amendment. The Federal Administration, and specifically the Director of the NIH, was surprised by the amendment and very much against the idea of nursing research at the institutes. There were also several medical groups that came forward against nursing research at the NIH, arguing that it is not a "good fit" with biomedical research.

It was only after Congressman Madigan became interested in the legislation that the measure began to move out of the Committee. In the Senate, there was more interest in an arthritis institute, but other controversial issues such as research using fetal tissue, was holding the reauthorization back. The issue became how best to move the reauthorization forward in the House and Senate, with or without a NIN.

Knowledge and Research Development

The House version of the NIH reauthorization including a NIN was ultimately passed by the Congress but vetoed by President Regan. Congress was not in session, so no counteractions could be taken. This allowed nursing organizations and nurse researchers to educate their membership on the issues and explain the benefits of nursing research at the NIH. The ANA Cabinet on Nursing Research developed a plan of what an institute would look like. Concerns about the focus of nursing research and methodologies that could be funded were addressed. Some researchers were concerned that only biomedical models of research would be funded.

At the same time, there were efforts to educate officials at the NIH about nursing research. There was an NIH Task Force, chaired by the Director of the Institute on Aging, Frank Williams, MD, to study nursing research funded at the NIH. The charge to the NIH Task force on Nursing Research was the following:

- To assess the NIH current support of nursing research;
- To evaluate the feasibility of increasing NIH support of nursing research consistent with the NIH mission; and
- To examine nurses' current and potential role on NIH peer review groups, advisory committees, councils, and boards.

The NIH Task Force found 64 applications assigned to institutes at the NIH from schools, departments, or colleges of nursing in 1984. Forty-one of the applications were competing, with 16 of 41 approved and 6 ultimately funded. The Task Force concluded that (1) the research funded did fit the mission of the NIH and (2) the nursing research environment could be enhanced at the NIH by strengthening and targeting specific programs as well as encouraging more collaborative and interdisciplinary research and training (Task Force on Nursing Research, 1984).

The Assistant Secretary for Health established a Public Health Service (PHS) Task Force on Nursing Research. A contract was issued to assess the organizational locus for PHS nursing research activities. The Lewin group interviewed a variety of stakeholders and considered several options for supporting nursing research. The report concluded that nursing research should be provided more visibility and be housed within the HRSA (Gornick & Lewin, 1985).

The third study that was conducted at the request of the Administration was a report undertaken by the IOM in 1984, entitled *Responding to Health Needs and Scientific Opportunity: The Organizational Structure of the National Institutes of Health*. The report suggested that certain criteria needed to be met by any proposed NIH institute: (1) compatible with the research and research training mission of the NIH, (2) the proposed research area is not already receiving adequate attention, (3) reasonable prospects for scientific growth and funding, and (4) the change would improve communication, management priority setting, and accountability. The nursing leaders declared that the NIN would meet these criteria.

Public Awareness

Initially, there was little public awareness of the contributions of nursing research to patient care and public health. However, there was general awareness that nursing research needed to be provided visibility and resources. Representatives of the Tri-Council for Nursing met with the Assistant Secretary for Health, the Director of the NIH, and other PHS leaders to explore the establishment of a nursing institute. They were told that the Secretary of the Health and Human Services would announce the establishment of an entity for nursing research at the HRSA.

The ANA and its Congressional Staff Office (Director, Jan Heinrich) began working with over 70 specialty nursing organizations to encourage their support of a nursing institute at the NIH. Several of these nursing organizations supported nursing research programs, such as the oncology nurses, and represented large numbers of professionals, such as the operating room nurses and critical care nurses. There was enthusiastic support by all of the nursing organizations for nursing research moving into the mainstream of biomedical and behavioral research.

Political Engagement

The ANA Cabinet on Nursing Research provided leadership, developing communication materials to educate the public, the U.S. Congress, and other nursing organizations about nursing research. Clear definitions and classifications of the research types that informed practice were developed. In 1985, the Cabinet published an overarching plan, Directions for Nursing Research: Towards the Twenty-First Century, used by nurse researchers and ANA staff to explain to members of the Congress how patient care could be improved by moving nursing research to the NIH. In response to the assertion that nursing research did not fit within the existing NIH structure, as claimed by some medical organizations and elected officials, leaders stated that nursing research is not a disease or body part, as is the focus of many NIH institutes, but does address processes for improving care, using biomedical and behavioral interventions. Some of the specific examples of nursing research used to educate elected and appointed officials included the following:

- Measurement and management of the pain experience; anticipatory preparation (Johnson, Rice, Fuller, & Endress, 1978);
- Patient and family adaptation to life-threatening illnesses, such as breast cancer (Benoliel & McCorkle, 1983);
- Parent-child interaction as predictor of cognitive and language development (Barnard, Bee, & Hammond, 1984); and
- Family care giving and implications for middle-aged women (Archbold, 1983).

Another strategy used by leaders of the ANA Cabinet on Nursing Research working closely with the ANA government relations staff was to identify champions within the House and Senate, elected officials who were willing to work on the authorizing legislation and on increasing appropriations for nursing research. On the House side, there was Congressman Ed Madigan (R-Illinois), who sponsored the authorizing language for the

NIN, and Congressman Carl Purcell (R-Michigan), who worked on appropriations. In the Senate, there was Senator Ted Kennedy (D-Massachusetts) and Senator Mark Hatfield (R-Oregon), who supported authorizing language, and Senator Daniel Inouye (D-Hawaii), who provided assistance with appropriations. Senator Orin Hatch (R-Utah) sponsored legislation that recognized nursing research but established an entity within the HRSA, although later, he supported the establishment of an NCNR at the NIH. Nursing leaders from each member's individual state and district formed strong relationships with these members of Congress and continued working with them and supporting them over time. For example, there was a large cadre of nurses from the University of Michigan that formed to support Congressman Purcell.

The ANA established a grassroots educational campaign, which included a nurse in almost every Congressional District in the United States, that could be activated when ever-important votes were taking place in the House and Senate. This outreach system, developed and coordinated by Pat Ford-Roegner of the ANA Government Relations staff, was instrumental in organizing calls and telegrams to offices of elected officials in support of the NIN at the NIH. The grassroots network was provided with concrete examples of nursing research by the Cabinet on Nursing Research to educate their elected officials.

The ANA coordinated outreach efforts with other nursing organizations, including the Tri-Council and the more than 70 specialty nursing organizations. This effort included sharing educational materials about nursing research. It also involved including the organizations in the communications on alerts when it was necessary to actively call elected officials on Capitol Hill.

The Arthritis Foundation was very eager to support a new institute at the NIH to address arthritis and other muscle and skeletal diseases. The foundation was working closely with Senator Barry Goldwater (R-Arizona), whose wife suffered from severe arthritis. The ANA reached out to the groups supporting the new Arthritis Institute, which also included the American Association for Retired Persons (AARP), to align interests in passing NIH reauthorization with the two new institutes. This provided an opportunity to educate a large group of people outside of nursing to the value and potential contributions of nursing research in caring for people with a common chronic disease. The alliance also increased the strength and impact of the message to members of the Congress. There were many reports from staff on Capitol Hill of receiving hundreds of letters from individuals with shaky handwriting supporting the arthritis and nursing institutes at the NIH.

MOVING INTO ACTION

Interest Group Activation

Interest group activation existed primarily through the unified front developed within nursing and its professional organizations and the multiple coalitions formed with interdisciplinary and health consumer organizations. The formation and collaboration among the Tri-Council of general nursing organizations was the foundation leader in activating the numerous interest groups. Multiple professional association members visited and spoke with their Congressional members about the importance of the NIN and building the research base for evidence-based nursing practice. Nursing addressed the Congress as a unified body with one clear message: the importance and need for nursing to build a strong scientific body of knowledge for practice. This unification strategy was crucial to the broad base of congressional support that was required for the NIN legislation to pass. Such unification is rare in the history of the nursing profession.

As a first step for Moving Into Action, the activation of numerous interest groups, particularly the unification of the nursing organizations, was critical. However, the multiple coalitions formed that were supportive of the NIN made nursing's claim for a nursing research entity much more visible and credible.

Public Policy Deliberation and Adoption

During the two different legislative processes attempting to amend the NIH Reauthorization Law, there were multiple opportunities for public policy discussion. A number of forums, conferences, and studies fostered public policy deliberation concerning the legislation involving the establishment of the NIN, ultimately to be the NCNR, at its beginning.

Several studies provided opportunity for public policy dialogue. In addition to the early IOM (1983) study panel and report from 1983 that recommended "an establish(ed) entity for nursing research in the mainstream of scientific investigation," three other studies provided forums for policy deliberation. Two of these studies were specific to nursing research and one, more general, addressed the proliferation of NIH Institutes (Gornick & Lewin, 1985; IOM, 1984; Task Force on Nursing Research, 1984). Shamian et al. (2003) suggest that public policy debate and discussion occur when public interest and support are strongly engaged, and thus, such deliberation surfaces issues and information for considering new policy and policy program adoption.

The two studies specific to nursing research raised two major issues: Does there need to be a separate entity for nursing research? And where should it be placed? An NIH Task Force study, chaired by the Director of the National Institute of Aging, raised the question of how much nursing research was already conducted by the institutes and how the NIH could support nursing research within the current institutes. Thus, inherently, the suggestion was that a separate entity might not be needed. A relatively narrow view of nursing research was taken by the NIH in its study of the institutes grant portfolios in estimating the amount of nursing research being conducted, and the results showed that the NIH supported relatively little nursing research. The Task Force recommended seven areas through which the NIH could increase nursing research support (Task Force on Nursing Research, 1984). During the study, a number of national consultants were interviewed and worked with the NIH Task Force, providing an important forum for policy discussion regarding the definition of nursing research and the fit within the mainstream of biomedical and behavioral research.

The second study was initiated by the Assistant Secretary of Health, with the purpose to assess essentially four different possibilities for the structure and organization of nursing research within the Department of Health and Human Services (DHHS; Gornick & Lewin, 1985). From this study, the Secretary of HHS created a Center for Nursing Research in the Division of Nursing at the HRSA. Again, public discourse was sought, with interviews of nursing and nonnursing leaders and governmental administrators, thus allowing for public policy deliberation of whether to establish a nursing research entity and where.

Nursing leaders, who were advocating for the legislation that would establish a NIN at the NIH, used the results of the NIH Task Force as evidence for the need of a separate entity for nursing research since it was not being conducted in other institutes. The proposed Center for Nursing Research at the HRSA was lauded as a step in the right direction of increasing the visibility and resources for nursing research, but essentially it was ignored, as the nursing professional organizations were focused on creating a NIN within the mainstream of biomedical research.

The third study that promoted public discourse was a panel and report undertaken by the IOM in 1984, entitled *Responding to Health Needs and Scientific Opportunity: The Organizational Structure of the National Institutes of Health.* Forums were held for public testimony, and an expert panel debated the issues and criteria for some months. Nursing leaders make systematic arguments for how a NIN met all the recommended criteria, especially the second one, since the NIH Task Force had found little funding of nursing research (IOM, 1984).

Thus, multiple opportunities were provided for public deliberation of the legislation surrounding the creation of new institutes at the NIH in the mid-1980s. The establishment of a nursing research entity was given particular scrutiny because the concept and its outcomes for health and healthcare were relatively unknown.

Cookies and Compromise

Public policy deliberation and adoption often include rethinking the policy issue or program and creating compromises that make a new policy or program acceptable to all parties. In the case of establishing a nursing research institute at the NIH, the concern was not only the proliferation of institutes but also the NIH's difficulty with creating an institute that was so much smaller than the others and which would have only part of the programs generally expected of an institute. In October of 1985, the "Cookies and Compromise" telephone call from the President and Congressional Staff Director of the ANA to the members of the Cabinet of Nursing Research (Current Chair, Ada Sue Hinshaw) occurred. In the midst of baking Halloween cookies with this author's children, President Eunice Cole and Dr. Heinrich called to say that as an organization, the Cabinet members needed to decide what could be compromised in the NIN legislation. The congressional sponsors were interested in crafting a compromise that would be more acceptable to the administration and to the NIH. The legislation was systematically worded to replicate all the other institutes' authorization language. The decision was to compromise on the name of the entity, that is, change the NIN to the NCNR. However, not a word of the legislative language was to be changed. Thus, the authorizing legislation for the NCNR read like an institute and opened the future for transitioning to the NINR without all new legislation.

Regulation, Experience, and Revision

In this final stage of the policy process, the proposed action becomes a formal policy in law and is implemented within the federal system. According to Shamian et al. (2003), the policy becomes a new norm or value in the culture, which is experienced and revised over time. This was certainly evident with the establishment of the NCNR.

The NCNR was authorized under the Health Research Extension Act of 1985, Public Law 99-158. On April 16, 1986, Secretary Otis Bowen, the Secretary of the HHS, announced the establishment of the NCNR at the NIH. This new entity brought a different perspective to health science and policy. Reflecting the values of the nursing profession, the focus for research was on the patient, family, and community. The profession has a strong value for health promotion and disease prevention, preferring to prevent a health problem and promote healthy lifestyles. The orientation was to understanding the illness experience and handling its consequences and side effects in the form of symptom management. It became apparent that this perspective on health and healthcare research was a complement to biomedical research as favored by other colleagues. The two perspectives interacted and strengthened each other in terms of the science (Cabinet on Nursing Research, 1985; Hinshaw & Merritt, 1988; McBride, 1987). Several of the NINR themes, published almost 20 years later in 2004 (Grady, p. 97), reflect a similar perspective:

- Changing lifestyle behaviors for better health,
- Managing the effects of chronic illness to improve health and quality of life, and
- Enhancing the end-of-life experience for patients and their families.

Development of the NCNR

Several major agendas guided the development of the NCNR in its initial stage. One, the need to integrate the center into the values and culture of the NIH, for example, ensuring the quality and scientific rigor of the extramural research programs, was paramount. Two, providing interdisciplinary opportunities for nursing research was important. Three, educating NIH colleagues and policy makers about nursing research was critical in terms of working together and obtaining additional resources. Four, systematically planning and implementing all the programs required for an institute were basic to ultimately moving the NCNR to institute status.

Integrating the NCNR Into the NIH

A major agenda for the NCNR was learning the values and culture of the NIH and actively pursuing activities and strategies for integration into the organization. The NIH values strategic planning and involving the scientific community in that process. Especially, with limited funding, that is, $16 million ($11 million from the HRSA and $5 million appropriated to start the NCNR) for research, research training, and center administration, it was critical to focus the investigator energy and research areas. In order to provide examples of research studies that would benefit the public in testifying to the Congress and working with NIH colleagues, clusters of studies around critical public health issues needed to be generated. The National Nursing Research Agenda was developed, initially consisting of seven nursing research priorities identified by the senior scholars and investigators in the field. This strategic plan, laying out research priorities, was consistent with other institute plans for guiding the research being developed in other disciplinary fields.

Another integration strategy was forming strong networks at each level of the organization and developing mentors for the multiple NIH activities and decisions. For example, for the new NCNR Director (Ada Sue Hinshaw), forming mentoring relationships with several other Directors for specific professional guidance was critical. Dr. Frank Williams and Dr. Ruth Kirschstein were mentors on what it meant to be an NIH Institute

Director and the types of issues that needed to be anticipated. Each provided feedback on various strategies such as developing an institute strategic plan, that is, the National Nursing Research Agenda. Dr. Williams was invaluable, since the National Institute of Aging was also a relatively young institute, in planning how to "market" the promise and value of nursing research in the early years before major research results were available to present to the Congress and the NIH administration. Dr. Doris Merritt, the courageous Acting Director of the NCNR in the first year, was an NIH veteran and a top "trouble shooter." She gave important advice on how to avoid the pitfalls in the new organization. Dr. Janet Heinrich, the Deputy Director and Extramural Program Director, formed a similar set of relationships with colleagues, as did each of the Program Directors. Many hours were spent understanding the "NIH Way" and deciding whether to adopt the norms and values and where to pursue other options.

A simple but long-term effective manner of integration was choosing to live on campus as the new NCNR Director. Social occasions with other Directors provided opportunities for many informal discussions about the NIH. These networks also provided excellent openings for NIH colleagues to learn about nursing research.

Interdisciplinary Collaboration for Research

Interdisciplinary collaboration for nursing research is critical for several reasons. Nursing practice, like other health professional practice, is complex and requires information from multiple fields in making decisions with and for patients and their families. The research questions about nursing practice are also quite complicated and usually require expertise from several disciplines to provide the necessary perspectives.

In addition, one of the values of having nursing research in the mainstream of health science at the NIH was taking advantage of the richness of the multiple perspectives available in such an environment. Interdisciplinary collaboration also facilitated integration into the NIH while it educated NIH colleagues about nursing research. Nursing learned many lessons through interdisciplinary collaboration on the cosponsorship of numerous research initiatives.

Interdisciplinary collaboration not only enriched the science developed for nursing practice but also increased the funding available for nursing research. In the initial years of minimal budgets, more nursing research could be funded by sharing the sponsorship with other institutes when the subject matter was appropriate. Jan Heinrich, as Director of Extramural Programs, was masterful at leveraging NCNR dollars through cofunding with other institutes, which not only extended the funding capacity but also educated NIH colleagues about the quality and contributions of nursing research.

Educating Congress and NIH Colleagues Regarding Nursing Research

A primary reason that the NCNR was established and supported by the Congress was that it represented a positive women's issue that was important to Representatives and Senators in the mid-1980s (Houser, 2004; Larson, 1984). The champions for nursing research, such as Representatives Madigan and Purcell, as well as Senators Inouye and Kennedy, understood its potential for contributions to the public's health. Representative Madigan (1986, p. 3) suggested that nursing research could "provide much of the needed data to enhance the provision of high quality effective and efficient care." However, a number of congressional members and NIH colleagues were curious but uninformed about nursing research. Thus, NCNR leaders spent countless hours in meetings, testimonies, and informal discussion defining nursing research through strategic plans, developing Requests for Applications and Proposals, and providing numerous examples of nursing research.

Building Institute Programs

While building the nursing research programs through extramural funding and ensuring the scientific rigor of the investigative processes through research training strategies, the ultimate goal of converting the Center to an Institute at the NIH was not lost. Initially, strong extramural programs of research needed to be developed with the nursing scientific community. Because of the breath of nursing research, a strategic plan was generated with senior nurse scientists from across the country that identified research priorities for focusing investigator energy and limited resources. By 1993, an NIH report on nursing research confirmed the generation and evolving body of knowledge around priority areas such as low-birth-weight mothers and infants, prevention and care of individuals with HIV, long-term care for older adults, symptom management interventions, and health promotion for children and adolescents. In addition, new priorities had been defined for the future (Office of Planning, Analysis and Evaluation, 1993; Director, Suzanne Feetham).

When the quality of the extramural programs of research and research training was assured, an Intramural Research Program was launched by Dr. Carolyn Murdaugh. This was the last program that was needed to qualify the NCNR for institute status. Although the programs were still small in relation to other NIH institutes, they were quality in nature and systematically focused on major public health issues that fulfilled the mission of the NIH, that is, to improve the nation's health through support of research and research training.

Redesignation of the NCNR to the NINR

As noted in the model of Shamian et al. (2003), the final step of Moving an Issue into Policy is one of regulation, experience, and revision. In June of 1993, the NINR was redesignated from the NCNR through two processes. The professional nursing community had begun to work with congressional champions for redesignation through amending the NIH reauthorization legislation, just as with the initial process. But with the process for redesignation, the NIH was an active leader in initiating and supporting the move through the Executive Branch of the DHHS. Dr. Bernadine Healy, the Director of the NIH at that time, was a strong supporter of nurses and of nursing research. When asked if the NIH and she could support the nursing professions' move to redesignate the NCNR to institute status, she not only was supportive but also then suggested that an Executive process be initiated. Dr. Healy wasted no time in obtaining the support of the Secretary of the Health and Human Services and the Assistant Secretary of Health. At a dinner meeting several nights after the initial discussion, Drs. Healy and Hinshaw joined a reception line to talk with the two officials about an executive branch process to redesignate the NCNR to an institute. They replied that the decision was Dr. Healy's and they had no difficulty with the move of nursing research to institute status. Thus, redesignation of the NCNR to the NINR occurred through two mechanisms, legislative and executive, with the support of the nursing leadership and professional community as well as the NIH and the DHHS.

The NINR legislation (NIH Revitalization Act of 1993) was passed in June of 1993. It was officially established as an institute 4 days later by Dr. Donna Shalala, the current Secretary of the DHHS (Houser, 2004). Representatives of the Tri-Council as well as the leadership of the NINR were in attendance. A decade after the 1983 hallmark recommendation of the IOM (1983, p. 19) study to "establish nursing research within the mainstream of scientific investigation" in this country, the nursing profession accomplished its goal of an NINR at the NIH.

SUMMARY

The establishment of the NINR provides a new perspective for scientific endeavors. Given the patient- and family-centered focus of the research and research training programs, and the emphasis on health promotion, symptom management, and strong interdisciplinary collaboration, nursing research shapes health policy from a different orientation. The very creation of the NINR has shaped science policy which, in turn, informs health policy. Certainly, being in the mainstream of scientific investigation has shaped the knowledge base for nursing practice.

REFERENCES

Archbold, P. G. (1983). The impact of parent-caring on women. *Family Relations, 32,* 39–45.

Barnard, K. E., Bee, H. L., & Hammond, M. A. (1984). Developmental changes in maternal interactions with term and preterm infants. *Infant Behavior and Development, 7,* 101–113.

Benoliel, J. Q., & McCorkle, R. (1983). Symptom distress, current concerns and mood disturbance after diagnosis of life threatening disease. *Social Science and Medicine, 17,* 431–438.

Cabinet on Nursing Research. (1985). *Directions for nursing research: Toward the twenty-first century.* Kansas City, MO: American Nurses' Association.

Gornick, J. C., & Lewin, L. S. (1985). *Assessment of the organizational locus of the Public Health Service nursing research activities.* Washington, DC: Office of Health Planning and Evaluation, Office of the Assistant Secretary for Health.

Gortner, S. R., & Nahm, H. (1977). An overview of nursing research in the U.S. *Nursing Research, 26*(1), 10–33.

Gortner, S. R., Bloch, D., & Phillips, T. (1976). Contributions of nursing research to patient care. *Journal of Nursing Administration, 6,* 222–228.

Grady, P. A. (2004). Setting future directions at the National Institute of Nursing Research (NINR). *Policy, Politics & Nursing Practice, 5*(2), 95–99.

Henderson, V. (1956). Research in nursing practice—when? (editorial). *Nursing Research, 4,* 99.

Hinshaw, A. S., & Merritt, D. H. (1988). Moving nursing research to NIH. *Perspectives in nursing 1987–1989* (pp. 93–103). New York: National League of Nursing.

Houser, B. P. (2004). Ada Sue Hinshaw. In B. P. Houser & K. N. Player, *Pivotal moments in nursing: Leaders who changed the path of a profession* (pp. 105–127). Indianapolis, IN: Sigma Theta Tau International Honor Society of Nursing.

Institute of Medicine. (1983). *Nursing and nursing education: Public policies and private actions.* Washington D.C.: National Academy Press.

Institute of Medicine. (1984). *Responding to health needs and scientific opportunity: The organizational structure of the National Institutes of Health.* Washington, DC: National Academy Press.

Johnson, J. E., Rice, V. H., Fuller, S. S., & Endress, M. P. (1978). Sensory information, instruction in coping strategy and recovery from surgery. *Research in Nursing and Health, 1,* 4–17.

Larson, E. (1984). Health policy and NIH: Implications for nursing research. *Nursing Research, 33*(6), 352–356.

Madigan, E. R. (Ed.) (1986). Nursing research to take its rightful place. *Nursing and Health Care, 7,* 3.

McBride, A. B. (1987). The National Center for Nursing Research: National Institutes of Health. *Social Policy Report: Society for Research in Child Development, II*(1), 5–5.

Office of Planning, Analysis and Evaluation. (1993). Nursing research at the National Institutes of Health 1989–1992. *Report to Congress from National Institute of Nursing Research at NIH.* Bethesda, MD: NINR.

Shamian, J., Skelton-Green, J., & Villeneuve, M. (2003). Policy is the lever for effecting change. In M. McIntyres, & E. Thomlison (Eds.), *Realities of Canadian nursing: Profession and practice power issues* (pp. 83–104). Philadelphia: Lippincott, Williams & Wilkins.

Task Force on Nursing Research, U. S. National Institutes of Health. (1984). *Report to the director.* Washington, D.C.: Department of Health and Human Services.

6

Using Evidence-Based Practice to Enhance Organizational Policies, Healthcare Quality, and Patient Outcomes

Bernadette Mazurek Melnyk and Kathleen M. Williamson

Although it is now well known that evidence-based practice (EBP) improves healthcare quality and patient outcomes and reduces morbidities, mortality, costs, and geographic variation of healthcare services, it is not standard practice in numerous health systems across the United States (McGinty & Anderson, 2008; Melnyk, 2007; Williams, 2004). Far too many clinicians in a multitude of settings across the care continuum continue to deliver care to their patients based upon tradition, information that was learned years before in their educational programs, and outdated policies and procedures that exist in institutions. In order to close the 17-year time gap between the generation of research findings and their translation into clinical practice to improve care and patient outcomes (Balas & Boren, 2000), intensive efforts must be placed on (a) educating both practicing clinicians and health professional students in the EBP process, with emphasis on the building of EBP skills, (b) creating cultures of EBP that provide resources and support to clinicians to engage in and sustain evidence-based care, (c) providing incentives for EBP, and (d) establishing evidence-based clinical practice guidelines (CPGs) and policies that are incorporated into technology (e.g., electronic health records) to facilitate best practice by clinicians at the point of care.

The primary purpose of this chapter is to discuss the EBP paradigm and how it can be used to guide and improve organizational policies, healthcare quality, and patient outcomes. The difference between external and internal evidence will be described, with an emphasis on how both types of evidence are important for changing institutional policies. In addition, outcomes management and types of data collection systems that can be used to inform organizational policies will be highlighted.

THE EBP PARADIGM

In the EBP paradigm, data-driven decisions and organizational policies make use of data from published rigorous research, unpublished research, evidence-based guidelines, outcomes management, quality improvement initiatives, and EBP implementation projects (Fineout-Overholt & Johnston, 2006). Translating outcome data that are collected, analyzed, and interpreted into useful information to guide best practices is essential in the redesign of healthcare systems, organizational policies, and changes in procedures (Block, 2006; Krumholz, 2008).

Patients should receive care that is based on the best evidence and delivered in a seamless, coordinated effort (Block, 2006; Institute of Medicine [IOM], 2001). When a healthcare system's policies for clinicians are evidence based and it provides care that is safe, effective, patient centered, timely, efficient, and equitable, it is far more successful in meeting patients' needs and improving healthcare outcomes (Block, 2006; IOM, 2001; Krumholz, 2008). Healthcare systems have a responsibility to provide evidence-based polices in order to achieve quality patient outcomes.

Evidence-based practice is a problem-solving approach to the delivery of healthcare that integrates the best evidence from well-designed studies (i.e., external evidence) with a clinician's expertise and patients' preferences and values (Melnyk & Fineout-Overholt, 2005; Sackett, Straus, Richardson, Rosenberg, & Haynes, 2000). Important components of clinical expertise in the EBP paradigm include (a) data gathered from a thorough patient assessment, (b) internal evidence generated from outcomes management, quality improvement initiatives, and EBP implementation projects, and (c) the evaluation of and use of available resources necessary to achieve desired patient outcomes (Melnyk & Fineout-Overholt, 2011). When all of these factors are integrated within a context of caring and a culture that supports EBP, the best evidence-based clinical decisions are made that lead to the highest quality of patient outcomes (see Figure 6.1).

Unfortunately, there are many interventions being implemented in healthcare systems across the United States that have little or no evidence to support them (e.g., routine vital

Evidence-Based Practice Organizational Culture

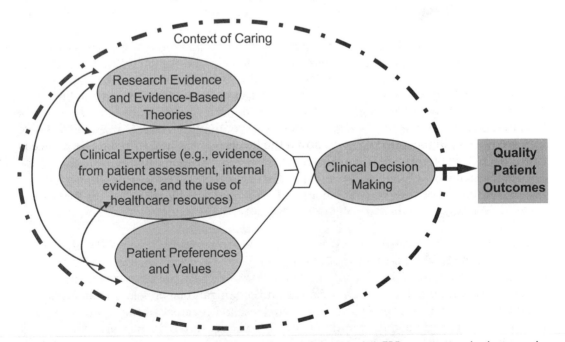

FIGURE 6.1 Evidence-based practice within a context of caring and an EBP organizational culture results in the highest quality of healthcare and patient outcomes. Copyright Melnyk & Fineout-Overholt, 2003.

signs and double checking of pediatric medications). On the other hand, there are numerous interventions that have been shown to be efficacious through rigorous randomized controlled trials (RCTs) and gold standard evidence-based screening recommendations (e.g., U.S. Preventive Services Task Force, 2008) that are not being used in clinical practice or routinely reimbursed by third-party payers.

Findings generated from rigorous research (e.g., RCTs and case-control studies) are ultimately intended to be generalized for use in healthcare settings across the nation. However, when external evidence from rigorous research is translated into clinical practice, it is important for clinicians to conduct some level of evaluation to determine whether the same results that were obtained from rigorous research can be achieved in the real-world practice setting (Gawlinski, 2007; Melnyk & Fineout-Overholt, 2011). Therefore, outcomes evaluation is important when translating research evidence into clinical practice and policies.

Researchers generate external evidence through rigorous research, and EBP provides clinicians the tools that they need to integrate that evidence with their clinical expertise and patient preferences to achieve optimal patient outcomes. However, there are many circumstances in the nursing profession where there is a paucity of external evidence from research to guide clinical practice. Therefore, clinicians must generate internal or practice-based evidence through outcomes management and EBP implementation projects in order to inform organizational policies and high-quality care for the patients in their own practice settings.

Levels of evidence have traditionally been used to guide clinical decision making in EBP (see Exhibit 6.1). Although there are various published tables of levels of evidence, there is consensus among them that the strongest level of evidence to guide clinical interventions or treatments is systematic reviews of RCTs. Systematic reviews are literature reviews that use rigorous methods to identify, critically appraise, and synthesize evidence from studies that were designed to answer the same research question. They provide an ability to manage huge volumes of information to develop best practices and are the heart of EBP (Stevens, 2011).

Many systematic reviews incorporate quantitative methods to summarize the results from multiple studies. These types of reviews are called meta-analyses. Unfortunately, the field of nursing has few systematic reviews of nursing interventions, in large part because nurses have been discouraged from conducting replication studies. If a systematic review is not available, then clinicians are encouraged to seek out Level II evidence (i.e., evidence from one RCT) to guide their intervention practices. If Level II evidence is not available, the search continues down the levels of evidence until some evidence is available that can guide practice. However, the evidence found must be critically appraised for quality before a decision is made regarding whether to implement the evidence in clinical practice. In EBP, the level of evidence plus the quality of that evidence gives clinicians the confidence to implement an EBP change or to revise institutional policies.

Multiple barriers exist in the current healthcare system that are imposing challenges for meeting the IOM's goal that, by 2020, 90% of clinical decisions will be evidence based (McClellan, McGinnis, Nabel, & Olsen, 2007). Some of the major barriers include (a) inadequate EBP knowledge and skills by clinicians, (b) a lack of EBP mentors in healthcare systems who can work with point-of-care providers in implementing evidence-based care, (c) lack of administrative support, (d) inadequate resources and tools at point of care, (e) negative attitudes of clinicians toward research, (f) misperceptions about EBP and the extent of time that it takes to implement, and (g) cultures that do not support EBP

EXHIBIT 6.1   *Rating System for the Hierarchy of Evidence for Intervention/Treatment Questions*

Level I: Evidence from a systematic review or meta-analysis of all relevant RCTs
Level II: Evidence obtained from well-designed RCTs
Level III: Evidence obtained from well-designed controlled trials without randomization
Level IV: Evidence from well-designed case-control and cohort studies
Level V: Evidence from systematic reviews of descriptive and qualitative studies
Level VI: Evidence from single descriptive or qualitative studies
Level VII: Evidence from the opinion of authorities and/or reports of expert committees

---

Note. RCT = randomized control trial.
Source: Melnyk, B. M. & Fineout-Overholt, E. (2011). *Evidence-based practice in nursing & healthcare: A guide to best practice (2nd ed.).* Philadelphia: Wolters Kluwer/Lippincott, Williams & Wilkins.

(Fineout-Overholt, Melnyk, & Schultz, 2005; Hannes et al., 2007; McGinty & Anderson, 2008; Melnyk et al., 2004; Melnyk, Fineout-Overholt, Feinstein, Sadler, & Green-Hernandez, 2008). Conversely, research has established facilitators of EBP, which include (a) EBP knowledge and skills, (b) strong beliefs about the value of EBP and the ability to implement it, (c) organizational cultures that support EBP, (d) EBP mentors who have in-depth knowledge and skills in evidence-based care and individual and organizational change, (e) administrative support, (f) EBP tools at the point of care, and (g) clinical promotion systems that incorporate EBP competencies (Melnyk, 2007; Melnyk et al., 2004; Melnyk, Fineout-Overholt, & Mays, 2008; Newhouse, Dearholt, Poe, Pugh, & White, 2007).

THE EBP PROCESS

There are seven steps in the EBP process (see Exhibit 6.2). The first step in EBP, Step 0, is cultivating a spirit of inquiry. Without a spirit of inquiry, clinicians will not question their current practices and organizational policies, and the quality and safety of care will be compromised (Melnyk & Fineout-Overholt, 2011). With a spirit of inquiry, clinicians routinely ask clinical questions and seek out evidence to answer those questions (e.g., "In adult preoperative patients, how does imagery versus deep breathing affect anxiety in the postoperative period?" and "In premature infants, how does music therapy versus light massage affect oxygen saturation in the neonatal intensive care unit?").

EXHIBIT 6.2   *The Steps of the EBP Process*

0. Cultivate a spirit of inquiry.
1. Ask the burning clinical question in PICOT format.
2. Search for and collect the most relevant best evidence.
3. Critically appraise the evidence (i.e., rapid critical appraisal, evaluation, and synthesis).
4. Integrate the best evidence with one's clinical expertise and patient preferences and values in making a practice decision or change.
5. Evaluate outcomes of the practice decision or change based on evidence.
6. Disseminate the outcomes of the EBP decision or change.

Note. EBP = evidence-based practice.
Source: Melnyk, B. M. & Fineout-Overholt, E. (2011). *Evidence-based practice in nursing & healthcare: A guide to best practice (2nd ed.).* Philadelphia: Wolters Kluwer/Lippincott, Williams & Wilkins.

The second step in EBP (i.e., Step 1) is placing the clinical question in PICO(T) (P = patient population, I = intervention or area of Interest, C = comparative intervention or comparison group, O = outcome, and T = time, if applicable). This step in EBP is key to the entire process, as questions formatted in PICO(T) will lead to streamlined searches instead of searches that are long and labor intensive. In the example regarding preoperative interventions that affect postoperative anxiety in the former paragraph, the P is adult preoperative patients, the I is imagery, the C is deep breathing, the O is anxiety, and the T is postoperative period.

The next step in EBP (Step 2) is searching for the best and latest evidence to answer the PICOT question. For the answer to intervention or treatment clinical questions, such as the one described above, clinicians should search first for systematic reviews of RCTs (i.e., Level I evidence) and evidence-based CPGs. The Cochrane Database of Systematic Reviews is an outstanding database that houses thousands of rigorous systematic reviews of RCTs that have been conducted by experts in the field.

Evidence-based CPGs are specific practice recommendations that have been grouped together, which are derived from a methodologically rigorous review of the best evidence on a specific topic. They are outstanding tools for clinicians to improve the quality of care, the process of care, and patient outcomes and reduce variation in care and unnecessary healthcare expenditures (Fein & Corrato, 2008). The American Medical Association and the Agency for Healthcare Research and Quality house thousands of evidence-based CPGs that are freely accessible at the National Guidelines Clearinghouse at www.guideline.gov. Healthcare institutions will often adopt some of these CPGs as their institutional policies for healthcare delivery.

In searching for the best evidence to answer the clinical question, each of the five key words from the PICO(T) question is entered one at a time in the database that is being searched (e.g., Medline or CINAHL). Then, in the final step, the five key words from the PICO(T) search are combined. Combining all five key words in the search will result in a yield of a few studies instead of hundreds of studies of which the far majority will be irrelevant to answering the PICO(T) question.

Once the evidence is found through the search process, the next step in EBP (i.e., Step 3) commences. Step 3 involves critical appraisal and synthesis of the evidence. Three key categories of questions are asked in the critical appraisal process, including the following (Melnyk & Fineout-Overholt, 2011): (1) Is the evidence valid (i.e., as close to the truth as possible), which involves evaluating the methods used to conduct the study and assessing whether the study was rigorously conducted? (2) Is the evidence reliable, which means did the intervention work in an RCT and can the clinician expect similar results if he or she implemented the intervention in his or her own practice setting? and (3) Will the results help me in caring for my patients (applicability)? Appraisal and synthesis of the evidence are a major component of a decision to make a change in practice or organizational policy.

Step 4 in the EBP process is the integration of the best evidence from the search and critical appraisal with a clinician's expertise and patient preferences and values to make a clinical decision. Patients desire to participate in the clinical decision-making process, and it is the ethical responsibility of the healthcare provider to involve patients in treatment decisions (Melnyk & Fineout-Overholt, 2006). Therefore, although organizational policies and the best evidence might direct the clinician to implement a certain treatment, it also is important to consider the patient's preferences and values in the EBP decision-making process.

Step 5 in the EBP process involves evaluating the outcomes of a new practice change or organizational policy based upon the best evidence. When evidence is transferred from rigorous research to a clinical practice setting, the results may be different in comparison with those from the rigorously conducted study because variables in the real-world setting often cannot be controlled as they were in rigorously conducted research. Therefore, when a new EBP, policy, or procedure is implemented, it is important to evaluate its outcomes to determine its positive impact in the clinical setting where it is being implemented.

The last step in the EBP process is disseminating the outcomes of the EBP change or policy. All too frequently, silos exist, even within the same healthcare institution. In addition, there is much geographic variation in standards of care. Therefore, disseminating and regularly communicating EBPs and policies are important to assure that clinicians are following them. However, dissemination of best practices and policies alone often does not change the behaviors of clinicians. Other key strategies must be present within institutions (e.g., EBP mentors, competencies built into clinical ladder promotion systems, an EBP culture) to facilitate change to consistent implementation of evidence-based practices and policies by clinicians.

AN EXAMPLE OF HOW THE EBP PROCESS INFORMS EVIDENCE-BASED ORGANIZATIONAL POLICIES

The EBP process can be used to inform, create, and change organizational policies. For example, a team composed of nurse EBP mentors, a librarian, and point-of-care staff at Cincinnati Children's Hospital recently revised 32 nursing policies and procedures to be evidence based (Long, Burkett, & McGee, 2009). For each of the 32 policies (e.g., central venous catheters and intramuscular injections), a PICO(T) question was formed (e.g., "Among hospitalized children [P], does use of chlorhexidine gluconate scrub [I] versus Betadine and alcohol scrub [C] decrease the incidence of catheter related infections [O]?" and "Among infants requiring intramuscular injections [P], does use of a long needle [I] versus a short needle [C] reduce localized reactions [O]?"). After formation of the PICO(T) questions, evidence searches were conducted by the team using databases such as CINAHL, Medline, and the National Guidelines Clearinghouse. Once the searches were conducted, the level of each evidence source was identified and an evidence grade was determined based upon critical appraisal of the quality of evidence found. New evidence-based policies and procedures were then created and forwarded to the Nurse Practice Council for review and approval. Each of the practice recommendations in a new policy was supported with the level and grade of evidence upon which it was based. Guidance regarding implementation of the new evidence-based policies and procedures also was included in each of the policies (e.g., how the policy or procedure would be implemented and by whom).

It also was decided upon by the team that these new evidence-based policies and procedures would be reviewed every 3 years at minimum. Once a new evidence-based policy or procedure was written, it was forwarded to the Nurse Practice Council for approval. Once approved by the council, the new policy was added to the policy and procedure manual. After approval, educational sessions were held across units to inform the point-of-care staff of the new evidence-based policies and procedures and how they were formulated, along with plans for implementation.

OUTCOMES MANAGEMENT AND DATA COLLECTION SYSTEMS INFORM ORGANIZATIONAL POLICIES

Health policies promote the welfare of citizens, institutional policies govern the workplace, and organizational policies are positions of organizations (Mason, Leavitt, & Chaffee, 2007). Individual patients are at the core of organizational as well as institutional policies, which provide the direction on how care is delivered (Traft & Nanna, 2008). Knowing how polices are generated by legislators and organizations as well as individuals in the work setting is important for learning how to affect policy at the system, local, state, national, and international levels (Mason, Leavitt, & Chaffee, 2007; Traft & Nanna, 2008).

Although external evidence from rigorous research is often used to drive organizational policies, it also is important to use internal evidence that is generated through outcomes management as well as EBP implementation and quality improvement projects to inform institutional policies. As previously described, an essential step in the EBP process is the evaluation of outcomes. Outcomes management will be further elaborated upon here because it is a key strategy for informing organizational policy within an institution. In order for organizational polices to change, evaluating outcomes of practice decisions or changes based on evidence is essential (Melnyk & Fineout-Overholt, 2005). To understand the impact of an EBP implementation or quality improvement project and how it can influence organizational policy or procedures, outcomes of the evidence-based change need to be collected, analyzed, and interpreted (Fineout-Overholt & Johnston, 2006). To produce organizational policies that positively impact patient, provider, and system changes in practice, clinical decision making using valid and reliable outcome data is essential.

A variety of outcomes can be collected in healthcare systems, including patients' clinical, physiological, psychological, and social outcomes as well as healthcare systems' outcomes, such as cost, access, and quality (Donabedian, 2003). Outcomes of EBP changes should be measured so that the positive impact of these changes can be documented and policies subsequently refined or changed.

Outcomes are often tied to reimbursement and regulatory issues by organizations, such as The Joint Commission, Centers for Medicare & Medicaid, and the American Nurses Credentialing Center's Magnet Recognition Program (Fineout-Overholt & Johnston, 2006). Because of their importance, outcome data are provided to healthcare professionals and institutions as well as consumers by a number of organizations and federal agencies (the Institute for Healthcare Improvement, the Agency for Healthcare Research and Quality, the Leapfrog Group, and Hospital Compare) so that determinations can be made of how healthcare institutions are comparing nationally on quality indicators (see Table 6.1).

Evaluation of outcomes is an essential step in the EBP process that helps the clinician to determine if the EBP implementation project was successful, effective, equitable, and timely and needs to be modified or discarded (Gawlinski, 2007). Outcomes flow from the PICO(T) question. An example is the following PICO(T) question, "In adult patients with

TABLE 6.1   *Name, Web site, and Description of Organizations That Collect Evidence/Outcome Data That Can Be Used to Inform Organizational Policies*

Name and Web Site	Description of Services Provided by Organizations
The Joint Commission (http://www.jointcommission.org/)	Not-for-profit organization that accredits and certifies healthcare organizations in the United States. It ensures that organizations provide safe patient care. The Joint Commission supports organizations in performance improvement and regulations that support quality of care.
Centers for Medicare & Medicaid Services (http://www.cms.hhs.gov/)	A federal organization that administers Medicare and Medicaid and other federal programs. They provide regulatory guidelines, research, statistics, large data sets, outreach, and education.
American Nurses Credentialing Center (ANCC; http://www.nursecredentialing.org/)	The ANCC is a subsidiary of the American Nurses Association. Healthcare organizations can receive recognition as a positive and safe institution through their Magnet Recognition Program.
Institute for Healthcare Improvement (IHI; http://www.ihi.org/ihi)	A not-for-profit organization that works to improve patient care and establish healthy communities and an effective workforce. The IHI provides educational programs and develops innovative programs that organizations can use and share to move the healthcare system toward patient safety and quality care.
Agency for Healthcare Research and Quality (AHRQ; http://www.ahrq.gov/)	This federal agency is part of the U.S. Department of Health and Human Services. It conducts research and specializes in quality improvement and patient safety, outcomes and effectiveness of care, technology, and systems. The AHRQ also provides training for researchers and the public to translate knowledge of what works and does not work into everyday practice and policy. In addition, it funds evidence-based practice centers for the purpose of conducting rigorous systematic reviews to inform the evidence-based gold standard screening recommendations by the U.S. Preventive Services Task Force.
The LeapFrog Group (http://www.leapfroggroup.org/)	This is a voluntary program in which hospitals provide data on safety and quality in their organizations. As a member, organizations become more transparent by providing consumers data about the care provided so they can compare institutions on quality indicators.
Hospital Compare (http://www.hospitalcompare.hhs.gov/)	A tool provided by Medicare where a healthcare consumer can compare quality of care hospitals provide on certain medical conditions or surgical procedures.

congestive heart failure (P), how does a structured education program at discharge (I) compared with pamphlets handed to patients at discharge (C) affect patient satisfaction, readmission rate, and patients' knowledge of congestive heart failure disease process and care (O)?" Outcomes selected should be (1) relevant to the EBP project's objective, (2) reflect what the clinician is aiming to accomplish, (3) achievable, and (4) measurable (i.e., the data on the outcome must be available; Block, 2006; Gawlinski, 2007). Evaluating the impact of an EBP implementation project in which a practice change is made based on a review of and critical appraisal of a body of evidence is important to determine whether the outcomes observed in studies are similar when applied to actual clinical practice (Gawlinski, 2007). Evaluation of outcomes from an EBP implementation project involves following up to determine whether the evidence-based actions or decisions implemented achieved the desired outcomes (Polit & Beck, 2008). Follow-up or continued monitoring of the project's outcomes includes continued data collection to track the project's success, developing an EBP guideline, and/or writing an evidence-based policy/procedure that reflects the change in practice. The collection of baseline data for the project is needed to understand the background and significance of the problem. During the postimplementation phase of the EBP project, baseline data are used to compare data collected after implementation to measure the impact of the EBP change on the outcome(s), which can then affect policy and/or procedure changes.

Healthcare organizations have their own systems that collect, maintain, and analyze data that can be used as internal evidence. Data are collected in a variety of categories, such as nurse vacancy rate, patient satisfaction, emergency room wait times, length of stay, failure to rescue, hospital-acquired infections, number of infant deliveries, fall rates, vital signs, and pain management to name just a few. Before starting an EBP implementation project, it is important to investigate and understand the structure of and data collection procedures of the organization (e.g., Where is the data housed? Who generates the data? How are data used?). Determining the appropriate outcomes that can be measured to evaluate the impact of an EBP implementation project that will influence a change in organizational policy is an important step. In addition, knowing the advantages and disadvantages of using various data sources and types of collection methods is important for success in effectively and efficiently implementing an EBP project (Ransom, Joshi, Nash, & Ransom, 2008). Another strategy for locating outcomes is through prior research (external evidence) on the issue and determining what is expected to change as a result of the evidence-based implementation project (Gawlinski, 2007).

Once the outcomes for a project are identified, it is important to determine how to measure them. Before conducting an EBP implementation project, the selection of tools to measure outcomes of the EBP change needs to be determined, including the cost of the tool(s), time for administration of the tool(s), how the data will be collected, and who will be involved in collection of the data (Ransom et al., 2008). According to Gawlinski (2007), it is best to use instruments from the original research that are short, concise, user-friendly, and easy to complete, rather than developing new ones. It also is important to determine how long after the EBP change is implemented that outcomes will continue to be measured, as sustainability of positive outcomes is becoming increasingly important in healthcare systems (Gawlinski, 2007; Melnyk & Fineout-Overholt, 2005).

Data collection should be driven by the outcomes in the EBP implementation project. It is important to ask the right questions and be clear about the request for data. Sources of internal evidence, which is locally obtained data or information, can be found in many areas in an organization (Stetler & Caramanica, 2007). Table 6.2 lists a variety of sources of outcome data that can be used as internal evidence in making EBP organizational policy changes.

Data can stimulate discussions about (a) what practices need improvement, (b) the need to change existent policies, (c) the importance of implementing EBP implementation and outcomes management or quality improvement projects, (d) what groups of patients are at high risk for adverse outcomes, and (e) the most pressing priorities in a healthcare system. Measuring outcomes and linking them to nursing actions are critical in developing EBP policies or procedures and in providing quality patient care (Polit & Beck, 2008).

TABLE 6.2   *Outcome Data Sources that Provide Internal Evidence*

Data Collection Sources	Types of Data Generated, Collected, and Accessed
Quality management data	Incident reports, sentinel events, patient satisfaction, and regulatory/accreditation requirements
Finances	Billing and diagnosis-related groups, charges for medications, equipment, patient days, and demographic data on patients
Human resources	Employee and payroll systems, turnover rate, staff education level, salaries, and labor laws
Clinical systems	Laboratory and pharmacy point-of-care outcomes
Administration	Dashboards, bed flow, patient complaints, and management policies
Electronic Medical Records	Patient records (vital signs, documentation of care provided, and clinical interventions)
Data collected from outside sources	Agency for Health Research and Quality, National Database of Nursing Quality Indicators, Centers for Medicare & Medicare, state discharge databases, etc.

IMPLEMENTING EVIDENCE-BASED ORGANIZATIONAL POLICIES IN CLINICAL PRACTICE

Translating evidence and evidence-based organizational policies into routine clinical practice remains a major challenge for healthcare systems. It is well known that dissemination of evidence alone does not typically lead to a sustainable change to EBP in clinicians. Providing an organizational culture that supports EBP (e.g., up-to-date resources and tools, ongoing EBP knowledge and skills building workshops, and EBP mentors at the point of care) is necessary for clinicians to consistently make evidence-based decisions (Melnyk, 2007; Melnyk & Fineout-Overholt, 2011; Rudd & Williams, 2009).

Interdisciplinary healthcare professionals and administrators should be involved when planning and implementing evidenced-based organizational policies and projects. Necessary training and resources, such as EBP education, technology infrastructure, data mining, and statistical analysis support for successful EBP implementation, and the protocol of how to change organizational policies should be provided to point-of-care clinicians. Healthcare organizations also need to provide the right information, at the right time, in the right format to support patient care and evidence-based policy decisions.

Point-of-care and advanced practice nurses need to connect with change agents, administrators, leaders, and policy makers in an organization to facilitate policy changes. Furthermore, nurses must disseminate the results of their EBP implementation projects to key stakeholders so that current policies are placed on an agenda for review and change. If the dissemination of outcomes does not take place, the chance of an organizational policy change lessens.

Clinicians cannot shy away from technology and need to contribute and be part of the process to establish their contributions to improved patient outcomes (Simpson, 2006). The use of electronic health records and dashboards are information-rich resources that can provide clinicians with searchable databases to locate outcomes in order to (1) assess whether a problem exists, (2) obtain baseline data before implementing an EBP project, and (3) collect important data to evaluate a project's outcomes that could influence a change in organizational policies. To determine if an EBP implementation project is successful in positively impacting patients, outcomes must be measured. The measurement of outcomes (i.e., internal evidence) along with external evidence from rigorous research will result in the best evidence-based organizational policies to guide the highest quality of care in healthcare institutions.

CONCLUSIONS

In conclusion, in order to facilitate the highest quality of care and best patient outcomes, organizational policies need to be evidence based. Healthcare leaders need to be involved in promoting and utilizing EBP by removing barriers, providing resources, securing technology adoption, and serving as champions for quality care (Ransom et al., 2008). External evidence from rigorous research and internal evidence from outcomes management and EBP implementation projects need to be integrated into organizational policies to achieve the best outcomes for patients. Dissemination of organizational policies alone is not enough to ensure that clinicians are consistently implementing EBPs. Evidence-based organizational policies must be combined with ongoing initiatives directed to building clinicians' EBP knowledge and skills and creating organizational cultures with key resources that support evidence-based care if this paradigm is to sustain and we are to reach the IOM goal of 90% of clinical decisions being evidence based by 2020.

REFERENCES

Balas, E. A., & Boren, S. A. (2000). *Managing clinical knowledge for healthcare improvements.* Germany: Schattauer Publishing Company.

Block, D. (2006). *Healthcare outcomes management: Strategies for planning and evaluation.* Sudbury, MA: Jones and Bartlett.

Donabedian, A. (2003). *An introduction of quality assurance in health care.* New York: Oxford University Press.

Fein, I. A., & Corrato, R. R. (2008). Clinical practice guidelines: Culture eats strategy for breakfast, lunch, and dinner. *Critical Care Medicine, 36*(4), 1360–1361.

Fineout-Overholt, E., & Johnston, L. (2006). Evaluation: An essential step in the EBP process. *Worldviews on Evidence-Based Nursing, 4*(1), 54–59.

Fineout-Overholt, E., Melnyk, B. M., & Schultz, A. (2005). Transforming health care from the inside out: Advancing evidence-based practice in the 21st century. *Journal of Professional Nursing, 21*(6), 335–344.

Gawlinski, A. (2007). Evidence-based practice changes: Measuring the outcome. *AACN Advanced Critical Care, 18*(3), 320–322.

Hannes, K., Vandersmissen, J., De Blaeser, L., Peeters, G., Goedhuys, J., & Aertgeerts, B. (2007). Barriers to evidence-based nursing: A focus group study. *Journal of Advanced Nursing, 60*(2), 162–171.

Institute of Medicine. (2001). *Crossing the quality chasm: A new health system for the 21st century.* Washington, DC: National Academy Press.

Krumholz, H. M. (2008). Outcomes research: Generating evidence for best practice and policies. *Circulation, 118,* 309–318.

Long, E. L., Burkett, K., & McGee, S. (2009). Promotion of safe outcomes: Incorporating evidence into policies and procedures. *The Nursing Clinics of North America, 44*(1), 57–70.

Mason, D. J., Leavitt, J. K., & Chaffee, M. W. (2007). *Policy & politics in nursing and health care.* St Louis, MO: Elsevier.

McClellan, M. B., McGinnis, M., Nabel, E. G., & Olsen, L. M. (2007). *Evidence-based medicine and the changing nature of health care.* Washington, DC: The National Academies Press.

McGinty, J., & Anderson, G. (2008). Predictors of physician compliance with American Heart Association Guidelines for acute myocardial infarction. *Critical Care Nursing Quarterly, 31*(2), 161–172.

Melnyk, B. M. (2007). The evidence-based practice mentor: A promising strategy for implementing and sustaining EBP in healthcare systems. *Worldviews on Evidence-Based Nursing, 4*(3), 123–125.

Melnyk, B. M., & Fineout-Overholt, E. (2011). *Evidence-based practice in nursing & healthcare. A guide to best practice* (2nd ed.). Philadelphia: Wolters Kluwer/Lippincott, Williams & Wilkins.

Melnyk, B. M., & Fineout-Overholt, E. (2005). *Evidence-based practice in nursing & healthcare. A guide to best practice* (1st ed.). Philadelphia: Wolters Kluwer/Lippincott, Williams & Wilkins.

Melnyk, B. M., & Fineout-Overholt, E. (2006). Consumer preferences and values as an integral key to evidence-based practice. *Nursing Administration Quarterly, 30*(1), 123–127.

Melnyk, B. M., Fineout-Overholt, E., Feinstein, N. F., Li, H., Small, L., Wilcox, L., et al. (2004). Nurses' perceived knowledge, beliefs, skills, and needs regarding evidence-based practice: Implications for accelerating the paradigm shift. *Worldviews on Evidence-Based Nursing, 1*(3), 185–193.

Melnyk, B. M., Fineout-Overholt, E., Feinstein, N. F., Sadler, L. S., & Green-Hernandez, C. (2008). Nurse practitioner educators' perceived knowledge, beliefs, and teaching strategies. *Journal of Professional Nursing, 24*(1), 7–13.

Melnyk, B. M., Fineout-Overholt, E., & Mays, M. (2008). The evidence-based practice beliefs and implementation scales: Psychometric properties of two new instruments. *Worldviews on Evidence-Based Nursing, 5*(4), 208–216.

Newhouse, R. P., Dearholt, S., Poe, S., Pugh, L., & White, K. M. (2007). Organizational change strategies for evidence-based practice. *Journal of Nursing Administration, 37*(12), 552–557.

Polit, D. F., & Beck, C. T. (2008). *Nursing research: Generating and assessing evidence for nursing practice.* Philadelphia: Lippincott Williams & Wilkins.

Ransom, E. R., Joshi, M. J., Nash, D. B., & Ransom, S. B. (2008). *The healthcare quality book* (2nd ed.). Chicago: Health Administration Press.

Rudd, A. G., & Williams, L. S. (2009). Advances in health policy and outcomes. *Stroke, 40*, e301–e304.

Sackett, D. L., Straus, S. E., Richardson, W. S., Rosenberg, W., & Haynes, R. B. (2000). *Evidence-based medicine: How to practice and teach EBM.* London: Churchill Livingstone.

Simpson, R. (2006). Automation: The vanguard of EBN. *Nursing Management, 37*(6), 13–14.

Stetler, C. B., & Caramanica, L. (2007). Evaluation of an evidence-based practice initiative: Outcomes, strength and limitations of a retrospective, conceptually-based approach. *Worldviews on Evidence-Based Nursing, 4*(4), 187–199.

Stevens, K. R. (2011). Critically appraising knowledge for clinical decision making. In B. M. Melnyk & E. Fineout-Overholt (Eds.), *Evidence-based practice in nursing & healthcare. A guide to best practice.* Philadelphia: Wolters Kluwer/Lippincott, Williams & Wilkins.

Traft, S. H. & Nanna, K. M. (2008). What are the sources of health policy that influence nursing practice? *Policy, Politics & Nursing Practice, 9*(4), 274–287.

U.S. Preventive Services Task Force. (2008). *Guide to clinical preventive services, 2008.* Rockville, MD: Agency for Healthcare Research and Quality. Available at http://www.ahrq.gov/clinic/pocketgd.htm

Williams, D. O. (2004). Treatment delayed is treatment denied. *Circulation, 109*, 1806–1808.

7

From Bedside to Bench to Practice

Norma A. Metheny

Tube feedings are administered to millions of people worldwide who are unable to take nourishment by mouth. Compared with the parenteral route for introducing nutrients, the enteral route is more physiologic, is less costly, and has fewer complications. However, serious complications are possible, including misplacement of feeding tubes into the respiratory tract and pulmonary aspiration of gastric contents. The purpose of this chapter is to describe a series of clinical and laboratory studies funded by the National Institute of Nursing Research (NINR) that have influenced healthcare policy and improved outcomes for tube-fed patients. Publications from these studies have been cited in a variety of documents offering information to clinicians to improve patient care (see Table 7.1 for three examples). In addition, hundreds of textbooks include findings from the studies and thus encourage adoption of research-based information by nurses, physicians, and allied healthcare workers to promote safe tube-feeding practices. See Table 7.2 for examples of a variety of textbooks that have cited research findings from the previously mentioned clinical and laboratory studies.

ASSESSMENT OF FEEDING TUBE PLACEMENT

Determining correct tube placement is a vital component of tube-feeding protocols; however, little research-based data were available on this procedure until the late 1980s. When a feeding tube is blindly inserted, the most important initial assessment is distinguishing between respiratory and gastric placement. After respiratory placement has been ruled out, the next assessment is determining if the tube is positioned in the correct segment of the gastrointestinal tract (either the stomach or small bowel, depending on individual patient needs). Finally, after feedings have been started, it is necessary to assure that the tube has remained in the desired position. Reported below are a series of nursing research studies conducted over the past two decades to evaluate a variety of methods to determine tube location. Findings from these studies are widely cited in textbooks and hospital protocols to help clinicians assure correct positioning of feeding tubes.

TABLE 7.1   *Examples of Policy Statements or Recommendations That Have Cited Findings From Tube-Feeding Studies Funded by the National Institute of Nursing Research*

Policy Statement or Recommendations	Citations
American Society for Parenteral and Enteral Nutrition: Enteral nutrition practice recommendations. Bankhead et al. (2009), *Journal of Parenteral & Enteral Nutrition, 33*(2)	Metheny, N. A., Schallom, L., Oliver, D. A., et al. (2008). Gastric residual volume and aspiration in critically ill patients receiving gastric feedings. *American Journal of Critical Care, 17,* 512–519. Metheny N. A. (2006). Preventing respiratory complications of tube feedings: Evidence-based practice. *American Journal of Critical Care, 15,* 360–369. Metheny, N. A., Clouse, R. E., Chang, Y. H., et al. (2006). Tracheobronchial aspiration of gastric contents in critically ill tube-fed patients: Frequency, outcomes, and risk factors. *Critical Care Medicine, 34,*1007–1015. Metheny, N. A., Dahms, T. E., Stewart, B. J., et al. (2005). Verification of inefficacy of the glucose method in detecting aspiration associated with tube feedings. *MEDSURG Nursing, 14,* 112–121. Metheny, N. A., Stewart, J., Nuetzel, G., et al. (2005). Effect of feeding tube properties on residual volume measurements in tube-fed patients. *JPEN, 29,* 192–197. Metheny, N. A., Schnelker, R., McGinnis, J., et al. (2005). Indicators of tube site during feedings. *Journal of Neuroscience Nursing, 37,* 320–325. Metheny, N. A., Dahms, T. E., Stewart, B. J., et al. (2002). Efficacy of dye-stained enteral formula in detecting pulmonary aspiration. *CHEST, 122,* 276–281. Metheny, N. A., & Meert, K. L. (2004). Monitoring feeding tube placement. *Nutrition in Clinical Practice, 19,* 487–495. Metheny, N. A. (2002). Risk factors for aspiration. *JPEN, 26*(Suppl), S26–S31. Metheny, N. A., & Titler, M. G. (2001). Assessing placement of feeding tubes. *American Journal of Nursing, 101,* 36–45. Metheny, N., Smith, L., & Stewart, B. (2000). Development of a reliable and valid bedside test for bilirubin and its utility for improving prediction of feeding tube location. *Nursing Research, 49,* 302–309. Metheny, N. A., Aud, M. A., Ignatavicius, D. D. (1998). Detection of improperly positioned feeding tubes. *Journal Healthcare Risk Management, 18,* 37–48. Metheny, N. A., Stewart, B. J., Smith, L., et al. (1997). pH and concentrations of pepsin and trypsin in feeding tube aspirates as predictors of tube placement. *JPEN, 21,* 279–285. Metheny, N., Reed, L., Berglund, B., et al. (1994). Visual characteristics of aspirates from feeding tubes as a method for predicting tube location. *Nursing Research, 43,* 282–287.
American Association of Critical Care Nurses Practice Alert: Verification of Feeding Tube Placement (2005)	Metheny, N. A., Reed, L., Wiersema, L., et al. (1993) Effectiveness of pH measurements in predicting feeding tube placement: An update. *Nursing Research, 42,* 324–331. Metheny, N., Dettenmeier, P., Hampton, K., et al. (1990). Detection of inadvertent respiratory placement of small-bore feeding tubes: A report of 10 cases. *Heart Lung, 19,* 631–638. Metheny, N., McSweeney, M., Wehrle, M. A., et al. (1990) Effectiveness of the auscultatory method in predicting feeding tube location. *Nursing Research, 39,* 262–267. Metheny, N. A., & Meert, K. (2004). Monitoring feeding tube placement. *Nutrition in Clinical Practice, 19*(5), 487–496. Metheny, N. A. (2002). Inadvertent intracranial nasogastric tube placement. *American Journal of Nursing, 102*(8), 25–27.

Continued

TABLE 7.1 *Continued*

Policy Statement or Recommendations	Citations
	Metheny, N. A., & Stewart, B. J. (2002). Testing feeding tube placement during continuous tube feedings. *Applied Nursing Research, 15*(4), 254–258.
	Metheny, N. A., Stewart, B. J., Smith, L., et al. (1999). pH and concentration of bilirubin in feeding tube aspirates as predictors of tube placement. *Nursing Research, 48*(4), 189–197.
	Metheny, N. A., Stewart, B. J., Smith, L., et al. (1997). pH and concentrations of pepsin and trypsin in feeding tube aspirates as predictors of tube placement. *JPEN, 21*(5), 279–285.
	Metheny, N. A., Clouse, R. E., Clark, J. M., et al. (1994). pH testing of feeding tube aspirates to determine placement. *Nutrition in Clinical Practice, 9*(5), 185–190.
	Metheny, N., Reed, L., Berglund, B., et al. (1994). Visual characteristics of aspirates from feeding tubes as a method for predicting tube location. *Nursing Research, 43*(5), 282–287.
	Metheny, N. A., Reed, L., Worseck, M., et al. (1993). How to aspirate fluid from small-bore feeding tubes. *American Journal of Nursing, 93*(5), 86–88.
	Metheny, N., Williams, P., Wiersema, L., et al. (1989) Effectiveness of pH measurements in predicting feeding tube placement. *Nursing Research, 38*(5), 280–285.
U.S. Food and Drug Administration Public Health Advisory: Subject: Reports of Blue Discoloration and Death in Patients Receiving Enteral Feedings Tinted With the Dye, FD&C Blue No.1, September 29, 2003	Metheny, N. A., et al. (2002). Efficacy of dye-stained formula in detecting pulmonary aspiration. *CHEST, 122*(1), 276–281.
	Metheny, N. A. (2002). Risk factors for aspiration. *Journal of Parenteral & Enteral Nutrition, 26*(6 Suppl), S26–S31.
	Metheny, N. A., Aud, M., & Wunderlich, R. (1999). A survey of bedside methods used to detect pulmonary aspiration of enteral formula in intubated tube-fed patients. *American Journal of Critical Care, 8*(3), 160–167.

Respiratory Versus Gastric Placement of Newly Inserted Feeding Tubes

It is difficult to determine how often feeding tubes are placed in the respiratory tract because these events are not recorded in a central location. Reports range from as low as 0.3% to as high as 5.4% of all new tube insertions (Aronchick, Epstein, Gefter, & Miller, 1984; Valentine & Turner, 1985). A blindly placed tube may easily take the wrong course into the trachea instead of the esophagus, especially in patients with a low level of consciousness and poor cough and gag reflexes. Because potentially lethal complications may follow, the Joint Commission of Healthcare Organizations (2000) has identified nasogastric feeding tube insertion into the trachea or bronchus as a sentinel event.

The type and severity of pulmonary complications resulting from a malpositioned tube depend on the placement site and whether feedings have been started. For example, a tube inadvertently placed in the tracheobronchial tree will usually cause no damage if it does not perforate the pleura and is quickly recognized and removed. On the other hand, a tube that perforates the pleura may cause pneumothorax, bronchopleural fistula, hemothorax, pleural effusion, or other complications (especially if nutrients are administered through the tube). For example, empyema and fatal sepsis occurred in a patient

TABLE 7.2   *Examples of Textbooks That Cite Publications From Tube-Feeding Studies Funded by the National Institute of Nursing Research*

Category	Examples of Publications
Fundamentals of nursing textbooks	Kozier, B., Erb, B., & Snyder, S. (2003). Kozier & Erb's *Techniques in clinical nursing: Basic to intermediate skills* (5th ed.). Prentice Hall. Potter, P. A., & Perry, A. G. (2006). *Basic nursing: Essentials for practice,* (6th ed.). Elsevier Health Sciences. White, L. (2004). *Foundations of basic nursing* (2nd ed.). Cengage Learning.
Medical-surgical nursing textbooks	Black, J. M., & Hawks, J. H. (2004). *Medical-surgical nursing: Clinical management for positive outcomes* (7th ed.). Elsevier Health Sciences. Lewis, S. L., Heitkemper, M. M., & Dirksen, S. R. (2007). *Medical-surgical nursing assessment and management of clinical problems* (7th ed.). Elsevier Health Sciences. Day, R., & Paul, P. (2009). *Brunner and Suddarth's Textbook of Canadian Medical-Surgical Nursing.* Wolters Kluwer Health.
Nutrition textbooks	Gottschlich, M. M., & Fuhrman, P. (2000). *The science and practice of nutrition support: A case-based core curriculum.* Kendall/Hunt Publishing Co. Alpers, D. H., et al. (2008). *Manual of nutritional therapeutics* (5th ed.). Lippincott Williams & Wilkins. Williams, S. R., & Schlenker, E. D. (2002). *Essentials of nutrition and diet therapy* (8th ed.). Elsevier Health Sciences.
Critical care nursing textbooks	Elliott, D., Aitken, L., & Chaboyer, W. (2007). *ACCCN's critical care nursing.* Elsevier Health Sciences. Urden, L.D., Stacy, K. M., & Lough, M. E. (2007). *Priorities in critical care nursing* (5th ed.). Elsevier Health Sciences. Carlson, K. (2008). *AACN Advanced Critical Care Nursing.* Elsevier Health Sciences.
Critical care medical textbooks	Hall, J. B., Schmidt, G. A., & Hogarth, K. (2007). *Critical care medicine: Just the facts.* McGraw-Hill Medical. Kruse, J. A., Fink, M. P., & Carlson, R. W. (2002). *Saunders manual of critical care.* Elsevier Health Sciences. Marino, P. L., & Sutin, K. M. (2006). *The ICU book* (3rd ed.). Lippincott Williams & Wilkins.
Pediatric textbooks	Bowden, V. R., & Greenberg, C. S. (2007). *Pediatric nursing procedures* (2nd ed.). Lippincott Williams & Wilkins. MacDonald, M.G. (Editor) (2007). *Atlas of procedures in neonatology* (4th ed.). Lippincott Williams & Wilkins. Williams, C. & Asquith, J. (2000). *Pediatric intensive care nursing.* Elsevier Health Sciences.
Geriatric textbooks	Easton, K. L. (1999). *Gerontological rehabilitation nursing.* W.B. Saunders. Mauk, K. L. (2009). *Gerontological nursing: Competencies for care* (2nd ed.). Jones & Bartlett. Watson, R. R. (2000). *Handbook of nutrition in the aged* (3rd ed.). Taylor & Francis, Inc.
Oncology textbooks	Evans, P. H., Montgomery, P. Q., & Gullane, P. J. (2003). *Principles and practice of head and neck oncology.* Informa Healthcare. Itano, J., & Taoka, K. N. (2005). *Core curriculum for oncology nursing* (4th ed.) Elsevier Health Sciences. Snow, J.B., & Wackym, P.A. (2008) *Ballenger's otorhinolaryngology head and neck surgery* (17th ed.). PMPHUSA
Medical specialty textbooks	DeLegge, M. H. (2007). *Nutrition and gastrointestinal disease.* Springer-Verlag. Wilson, W. C., Grande, C. M., & Hoyt, D. B. (2006) *Trauma: Critical Care,* Volume 2. Taylor & Francis, Inc. Wijdicks, E.G. (2010). *The practice of emergency and critical care neurology.* Oxford University Press.

who received 4 L of formula through a tube inadvertently placed in the left pleural cavity (Torrington & Bowman, 1981).

A reliably obtained and interpreted radiograph provides the best evidence of correct placement (Bankhead et al., 2009; Metheny, Meert, & Clouse, 2007). Thus, radiographic confirmation of correct placement is recommended before a blindly placed tube is initially used for feedings or medication administration (Agency for Healthcare Research and Quality Commentary, 2008; American Association of Critical-Care Nurses [AACN], 2005b; Baskin, 2006; Metheny et al., 2007). A variety of bedside methods (described in the following sections) have been evaluated for use at the time of tube placement, prior to obtaining the confirmatory radiograph. If results from these tests do not support correct position, the tube is removed and reinserted; proper use of bedside tests as a precursor to radiography can limit the required number of radiographs to one, thus reducing healthcare costs.

pH Method

Measuring the pH of fluid withdrawn from a newly inserted feeding tube is the most helpful bedside test for distinguishing between tube placement in the stomach and that in the lung, especially when gastric pH is low (Metheny, Aud, & Ignatavicius, 1998; Metheny & Meert, 2004; Metheny, Reed, Wiersema, McSweeney, Wehrle, & Clark, 1993; Metheny, Stewart et al., 1999; Metheny et al., 1989). In a report of more than 1,000 gastrointestinal and respiratory secretions from fasting adult patients, researchers found that 60% of the gastric aspirates had pH readings of ≤ 4, whereas none of the respiratory secretions had pH values less than 6 (Metheny, Wehrle, Wiersema & Clark, 1998). Over two thirds of the patients in this sample were receiving some type of a gastric-acid-inhibiting drug. Other investigators have found that gastric pH readings are often low despite the administration of gastric-acid-inhibiting agents (Griffith et al., 2003). Investigators who evaluated gastric pH in critically ill children found that fasting gastric pH was similar to that observed in adults (Gharpure, Meert, Sarnaik, & Metheny, 2000).

In a prospective study of tube-fed patients, 10 cases were identified in which feeding tubes had been inadvertently placed into the respiratory tract (Metheny, Dettenmeir, Hampton, Wiersema, & Williams, 1990). In five of the cases, the pH of the aspirates was tested and found to range between 6.7 and 8.4. Pleural fluid generally has a pH of 7.6, although it may range from 7.0 to 7.3 in malignancies and even 6 when esophageal rupture has occurred (Sahn, 1988). Tracheobronchial secretions most likely have pH values of 7.4 or greater. Despite the pH method's obvious clinical utility in validating feeding tube position, there are drawbacks to its use. For example, when gastric pH is ≥ 6, it is impossible to differentiate between gastric and respiratory placement on the basis of pH alone.

Aspirate Appearance

Clinicians often try to determine if a tube is in the stomach or respiratory tract on the basis of the appearance of fluid withdrawn from the tube. However, no research-based data on this method were available until the early 1990s, when investigators systematically described the appearance of gastric and respiratory fluids from a large group of acutely ill, fasting adults (Metheny, Reed, Berglund, & Wehrle, 1994). Most of the fluids withdrawn from gastric tubes were clear and colorless, green, or light yellow. Tracheobronchial secretions were usually off-white mucus-containing fluid, whereas pleural fluid was usually straw-colored with a watery appearance (often with tinges of blood due to pleural perforation). Investigators asked a group of 30 staff nurses to identify photographs of six respiratory samples (either tracheobronchial secretions or pleural fluid) interspersed with 14 photographs of fasting gastric samples (Metheny, Reed et al., 1994). Less than half of the photographs were correctly identified. These findings, coupled with reports in the literature of visual misidentification of fluids withdrawn from feeding tubes in the lung, indicate that aspirate appearance is not reliable in distinguishing between gastric and respiratory tube placement (Balogh et al., 1983; Hand, Kempster, Levy, Rogol, & Spirn, 1984; Nakao, Killam, & Wilson, 1983; Theodore, Frank, Ende, Snider, & Beer, 1984).

Despite difficulty in distinguishing between gastric and respiratory secretions solely on the basis of appearance of fluid withdrawn from feeding tubes, it was concluded that aspirate appearance could be used in combination with aspirate pH to increase the probability of distinguishing between respiratory and gastric placement (Metheny, Reed et al, 1994). For example, a green aspirate with a low pH is likely gastric in origin, while a straw-colored, watery blood-tinged fluid with a high pH is likely pleural in origin.

Auscultatory Method

In the past, clinicians placed a stethoscope over the epigastric region and listened for a "whooshing" or "gurgling" sound while injecting air through a feeding tube; if the sound was heard, it was assumed that the tube was in the stomach instead of the lung. However, there are numerous anecdotal reports in which the auscultatory method failed to identify tubes malpositioned in the respiratory tract (El Gamel & Watson, 1993; Hendry, Akyureki, McIntyre, Quarrington, & Keon, 1986; Kolbitsch, Pomaroli, Lorenz, Gassner, & Luger, 1997; Lipman, Kessler, & Arabian, 1985; Metheny, Dettenmeir et al., 1990; Miller, Tomlinson, & Sahn, 1985; Schlorlemmer & Battaglini, 1984; Siemers & Reinke, 1976; Torrington & Bowman, 1981). For example, in a retrospective study of nine tubes inadvertently placed in the respiratory tract, clinicians (nurses and physicians) who used the auscultatory method reported hearing a whooshing sound at the epigastric region in eight of the nine cases (Metheny, Dettenmeir et al., 1990). Failure of the auscultatory method to identify a tube malpositioned in the lung has resulted in serious and even fatal outcomes (El Gamel & Watson, 1993; Hand et al., 1984; Harris & Huseby, 1988; Kolbitsch et al., 1997; Lipman et al., 1985; Metheny et al., 1998; Torrington & Bowman, 1981). The auscultatory method can also falsely predict that a tube is in the respiratory tract when it is actually in the stomach. For example, a recent study showed that the auscultatory method falsely predicted respiratory placement in 5 of 91 gastric cases (Elpern, Killen, Talla, Perez, & Gurka, 2007). Although less dangerous than a false-negative result, a false-positive prediction of respiratory placement causes unnecessary removal and reinsertion of a feeding tube. In a tragic case report, the auscultatory method failed to alert nurses that a large-bore nasogastric tube had been inadvertently inserted through an elderly patient's sphenoidal sinus into her brain (Metheny, 2002).

For all of these reasons, the auscultatory method has fallen from favor, and guidelines caution against relying on it to rule out respiratory placement of a feeding tube (Bankhead et al., 2009; AACN, 2005b).

Gastric Versus Small Bowel Placement of Newly Inserted Feeding Tubes

After respiratory placement has been ruled out and gastric placement is confirmed, it may be necessary to advance the tube into the small bowel to reduce risk for aspiration. Small bowel feedings are commonly recommended for patients who have significantly slowed gastric emptying (McClave et al., 2002). As indicated earlier, no bedside method is as accurate as radiography in determining tube location. Thus, guidelines recommend radiographic confirmation of desired tube location (gastric or small bowel) prior to the initial infusion of formula or medications through a blindly inserted feeding tube (AACN, 2005b). Several bedside tests have been evaluated as precursors to radiography to distinguish between gastric and small bowel tube placement. There is evidence that proper use of these tests can usually reduce the number of radiographs required to confirm tube placement to one (Gharpure et al., 2000; Metheny, Clouse et al., 1994; Welch, 1996).

pH Method

The pH method is helpful in distinguishing between gastric and small bowel placement because fasting gastric juice typically has a much lower pH than does small bowel juice. For example, in a study of over 1,000 gastrointestinal secretions from acutely ill adults, 94% of the small bowel aspirates had pH values ≥ 7, whereas only 22% of the gastric aspirates had pH values this high (despite the fact that two thirds of the population was receiving some type of gastric-acid-inhibiting agent; Metheny, Wehrle et al., 1998). The mean difference in gastric pH was not large between patients receiving and not receiving gastric acid inhibitors (4.3 vs. 3.3, respectively). Testing the pH of fluid withdrawn from a tube during the insertion procedure has been shown to be helpful in detecting when passage from the stomach into the small bowel has occurred (Gharpure et al., 2000; Metheny, Clouse et al., 1994; Welch, 1996).

Descriptions of usual gastrointestinal pH values are included in guidelines to assist clinicians in differentiating between gastric and small bowel tube placement at the time of new tube insertions (AACN, 2005b; Bankhead et al., 2009). While a high pH should not be used as the sole indicator of small bowel versus gastric tube placement, it is a reasonable indication that it is time to obtain a radiograph to establish small bowel placement.

Aspirate Appearance

Clinicians often try to determine if a newly inserted feeding tube is in the stomach or small bowel on the basis of the appearance of fluid withdrawn from the tube. However, there were no research-based data on this method until the early 1990s, when a group of researchers described the appearance of fasting aspirates from almost 900 patients with newly inserted feeding tubes (Metheny, Reed et al., 1994). The gastric aspirates were most often classified as green and cloudy, clear and colorless, or light yellow. In contrast, the small bowel aspirates were most often classified as golden to bile colored, having a thicker consistency than do gastric secretions. A group of 30 staff nurses viewed a sample of 100 photographs of feeding tube aspirates and were able to correctly identify 91% of the gastric aspirates and 72% of the small bowel aspirates. Descriptions of typical fasting gastric and small bowel secretions are included in guidelines to assist nurses in differentiating between gastric and small bowel tube placement at the time of new tube insertions (AACN, 2005b). As indicated in the guidelines, a combination of a low pH with a gastric color increases the probability of gastric placement (while a combination of a high pH with a small bowel aspirate color increases the probability of small bowel placement). Use of this combination of indicators can usually reduce the number of radiographs required to document correct positioning of a newly inserted feeding tube to one.

Auscultatory Method

In a study in which air was injected through the feeding tubes of 85 acutely ill adults, a group of advanced practice nurses was unable to distinguish between gastric and small bowel placement in almost two thirds of the attempts (Metheny, McSweeney, Wiersema, & Wehrle, 1990). Also, there are anecdotal reports of an inability of the auscultatory method to detect when a feeding tube's tip is located in the esophagus (Metheny, Clouse et al., 1994; Metheny et al., 2007). On the basis of these findings, the auscultatory method is not recommended to assess where a feeding tube's tip is located in the gastrointestinal tract (Metheny & Meert, 2004).

Gastric Versus Small Bowel Placement During Feedings

Feeding tubes frequently become dislocated during feedings, usually by being partially pulled out by agitated patients or by being subjected to tension during care (Metheny, Spies, & Eisenberg, 1986). Introducing feedings through a dislocated tube can result in serious complications; thus, it is important to monitor tube location at regular intervals (usually every 4 hours). Obviously, radiographs cannot be obtained several times a day to confirm that a tube has remained in the correct position; therefore, researchers evaluated a series of bedside methods to aid in this determination (Metheny, Schnelker et al., 2005). Among these were the following:

- Determining if the external length of the tubing has changed since the time of the initial confirmatory radiograph
- Observing for changes in fluid volume withdrawn from the tube
- Observing for changes in the appearance of fluid withdrawn from the tubes
- Observing for changes in the pH of fluid withdrawn from the tubes

The efficacy of these indicators was evaluated five times daily over a period of 2 to 3 days in a population of 201 critically ill tube-fed patients receiving continuous tube feedings. At the time of entry into the study, 85 patients had gastric feeding tubes and 116 patients had small bowel feeding tubes. Over 2,700 concurrent measurements of the variables were attempted; sufficient fluid for pH testing and color description was obtained in almost three fourths of the attempts from gastric tubes and in almost two thirds of the attempts from small bowel tubes. The technique used to increase the probability of withdrawing fluid from a feeding tube involved injecting approximately 30 ml of air through the tube and then applying slow and steady negative pressure with a 60-ml syringe (Metheny, Reed, Worseck, & Clark, 1993). During the study, 25 tubes became displaced: 23 tubes dislocated from the small bowel into the stomach and 2 tubes dislocated into the esophagus (1 from the stomach and 1 from the small bowel).

Change in External Tube Length

In order to assess for a change in external tube length, it was necessary to mark each tube's exit site from the nose or mouth at the time of the initial confirmatory radiograph. The external length of the tubing was also measured at this time with a centimeter tape; subsequent comparisons of external tubing length were made at 4-hour intervals. The distal tip of one of the small bowel tubes dislocated upward into the stomach with no change in its external length; however, the remaining 24 tubes that became dislocated had significantly greater mean increases in their external length than did the tubes that remained correctly positioned (14 vs. 2 cm, respectively; Metheny, Schnelker et al., 2005).

Change in Aspirate Volume

In the study described previously, the volume of fluid that could be withdrawn from the feeding tubes was also evaluated at 4-hour intervals (Metheny, Schnelker, et al., 2005). The mean volume of fluid that could be withdrawn from feeding tubes in the stomach was almost four times greater than the mean volume aspirated from small bowel tubes (26 vs. 7 ml, respectively). This is because motility in the small bowel typically propels intestinal contents forward rapidly. Thus, it was reasonable to hypothesize that a significant increase in aspirate volume from a small bowel feeding tube could signal its upward displacement into the stomach. A significant increase in aspirate volume was observed in 17 of the 23 cases in which small bowel tubes displaced upward into the stomach (range, 10 to 330 ml). Only minute quantities of fluid could be withdrawn from the two tubes displaced into the esophagus.

Change in Aspirate Appearance

Due to the continuous infusion of formula, approximately three fourths of the feeding tube aspirates had the appearance of unchanged formula (regardless of tube location in the stomach or small bowel). Thus, aspirate appearance was helpful in only a few cases in which patients were receiving continuous tube feedings.

Change in Aspirate pH

Most tube-feeding formulas have a pH of 6.6 and can thus buffer the pH of local gastrointestinal secretions. Nonetheless, 11 of the 23 cases in which small bowel tubes displaced upward into the stomach were accompanied by a decrease in the pH of the feeding tube aspirate to five or less.

Combination of Bedside Methods

When the investigators entered results from all four of the tests into a logistic regression analysis, it was found that correct classification of tube location was possible in 81% of the 201 patients. In summary, using a combination of the above indicators is more helpful than using a single indicator. Applying nursing judgment to the findings, it is possible to limit the need for radiographic confirmation that a feeding tube has remained in correct position during feedings.

Development of New Tests to Determine Tube Placement

In the mid-to-late 1990s, researchers evaluated new tests to use in conjunction with the pH method to distinguish between respiratory, gastric, and small bowel tube location. Among these were the analyses of enzyme and bilirubin concentrations in respiratory and gastrointestinal secretions (Metheny, Smith, & Stewart, 2000; Metheny et al., 1997; Metheny, Stewart et al., 1999). It was hypothesized that pepsin would be plentiful in gastric juice but lacking in respiratory and small bowel secretions. It was further hypothesized that trypsin and bilirubin would be plentiful in small bowel secretions but absent in gastric and respiratory secretions. Thus, theoretically, assays of these constituents in fluid withdrawn from feeding tubes could be used to predict tube location.

pH and Enzyme Concentrations in Aspirates

In a prospective clinical study, over 700 fasting gastrointestinal feeding tube aspirates were tested for pH and enzyme concentrations (Metheny et al., 1997). Also tested were aspirates from two feeding tubes inadvertently positioned into the lung (one in the pleural space and one in the tracheobronchial tree) and over 100 samples of tracheobronchial and pleural fluids collected by other methods. Fasting gastric fluid had a low mean pH (4), a high mean pepsin concentration (349 μg/ml), and a low mean trypsin concentration (19 μg/ml). In contrast, fasting intestinal fluid had a high mean pH (7.4), a high mean trypsin concentration (140 μg/ml), and a low mean pepsin concentration (24 μg/ml). Respiratory samples also had a high mean pH (7.9) but contained little or no pepsin or trypsin. It was concluded that laboratory-determined enzyme concentrations in feeding tube aspirates are helpful in predicting tube location. Unfortunately, lengthy laboratory assays are impractical for routine clinical use.

pH and Bilirubin Concentrations in Aspirates

Researchers also explored the extent to which a combination of measurements of pH and bilirubin concentrations in gastrointestinal and respiratory secretions could be used to predict tube location (Metheny, Stewart et al., 1999). Almost 500 fasting gastrointestinal samples for concurrent pH and bilirubin testing were collected from acutely ill adult patients with newly inserted feeding tubes. Over 125 respiratory secretions (tracheobronchial and pleural fluid) were obtained during routine tracheal suctioning or when thoracentesis procedures were performed for treatment purposes. Bilirubin content in the fluids was measured in a research laboratory, and pH was measured with a pH meter. Mean pH levels in the lung (7.7) and intestine (7.4) were significantly higher than the mean pH level in the stomach (3.9). Mean bilirubin levels in the lung (0.08 mg/dl) and stomach (1.3 mg/dl) were significantly lower than the mean bilirubin level in the intestine (12.7 mg/dl). The results were dichotomized to develop a predictive algorithm. A pH >5 and a bilirubin value <5 mg/dl correctly identified all of the respiratory cases, whereas a pH >5 coupled with a bilirubin level ≥ 5 mg/dl correctly identified three fourths of the intestinal cases. A pH ≤ 5 coupled with a bilirubin value <5 mg/dl correctly identified more than two thirds of the gastric cases. It was concluded that appropriate use of the proposed algorithm could significantly reduce the number of radiographs needed to exclude respiratory placement and to distinguish between gastric and intestinal placement.

Development of Bilirubin Test Strip

Because laboratory-determined bilirubin concentrations in feeding tube aspirates were found to be helpful in predicting tube location, researchers developed a bilirubin test strip that could be used at the bedside (Metheny et al., 2000). To evaluate the newly developed test strip, over 800 fasting gastrointestinal and respiratory specimens were obtained from acutely ill adults for concurrent bilirubin and pH testing. Bilirubin concentrations were measured with a test strip incorporating the newly developed colorimetric visual bilirubin (VBIL) scale and by a laboratory assay. pH was measured with a test strip and a pH meter. Results from the bilirubin and pH tests were read by research assistants and staff nurses and compared with tube location as determined by radiography. The correlation between readings made from the five-point VBIL scale and the laboratory bilirubin assay was 0.9. A pH >5 and a bilirubin value <5 mg/dl successfully identified 100% of the respiratory cases. In the category of pH ≤ 5 and bilirubin <5 mg/dl, 98% of the cases were gastric cases. In the category of pH >5 and bilirubin ≥ 5 mg/dl, nearly 88% of the cases were intestinal cases. Dichotomized readings from the VBIL test strip, used in combination with a pH test strip, improved the ability to predict correct tube location (when compared with the use of pH alone or bilirubin alone). Unfortunately, the VBIL test has not undergone the testing procedure required by the Federal Drug Administration for application in clinical practice.

ASSESSMENT FOR ASPIRATION DURING TUBE FEEDINGS

Pulmonary aspiration of gastric contents is a dreaded complication of tube feedings and can produce serious consequences, including hypoxemia, chemical pneumonitis, and potentially life-threatening pneumonia. While a few tube-fed patients experience a large-volume aspiration event (accompanied by coughing and choking), most will experience a series of clinically silent, small-volume aspirations (sometimes referred to as microaspirations). If not detected early and corrected, repeated microaspirations can lead to pneumonia. Unfortunately, an effective bedside test for aspiration is not available, and thus, it is difficult for clinicians to evaluate aspiration. Described in the following sections are bedside tests used in the past to detect aspiration, as well as a series of studies conducted by investigators to attempt to identify effective methods to detect aspiration and reduce aspiration risk.

Aspiration Detection Methods

Blue Dye Method

Until the past decade, the most commonly used bedside method to detect aspiration in tube-fed patients consisted of adding FD&C Blue Dye No. 1 to enteral formula delivered to the patient. If a blue discoloration was found in the patient's tracheobronchial secretions, an assumption was made that the patient had aspirated the dye-stained enteral formula. In a survey conducted in 1998, it was found that over 85% of hospitals in the United States used dye to monitor for aspiration in mechanically ventilated, tube-fed patients (Metheny, Aud et al., 1999). However, the respondents reported great variability in the amount of dye used for this purpose (ranging from a few drops to over 10 ml per bag of formula). Although it appeared logical to use a high concentration to increase the visibility of the dye, there were important reasons for using the smallest effective amount. For example, dye-stained enteral formula can result in generalized discoloration of patients' skin, stool, urine, and serum after absorption from the gastrointestinal tract and can lead to potentially lethal events in some types of patients (Metheny & Clouse, 1997; U.S. Food and Drug Administration [FDA], Center for Food Safety and Nutrition, 2003).

Glucose Method

About 14% of hospitals included in the previously mentioned survey used the glucose method to monitor for aspiration (Metheny, Aud & Wunderlich, 1999). The premise of this method is that tracheal aspirates normally contain less than 5 mg/dl of glucose; thus, a higher than expected level of glucose could indicate the aspiration of glucose-rich formula. Proponents of this method use glucose oxidase reagent strips to test for glucose in tracheal secretions, using the protocol outlined for testing capillary blood (Winterbauer, Durning, Barron, & McFadden, 1981). The specificity of the glucose method was questioned by investigators, who found high glucose concentrations in tracheal secretions from patients who were not receiving tube feedings (Kinsey, Murray, Swensen, & Miles, 1994). Even investigators who favored the glucose method to detect aspiration cautioned that it may be ineffective if low to moderate glucose-containing formulas were used (Winterbauer et al., 1981).

Pepsin Method

Because pepsin is the major gastric enzyme, and because it is not normally present in the respiratory tract, pepsin is a reasonable marker for the pulmonary aspiration of gastric contents. A group of researchers developed a laboratory assay for pepsin and developed a human pepsin antibody to increase the assay's sensitivity and specificity (Metheny et al., 1997). This was necessary for the assay to detect the small quantities of pepsin expected after microaspirations of gastric contents into the respiratory tract. The human pepsin antibody was developed by purifying human pepsin from gastric secretions and injecting it into roosters to produce polyclonal antibodies. Blood from the animals was subsequently obtained, and purified antibody was extracted.

Animal Model Study to Compare Aspiration Detection Methods

Controlled studies of aspiration can be conducted only in an animal model. Thus, between 1999 and 2002, a group of investigators undertook an animal model study to evaluate three aspiration detection methods: the blue dye bedside method, the glucose oxidase reagent strip bedside method, and a laboratory assay for the gastric enzyme pepsin (Metheny et al., 2002; Metheny, Dahms, Stewart, Stone, Frank et al., 2005; Metheny et al., 2004).

Study Design and Methods

An $8 \times 2 \times 3$ (formula type × dye concentration × time) experimental design was used. Eight enteral formulas (three with low glucose concentration, two with moderate glucose concentration, and three with high glucose concentration) were used, along with two dye concentrations (0.8 and 1.5 ml/L). The study was conducted in an animal research laboratory and used 182 New Zealand white rabbits (161 experimental animals and 21 control animals). Gastric juice was collected from 161 acutely ill humans and mixed half and half with one of the eight enteral formulas stained with one of two dye concentrations. The animals were anesthetized, tracheally intubated, and mechanically ventilated. The appropriate mixture of gastric juice mixed with dye-stained enteral formula was delivered via a small catheter positioned in a crease in the animals' endotracheal tube cuff over a 30-minute period at baseline, Hour 2, and Hour 4. The infusion was stopped for 90 minutes after each bolus administration and tracheal suctioning was performed. Only isotonic saline was infused into the tracheas of the 21 control animals, using the same protocol described for the experimental animals. Outcome measures (visibility of dye, glucose readings, and pepsin readings) were made every 2 hours for a total of three times. Dye was recorded as visible or not visible. Tracheal glucose concentrations were recorded as ≥ 20, ≥ 40, ≥ 60, or ≥ 80 mg/dl. The concentration of pepsin found in the tracheal secretions was reported in µg/ml. At the conclusion of the experiment, the animals were sacrificed.

Results

Dye Method. Dye was visible in less than half (125/270) of the tracheal secretions collected from the experimental animals (Metheny et al., 2002). The concentration of dye did not produce a significant effect on dye visibility at any of the time points; however, dye was less visible at the second and third aspiration events than at the first event. Dye was not observed in any of the secretions from the control animals. The dye method is no longer recommended because it is not sensitive and has potential for harm (AACN, 2005a; McClave et al., 2002; Maloney & Metheny, 2002).

Glucose Method. Glucose was found in a concentration of at least 20 mg/dl in about half of the tracheal secretions collected from the control animals who had received only isotonic saline intratracheally (Metheny, Dahms et al., 2005). Tracheal glucose concentrations were also high in the experimental animals, regardless of the type of enteral formula (low, moderate, or high glucose) used. The major predictor of tracheal glucose in all of the animals was their arterial glucose concentrations.

Pepsin Method. The pepsin detection method had a sensitivity of 93% and a specificity of 100% (Metheny et al., 2004). Pepsin was present in all of the tracheal secretions from 149 of the 161 experimental animals. At Hour 2, the mean pepsin concentration in the tracheal secretions was 141µg/ml; at Hour 4, it was 127µg/ml; and at Hour 6, it was 116 µg/ml. In contrast, no pepsin was found in any of the tracheal secretions from the 21 control animals.

As indicated above, the laboratory pepsin assay was highly effective in detecting aspiration in the animal model study. In the next study reported, researchers used the laboratory pepsin assay to assess for aspiration in a clinical study.

Descriptive Clinical Study of Aspiration

Between 2002 and 2005, investigators used the pepsin immunoassay previously discussed to describe the frequency of aspiration in a population of 360 critically ill, mechanically ventilated adult patients (Metheny et al., 2006). Inclusion criteria were mechanical ventilation and tube feedings; an exclusion criterion was physician-diagnosed pneumonia at the time of enrollment. Research nurses were present daily from 8:00 a.m. through 12 midnight to prospectively collect data for three consecutive days for each patient enrolled in the study.

Bedside nurses collected tracheobronchial secretions in sputum traps when suctioning was performed for therapeutic purposes. The secretions were saved and given to the investigators for transport to a research laboratory where they were assayed for pepsin.

The mean age of the patients included in the study was 52 years; a higher percentage (60%) of men participated (presumably because the study site was a Level I Trauma Center). Five intensive care units were used and consisted of trauma/surgery, neurosurgery/neuromedicine, general medicine, cardiac surgery, and cardiac medicine. Approximately half of the patients received gastric feedings; the majority of the rest received feedings in the proximal duodenum. Only 38% of the patients had a mean head-of-bed elevation of ≥30° throughout the 3-day study period.

Almost 6,000 tracheal secretions were collected and assayed for pepsin; of these, over 31% were positive. At least one microaspiration event was identified in 320 (89%) of the patients. Patients whose tracheal secretions were positive for pepsin in 25% or more of the observations were classified as frequent aspirators; those with less than 25% of their secretions positive for pepsin were classified as infrequent aspirators. Patients who developed pneumonia while participating in the study were four times more likely to be in the frequent aspiration group.

Risk factors identified as significant for aspiration included a mean head-of-bed elevation less than 30°, a Glasgow Coma Scale score less than 9, gastric feedings (as opposed to small bowel feedings), vomiting, and gastroesophageal reflux disease. The most significant risk factors for pneumonia were aspiration and heavy sedation. To determine the effect of gastric residual volume on aspiration, only the 182 patients who were consistently fed in the stomach were included in the analysis. Two or more gastric residual volumes ≥200 ml were observed in 20 (11%) of the 182 gastric-fed patients during the 3-day observation period. Of these 20 patients, 15 were in the frequent aspiration group. A subsequent study by the same investigators also identified gastric residual volumes ≥200 ml as a risk factor for aspiration (Metheny, Schallom, Oliver, & Clouse, 2008).

Hospital and intensive care unit lengths of stay were each approximately 2 days longer in the frequent aspiration group, while the need for ventilator support was approximately 2.6 days longer. Hospital length of stay was about 3.5 days longer in patients with pneumonia, whereas intensive care unit length of stay was about 3.8 days longer, and the need for ventilator support was 4.3 days longer. It was concluded that aspiration is a major risk factor for pneumonia and that it significantly increases use of hospital resources. It was also concluded that modifiable risk factors for aspiration (such as head-of-bed elevation, gastric feeding site, and high gastric residual volumes) need to be addressed.

Study of Interventions to Reduce Aspiration

Between 2006 and 2008, researchers studied the effect of an aspiration risk reduction protocol (ARRP) in a population of 145 critically ill, mechanically ventilated patients (Metheny, Davis-Jackson, & Stewart, 2010). The ARRP consisted of a series of components, including maintaining the head-of-bed angle at 30° or higher and placing feeding tubes in the distal small bowel when deemed necessary by attending physicians. An advanced practice nurse was present 40 hours per week during the study to encourage the staff to implement the interventions. Findings were compared with a usual care group (*n* = 329) in an earlier study conducted in the same intensive care units (Metheny et al., 2006). Eighty-eight percent of the patients in the ARRP group had mean head-of-bed elevations of 30° or higher as compared with only 38% of the patients in the usual care group. Almost three fourths of the patients in the ARRP group had feeding tubes placed in the small bowel, as compared with less than 50% in the usual care group. Furthermore, over one half of the small bowel tubes in the ARRP group were placed in the mid-to-distal small bowel (as opposed to only 16% placed in the mid-to-distal small bowel in the usual care group). The percentage of patients who aspirated at least once was much lower in the ARRP group than in the usual care group (39% vs. 89%, respectively). Similarly, aspiration-related pneumonia was much lower in the ARRP group than in the usual care group (19% vs. 48%, respectively). Findings from this study suggest that a combination of an elevated head-of-bed position to at least 30° and use of a mid-to-distal small bowel feeding site can dramatically reduce the incidence of aspiration and aspiration-related pneumonia in critically ill, tube-fed patients.

CONCLUSION

Inclusion of findings from the previously described tube-feeding research studies in recommendations provided by national-level groups has been highly instrumental in improving the care of tube-fed patients, both in the United States and abroad. For example, the American Society for Parenteral and Enteral Nutrition (ASPEN) Enteral Nutrition Practice Guidelines (Bankhead et al., 2009) are followed closely by acute care and long-term care facilities throughout the world in determining standard of care for tube-fed patients. As noted in Table 7.1, the Enteral Nutrition Guidelines include multiple NINR-funded studies pertaining to methods to determine feeding tube placement.

Similarly, multiple research studies funded by the NINR are cited in the AACN's Practice Alert: Verification of Feeding Tube Placement (American Association of Critical Care Nurses, 2005b). The Practice Alert is available online and is regularly consulted by critical care nurses and nurses in other realms of patients care. Both the ASPEN Enteral Nutrition Guidelines and the AACN Practice Alert provide nurses with research-based information to help them deliver the best possible care to patients in all types of settings.

The FDA issued an alert in September 2003 about possible dangers associated with the use of FD&C Blue Dye No. 1 (U.S. FDA, 2003). The FDA alert included a citation of a survey conducted by NINR-funded nurse researchers that found widespread use of the potentially harmful dye (Metheny et al., 1999). The FDA alert also included a citation of an animal model study conducted by the same principal investigator, demonstrating that the blue dye method is insensitive (Metheny et al., 2002). Although blue food dye was widely used in the past, it is rarely used today.

The principal investigator of the numerous tube-feeding studies cited in this chapter answers an average of two to three e-mails or telephone calls per week from nurses throughout the United States and in many foreign countries regarding enteral feeding issues. In this way, specific information tailored to individual questions is provided to caregivers to help them improve their ability to provide good care to tube-fed patients.

Although findings from the studies described in this chapter have had a significant and favorable impact on the care of tube-fed patients, nurse researchers are continuing their efforts to reduce risk for harmful outcomes in patients receiving tube feedings. For example, a study is currently underway to attempt to develop a rapid bedside assay for pepsin that nurses can use with minimal difficulty to assess for the pulmonary aspiration of gastric contents.

REFERENCES

Agency for Healthcare Research and Quality Commentary. (2008, September 10). Where's the feeding tube? Morbidity and mortality rounds on the Web. Retrieved March 8, 2009, from http://www.webmm.ahrq.gov/case.aspx?caseID=184

American Association of Critical Care Nurses. (2005a). Practice alert: Dye in enteral feedings. Retrieved March 8, 2009, from http://www.aacn.org/WD/Practice/Docs/Dye_in_Enteral_Feeding_4-2005.pdf

American Association of Critical Care Nurses. (2005b). Practice alert: Verification of feeding tube placement. Retrieved March 8, 2009, from http://www.aacn.org/WD/Practice/Docs/Verification_of_Feeding_Tube_Placement_05-2005.pdf

Aronchick J., Epstein, D., Gefter, W., & Miller, W. (1984). Pneumothorax as a complication of placement of a nasoenteric tube. *Journal of the American Medical Association, 252*, 3287–3288.

Balogh, G. J., Adler, S. J., Vander Woude, J., Glazer, H. S., Roper, C., & Weyman, P. J. (1983). Pneumothorax as a complication of feeding tube placement. *American Journal of Roentgenology, 141*, 1275–1277.

Bankhead, R., Boullata, J., Brantley, S., Corkins, M., Guenter, P., Krenitsky, J., Lyman, B., Metheny, N. A., Mueller, C., Robbins, S., Wessel, J., & the A.S.P.E.N. Board of Directors. (2009). ASPEN enteral nutrition practice recommendations. *Journal of Parenteral & Enteral Nutrition, 33*(2), 122–166.

Baskin, W. N. (2006). Acute complications associated with bedside placement of feeding tubes. *Nutrition in Clinical Practice, 21*, 40–55.

El Gamel, A., & Watson, D. C. (1993). Transbronchial intubation of the right pleural space: A rare complication of nasogastric intubation with a polyvinylchloride tube: A case study. *Heart Lung, 22*, 224–225.

Elpern, E. H., Killen, K., Talla, E., Perez, G., & Gurka, D. (2007). Capnometry and air insufflation for assessing initial placement of gastric tubes. *American Journal of Critical Care, 16*, 544–549.

Gharpure, V., Meert, K., Sarnaik, A., & Metheny, N. (2000). Indicators of post pyloric feeding tube placement in children. *Critical Care Medicine, 28*(8), 2962–2966.

Griffith, D. P., McNally, A. T., Battey, C. H., Forte, S. S., Cacciatore, A. M., Szeszycki, E., Bergman, G. F., Furr, C. E., Murphy, F. B., Galloway, J. R., & Ziegler, T. R. (2003). Intravenous erythromycin facilitates bedside placement of postpyloric feeding tubes in critically ill adults: A double-blind, randomized, placebo-controlled study. *Critical Care Medicine, 31*(3), 39–44.

Hand, R. W., Kempster, M., Levy, J. H., Rogol, P. R., & Spirn, P. (1984). Inadvertent transbronchial insertion of narrow-bore feeding tubes into the pleural space. *Journal of the American Medical Association,* (18), 2396–2397.

Harris, M., & Huseby, J. (1988). New feeding tube insertion technique prevents inadvertent placement in the lung [Abstract]. *American Review of Respiratory Disease, 137*, 216.

Hendry, P. J., Akyureki, Y., McIntyre, R., Quarrington, A., & Keon, W. J. (1986). Bronchopleural complications of nasogastric feeding tubes. *Critical Care Medicine, 14*, 892–894.

Joint Commission of Healthcare Organizations. (2000, February 4). Operative and post-operative complications: Lessons for the future. *Sentinel Event Alert, 12.* Retrieved March 9, 2009, from http://www.jointcommission.org/SentinelEvents/SentinelEventAlert/sea_12.htm

Kinsey, G. C., Murray, M. J., Swensen, S. J., & Miles, J. M. (1994). Glucose content of tracheal aspirates: Implications for the detection of tube feeding aspiration. *Critical Care Medicine, 22*, 1557–1562.

Kolbitsch, C., Pomaroli, A., Lorenz, I., Gassner, M., & Luger, T. J. (1997). Pneumothorax following nasogastric feeding tube insertion in a tracheotomized patient after bilateral lung transplantation. *Intensive Care Medicine, 23*, 440–442.

Lipman, T. O., Kessler, T., & Arabian, A. (1985). Nasopulmonary intubation with feeding tubes: Case reports and review of the literature. *Journal of Parenteral and Enteral Nutrition, 9*, 618–620.

Maloney, J., & Metheny, N. (2002). Controversy in using blue dye in enteral tube feeding as a method of detecting pulmonary aspiration. *Critical Care Nurse, 22*, 84–85.

McClave, S., DeMeo, M., DeLegge, M., DiSario, J., Heyland, D., Maloney, J., Metheny, N. A., Moore, F. A., Scolapio, J. S., Spain, D. A., & Zaloga, G. P. (2002). Consensus statement: North American Summit on aspiration in the critically ill patient. *Journal of Parenteral and Enteral Nutrition, 26*(6), S80–S85.

Metheny, N. (2002). Inadvertent intracranial nasogastric tube placement. *American Journal of Nursing, 102*(8), 25–27.

Metheny, N. A., Aud, M. A., & Ignatavicius, D. D. (1998). Detection of improperly positioned feeding tubes. *Journal of Healthcare Risk Management, 18*, 37–48.

Metheny, N., Aud, M., & Wunderlich, R. (1999). A survey of bedside methods used to detect pulmonary aspiration in intubated, tube-fed patients. *American Journal of Critical Care, 8*(3), 160–169.

Metheny, N. A., & Clouse, R. E. (1997). Bedside methods for detecting aspiration in tube-fed patients. *Chest, 111*(3), 724–731.

Metheny, N., Clouse, R., Chang, Y. H., Stewart, B., Oliver, D., & Kollef, M. (2006). Tracheobronchial aspiration of gastric contents in critically ill tube-fed patients: Frequency, outcomes and risk factors. *Critical Care Medicine, 34*(4), 1007–1015.

Metheny, N. A., Clouse, R. E., Clark, J. M., Reed, L., Wehrle, M. A., & Wiersema, L. (1994). pH testing of feeding tube aspirates to determine placement. *Nutrition in Clinical Practice, 9*, 185–190.

Metheny, N., Dahms, T., Chang, Y., Stewart, B., Frank, P., & Clouse, R. E. (2004). Detection of pepsin in tracheal secretions after three forced small-volume aspirations of gastric juice. *Journal of Parenteral and Enteral Nutrition, 28*(2), 79–84.

Metheny, N., Dahms, T., Stewart, B., Stone, K., Edwards, S., Defer, J., & Clouse, R. E. (2002). Efficacy of dye-stained enteral formula in detecting pulmonary aspiration. *Chest, 122*, 276–281.

Metheny, N., Dahms, T., Stewart, B., Stone. K., Frank, P., & Clouse, R. E. (2005). Verification of inefficacy of the glucose method in detecting aspiration associated with tube feedings. *Medsurg Nursing, 14*(2), 112–121.

Metheny, N. A., Davis-Jackson, J., & Stewart, B. J. (2010). Effectiveness of an aspiration risk-reduction protocol. *Nursing Research, 59*(5), 18–25.

Metheny, N., Dettenmeir, P., Hampton, K., Wiersema, L., & Williams, P. (1990). Detection of inadvertent respiratory placement of small-bore feeding tubes: A report of 10 cases. *Heart Lung, 19*(6), 631–638.

Metheny, N. A., & Meert, K. L. (2004). Monitoring feeding tube placement. *Nutrition in Clinical Practice, 19*, 487–495.

Metheny, N. A., Meert, K. L., & Clouse, R. E. (2007). Complications related to feeding tube placement. *Current Opinion in Gastroenterology, 23*, 178–182.

Metheny, N., McSweeney, M., Wiersema, L., & Wehrle, M. (1990). Effectiveness of the auscultatory method in predicting feeding tube placement. *Nursing Research, 39*(5), 262–267.

Metheny, N., Reed, L., Berglund, B., & Wehrle, M. (1994). Visual characteristics of aspirates from feeding tubes as a method for predicting tube location. *Nursing Research, 43*(5), 282–287.

Metheny, N., Reed, L., Wiersema, L., McSweeney, M., Wehrle, M., & Clark, J. (1993). Effectiveness of pH measurements in predicting feeding tube location: An update. *Nursing Research, 42*(6), 324–331.

Metheny, N. A., Reed, L., Worseck, M., & Clark, J. (1993). How to aspirate fluid from small-bore feeding-tubes. *American Journal of Nursing, 93*, 86–88.

Metheny, N., Schallom, L., Oliver, D. A., & Clouse, R. E. (2008). Gastric residual volume and aspiration in critically ill patients receiving gastric feedings. *American Journal of Critical Care, 17*, 512–520.

Metheny, N., Schnelker, R., McGinnis, J., Zimmerman, G., Duke, C., Merritt, B., Banotai, M., & Oliver, D. A. (2005). Indicators of tube site during feedings. *Journal of Neuroscience Nursing, 37*(6), 320–325.

Metheny, N., Smith, L., & Stewart, B. (2000). Development of a reliable and valid bedside test for bilirubin and its utility in predicting feeding tube location. *Nursing Research, 49*(6), 302–309.

Metheny, N., Spies, M., & Eisenberg, P. (1986). Frequency of nasoenteral tube displacement and associated risk factors. *Research in Nursing & Health, 9*(3), 241–247.

Metheny, N., Stewart, B., Smith, L., Yan, H., Diebold, M., & Clouse, R. (1997). pH and concentrations of pepsin and trypsin in feeding tube aspirates as predictors of tube placement. *Journal of Parenteral and Enteral Nutrition, 21*(5), 279–285.

Metheny, N., Stewart, B., Smith, L., Yan, H., Diebold, M., & Clouse, R. (1999). pH and concentration of bilirubin in feeding tube aspirates as predictors of tube placement. *Nursing Research, 48*(4), 189–197.

Metheny, N., Wehrle, M. A., Wiersema, L., & Clark, J. (1998). Testing feeding tube placement: Auscultation versus pH method. *American Journal of Nursing, 98*, 37–42.

Metheny, N., Williams, P., Wiersema, L., Wehrle, M., Eisenberg, P., & McSweeney, M. (1989). Effectiveness of pH measurements in predicting feeding tube placement. *Nursing Research, 38*(5), 280–285.

Miller, K. S., Tomlinson, J. R., & Sahn, S. A. (1985). Pleuropulmonary complications of enteral tube feedings: Two reports, review of the literature, and recommendations. *Chest, 88*, 230–233.

Nakao, M. A., Killam, D., & Wilson, R. (1983). Pneumothorax secondary to inadvertent nasotracheal placement of a nasoenteric tube past a cuffed endotracheal tube. *Critical Care Medicine, 11*, 210–211.

Sahn, S. (1988). State of the art: The pleura. *American Review of Respiratory Disorders, 138,* 184–234.

Schlorlemmer, G. R., & Battaglini, J. W. (1984). An unusual complication of nasoenteral feeding with small-diameter feeding tubes. *Annals of Surgery, 199,* 104–106.

Siemers, P. T., & Reinke, R. T. (1976). Perforation of the nasopharynx by nasogastric intubation: A rare cause of left pleural effusion and pneumomediastinum. *American Journal of Roentgenology, 127,* 341–343.

Theodore, A. C., Frank, J. A., Ende, J., Snider, G. L., & Beer, D. J. (1984). Errant placement of nasoenteric tubes: A hazard in obtunded patients. *Chest, 86,* 931–933.

Torrington, K., & Bowman, M. (1981). Fatal hydrothorax empyema complicating malpositioned nasogastric tube. *Chest, 79,* 240–242.

United States Food and Drug Administration. Center for Food Safety and Nutrition. (2003, September 29). *Discoloration and death in patients receiving enteral feedings tinted with the dye, FD & C Blue No. 1.* Retrieved March 8, 2009, from http://www.cfsan.fda.gov/~dms/col-ltr2.html

Valentine, R., & Turner, W. (1985). Pleural complications of nasoenteric feeding tubes. *Journal of Parenteral and Enteral Nutrition, 9,* 605–607.

Welch, S. K. (1996). Certification of staff nurses to insert enteral feeding tubes using a research-based procedure. *Nutrition in Clinical Practice, 11*(1), 21–27.

Winterbauer, R. H., Durning, R. B. J., Barron, E., & McFadden, M. C. (1981). Aspirated nasogastric feeding solution detected by glucose strips. *Annals of Internal Medicine, 95*(1), 67–68.

8

Translating Personal Challenges to Public Policy

Carolyn M. Sampselle

Incontinence is a personal challenge that imposes heavy consequences on individual quality of life and a high financial burden on national healthcare costs. Both women and men suffer with incontinence, but more women than men experience it, with a female-to-male ratio of 2.6 (McGrother et al., 2004). Smaller numbers of both sexes suffer from fecal incontinence. The scope of this chapter is limited to urinary incontinence (UI) in women, but similar factors influence policy affecting UI in men and fecal incontinence.

Historically, pharmacologic and surgical treatments have comprised the first line of therapy for UI in women, but a substantial body of research in the last two decades has shifted that paradigm to one of a first-line management strategy that is noninvasive, i.e., a strategy that emphasizes self-management. Nurses, physical therapists, and behavioral psychologists have been leaders in generating the research that has resulted in this paradigm shift. They are also leading in the more recent policy shift from treatment to prevention.

INCONTINENCE IS A MAJOR HEALTH PROBLEM

Urinary incontinence affects large numbers of women, but the reported numbers likely underestimate the true prevalence/incidence due to the very personal and socially stigmatized nature of the condition. Many women do not disclose a problem with UI to their healthcare provider because they are too embarrassed. Healthcare providers contribute to the hidden nature of incontinence by rarely including it as a component of routine screening. Patients are reluctant to initiate a discussion with providers until severity has reached life-altering levels. This is unfortunate because, as with other health problems, early detection and treatment favor better outcomes.

Prevalence and Severity

In 2005, Hunskaar and colleagues reviewed 36 general population studies to estimate the prevalence of UI in community-dwelling women across the lifespan (Hunskaar et al., 2005). Prevalence reports range from 5% to 69%, with most estimates falling into the range of 25% to 45%. Incontinence prevalence increases up to middle age, stabilizes somewhat at about 30% during the menopausal years, and then steadily increases as women get older, when it rises to levels of 40% and higher (Hunskaar et al., 2005). The Agency for Healthcare Quality Research supported a more recent review of Prevention of Fecal and Urinary Incontinence in Adults (2007). That report estimated the overall prevalence in women at somewhat lower proportions in the range of 16%–22% (ahrq. gov/downloads/pub/evidence/pdf/fuiad/fuiad.pdf). More severe levels of UI requiring the use of frequent changes of absorbent pads or clothing affect as high as 10% to 25% of women (Melville, Katon, Delaney, & Newton, 2005; Sampselle, Harlow, Skurnick, Brubaker, & Bondarenko, 2002). Clearly, even if the most conservative estimates are used, this is a problem that negatively affects the lives of large numbers of women.

Economic Cost of Incontinence

Estimates of the cost of UI include the direct costs of diagnosis, treatment such as medication or surgery, and routine care such as absorbent pads. (Importantly, the cost of protective absorbent supplies is often borne completely by the patient.) Other direct costs are related to the consequences of incontinence such as fall injuries (Brown, Vittinghoff et al., 2000), skin breakdown, and urinary tract infections. Incontinence is also a primary reason for nursing home admission (Thom, Haan, & Van Den Eeden, 1997). Indirect costs include the value of lost productivity in the form of early retirement or an incontinent employee's reduced capacity to work without distractions or interruptions. Due to the imprecision of calculating monetary value, most economic estimates exclude indirect costs and intangible costs, costs that are imputed from the personal and family distress caused by the condition.

Recent global estimates of direct costs of incontinence in the United States range from $16.3 billion to $19.5 billion per year (Hu et al., 2004; Wilson, Brown, Shin, Luk, & Subak, 2001). As seen in the disease-specific comparisons provided by the National Institutes of Health (NIH) in 2000 (Kirschstein, 2000), these costs exceed those imposed on the healthcare system by HIV/AIDS, asthma, or breast cancer (http://ospp.od.nih.gov/ecostudies/COIreportweb.htm).

Quality-of-Life Cost of Incontinence

Although a dollar figure cannot be placed on the emotional cost imposed on those who suffer from incontinence, its impact must be considered. Women suffering from stress UI and from an overactive bladder have reported greater levels of bother, lower levels of health-related quality of life, increased depression, and less enjoyment of sexual activity (Coyne et al., 2008). Not surprisingly, lower incontinence-related quality of life is significantly and independently associated with severity, nocturia, and length of time suffered prior to seeking treatment (Monz et al., 2007). Demographic factors have been associated with higher incontinence-related bother, with women in lower socioeconomic groups and those of Hispanic ethnicity reporting higher levels of bother (Tennstedt et al., 2007). In fact, the psychological distress imposed by UI in African American and Latina women exceeds that of women of European descent: adjusted odds ratio, 1.26 (95% confidence interval, 1.67) for African Americans and 5.70 (95% confidence interval, 12.05) for Latinas (Longworth, Davila, & Sampselle, 2003).

POPULATIONS AT INCREASED RISK OF INCONTINENCE

When considering policy implications, it is important to identify key populations that are at increased risk. With this knowledge, resources can be channeled into care and prevention programs that are better aligned with the risk group and thus more likely to yield the greatest benefit.

Obese Individuals

In addition to age, body mass index has been linked to UI in women. Among perimenopausal and postmenopausal women, each unit increase of body mass index was associated with a 5% increase in the odds of having UI (Sampselle et al., 2002) Weight loss in overweight and obese women covaried with UI episodes (Subak et al., 2009). In light of the obesity epidemic that is spreading in the United States, incontinence prevalence is likely to increase, adding to the healthcare cost burden in the coming years.

Specific Occupations

Some occupations constrain ready access to toilet facilities. Women who work on production lines come immediately to mind in this category, but school teachers, nurses, and women in the military also function in situations where ad lib toilet access may be limited. In work settings where there is limited allowance for self-initiated restroom breaks, women report using practices such as self-restriction of fluids, avoiding elimination during the work shift, and wearing absorbent pads to contain urine leakage for extended periods of time (Nygaard & Linder, 1997; Sherman, Davis, & Wong, 1997). These practices can increase urinary tract pathology and cause skin breakdown. Higher levels of UI and urinary tract infections have been reported by women in these circumstances; moreover, they indicate that restricted access hampers job performance (Davis et al., 1999; Fitzgerald, Palmer, Kirkland, & Robinson, 2002).

Childbearing Women

Changes during pregnancy, both hormonal and physical, increase women's risk of incontinence during the gestation period. Three-month postpartum incidence in primiparas ranges from 9.3% to 38.4% (Antonakos, Miller, & Sampselle, 2003; Burgio et al., 2003). Birth-related pelvic floor injury offers potential mechanisms to explain the relative risk that, compared with nulliparas, increases from 2.0 after the first vaginal birth to 2.6 after the third birth (Rortveit, Daltveit, Hannestad, & Hunskaar, 2003). Segments of the pelvic floor are at heightened risk during vaginal birth; the pubococcygeas, which is the shortest, most medial, and most ventral portion, stretches to 3.3 times its prebirth state (Lien, Mooney, DeLancey, & Ashton-Miller, 2004). Magnetic resonance images of women with a history of difficult birth demonstrate injury that is consistent with pelvic floor dysfunction (DeLancey et al., 2007).

Some clinicians favor making cesarean section available upon maternal request as a protective measure for incontinence. This practice was considered at a 2006 State-of-the Science conference on cesarean delivery, but the evidence did not support this recommendation (http://consensus.nih.gov/2006CesareanSOS027main.htm). Importantly, the predominant predictor of incontinence across the lifespan is history of one or more pregnancies, not mode of birth. Midlife women who had given birth exclusively via cesarean demonstrated no significant difference in incontinence prevalence when compared with women who had one or more vaginal births and they had 3.5 times the risk in comparison with their never-pregnant counterparts (Faudes, Guarisi, & Pinto-Neto, 2001). Furthermore, history of exclusive cesarean birth is not protective for severe incontinence; rather, the condition is related to history of any pregnancy carried beyond 20 weeks (MacLennan, Taylor, Wilson, & Wilson, 2001).

Because of the heightened risk of incontinence during the childbearing period, pregnant and postpartum women have been targeted as a special group that can benefit from knowledge of bladder health self-management practices. Persuasive evidence of benefits to continence status has resulted from the practice of these strategies (Morkved, Bo, Schei, & Salvesen, 2003; Sampselle et al., 1998). Thus, an important opportunity for prevention occurs for women seen by prenatal and postpartum healthcare providers.

Older Adults With Comorbid Conditions

Disease that affects motor capacity, such as multiple sclerosis, has been associated with rates of bladder dysfunction as high as 93% (Betts, D'Mellow, & Fowler, 1993). Diabetics, who experience microvascular changes that can damage detrussor innervation, are at significantly higher risk of urge incontinence (Brown et al., 2003). Arthritis and other diseases that decrease functional mobility have a pronounced effect on the individual's dexterity and mobility, thus increasing incontinence risk simply because of the reduced capacity to access the necessary facilities (Jakobsson & Hallberg, 2002). Cognitive deficits stemming from depression and Alzheimer's disease have also been associated with incontinence (Jumadilova, Zyczynski, Paul, & Narayanan, 2005).

Nursing Home Residents

Approximately 50% of nursing home residents suffer from incontinence (Aggazzotti et al., 2000; Ouslander, Kane, & Abrass, 1982). Although they typically suffer from some of the comorbid diseases associated with incontinence described in the previous section, there are system issues, as well, in the nursing home situation that contribute a further level of risk. These concerns include resident dependence on providers for timely and consistent assistance and inadequate signage that exacerbates congnitive wayfinding deficits (Schnelle et al., 2003). Since care providers are essential to the mediation of these system issues, policies that incentivize more effective and preventive toileting are warranted as opposed to the palliative bed linen and pad changes that too often occur in the contemporary situation (Watson, Brink, Zimmer, & Mayer, 2003).

EMPIRICAL BASIS FOR CONSERVATIVE MANAGEMENT OF UI

Stress, urge, and mixed incontinence are the most common types of UI in women. Stress incontinence results from increased intra-abdominal pressure that can occur during coughing, sneezing, lifting, or exercising. Urge incontinence is due to contraction of the detrussor muscle in the form of frequent urges to void; it may also arise without warning as a sudden, irrepressible strong urge that results in an incontinent episode. The term *overactive bladder* has gained popular usage as a description of the frequency that is experienced with or without accompanying incontinence.

Strong research support has accumulated in favor of choosing conservative approaches (conservative management, behavioral therapy, and self-management) as the first-line treatment for all three types of incontinence common in women. These practices include pelvic floor muscle training, bladder training, and the Knack Maneuver. All three strategies are characterized by their noninvasive nature and virtual absence of adverse events.

Pelvic Floor Muscle Training

Pelvic floor muscle training was introduced in the mid-20th century by Arnold Kegel and is often referred to as Kegel exercises. The goal of this regularly prescribed set of pelvic floor muscle contractions (typically tested in protocols that recommend 30–50 contractions per day) is to increase the diameter of and control over these voluntary, striated muscles. Positioned to support the pelvic organs and surround the urethra, the increased muscle capacity exerts greater opposing force, offsetting increased bladder pressure. This avoids leakage due to increased intra-abdominal pressure or detrussor contraction.

The efficacy of pelvic floor muscle training in decreasing or eliminating urine leakage has been demonstrated in women during the childbearing period and among older women. It is efficacious in the treatment of the three types of incontinence that are most common among women. Evidence from several well-conducted randomized controlled trials shows pelvic floor muscle training benefits continence (Goode et al., 2003; Hay-Smith, Berghmans, Burgio et al., 2009). It has yielded improvements in reported severity of leakage and in quality of life in up to 94% of women treated; ability to engage in daily activities improved more than 12-fold (Lagro-Janssen, Debruyne, Smits, & Van Weel, 1992).

Electromyography-assisted biofeedback in pelvic muscle training has demonstrated the strongest benefit to relative risk, with a more than 17-fold advantage (Aksac, Aki, Karan et al., 2003). Training provided in groups led by a skilled therapist is associated with the highest levels of cure (Bo, Talseth, & Holme, 1999). With respect to healthcare policy, these findings have clear implications for third-party payers.

After reviewing the extant literature in 17 randomized controlled trials on pelvic floor muscle training, expert panels such as the recent International Consultation on Incontinence Committee on Conservative Management in Adults (Hay-Smith, Berghmans, Burgio et al., 2009) concluded that the level of evidence was Grade A and recommended that "Supervised pelvic floor muscle training should be offered as first line conservative therapy for women with stress, urge, or mixed urinary incontinence."

Although the International Consultation on Incontinence recommendation is aimed at women who are experiencing UI, the underlying principles of these self-management practices can be reasonably expected to yield preventive effects as well. Thus, it is not surprising that the November 2007 NIH State of the Science Conference on Prevention of Fecal and Urinary Incontinence concluded that "simple, non-invasive self-management practices could prevent or greatly delay the development of UI" (Landefeld et al., 2008).

Bladder Training

Bladder training is also referred to as bladder retraining, bladder re-education, and bladder discipline. This self-management strategy aims to gradually increase the time interval between voidings to 3–4 hours and to decrease total voiding frequency during waking hours.

The International Consultation on Incontinence expert panel reviewed randomized controlled trials that evaluated bladder training as the sole intervention; statistically significant improvements were found for women who were taught bladder training (Fantl et al., 1999; Lagro-Janssen et al., 1992). The panel concluded that the level of evidence in support of bladder training was Grade A and recommended that "bladder training is an appropriate first line conservative therapy for UI in women" (Hay-Smith, Berghmans, Burgio et al., 2009).

When bladder training is combined with pelvic floor muscle training, it has demonstrated a consistent pattern of success in treating stress, urge, and mixed UI. Combined training reduced incontinence symptoms by more than 50% in 86% of women between the ages of 40 and 78 years regardless of incontinence type (Dougherty et al., 2002; Goode et al., 2003). The Prevention of Fecal and Urinary Incontinence in Adults report estimates that assessment of UI by nurses followed up with conservative advice on pelvic floor muscle and bladder training could avoid 121 cases of UI and 59 cases of severe incontinence among 1,000 treated women with pregnancy- and birth-related incontinence (ahrq.gov/downloads/pub/evidence/pdf/fuiad/fuiad.pdf).

The Knack Maneuver

Tested more recently and, thus, with less accumulated evidence than pelvic floor muscle training and bladder training, the Knack Maneuver (Miller, Ashton-Miller, DeLancey et al., 1998) is showing great promise as a brief intervention for UI. It is a preemptive pelvic muscle contraction to avert leakage that is well timed with events that challenge the continence mechanism. For example, if a woman experiences stress incontinence when she coughs, she can learn to execute the Knack Maneuver when she begins to cough. In many instances, this intentional well-timed contraction is sufficient to avoid urine leakage. The Knack Maneuver is also valuable in the avoidance of leakage due to urge incontinence. For example, women have learned to use it in situations such as immediately upon arrival home when the detrussor often contracts out of habit rather than due to a full bladder. In such situations, the simple performance of the Knack Maneuver, in conjunction with conscious relaxation and a slow as opposed to a hurried trip to the bathroom, enables many women to gain the control needed to avoid an incontinent episode.

The potential of the Knack Maneuver has been demonstrated with older women and women who are in the childbearing period. Women with demonstrated incontinence (some older and some pregnant) were instructed to cough without contracting the pelvic floor muscles and then to contract the muscles and cough. Reduction in urine leaked was seen in 77% of the older women, with 19% able to eliminate leakage entirely; in the pregnant women, 79% reduced the amount of leakage and 55% eliminated it completely (Miller, Sampselle, Ashton-Miller, Hong, & DeLancey, 2008). Instruction in this intervention is brief and it is easily comprehended. Women may need assistance incorporating it into their daily activities as a patterned response, i.e., a habituated response to a challenge to the continence mechanism, but once learned, women tend to sustain the practice (Hines et al., 2007).

Combined Pelvic Floor Muscle/Bladder Training and Knack

Each of the conservative self-management strategies outlined in the previous sections has demonstrated efficacy when tested independently. A recent randomized controlled trial with women 55 years or older tested a behavior modification program called the bladder health class. This self-management program to prevent UI was based on Bandura's sources of information to increase self-efficacy. Women were followed for 4 years postintervention. A group session presented an array of conservative strategies—pelvic floor muscle training, bladder training, and the Knack Maneuver. Results at 12 months postintervention demonstrated a twofold UI prevention effect, as well as increases in pelvic floor muscle strength and decreases in voiding frequency (Diokno et al., 2004).

Further findings from that study included high and sustained adherence: 82% at 3 months postintervention and 68% at 12 months; at 4 years follow-up, adherence was sustained at 70% and was predicted by self-efficacy immediately postintervention (Sampselle et al., 2005). We further observed synergistic effects between pelvic floor muscle and bladder training, suggesting that this combined approach may enhance overall adherence in this healthy, essentially asymptomatic population (Hines et al., 2007).

This intervention is novel because it enables women to adopt and sustain efficacious bladder health practices for incontinence prevention, whereas conservative management approaches to date have focused heavily on treatment. The major barrier to widespread dissemination and adoption is that the current model for providing this information and motivating women to adopt and sustain the practices is a 2-hour face-to-face classroom presentation to groups of approximately 25 women. This has obvious limitations with respect to cost, convenience, and time, entailing provider intensity and a special trip to the scheduled class on the part of participants. Ideally, this information would be available in a format that could be expeditiously provided during a brief clinic visit or in a Web-based format. Moving in that direction, we developed a 15-minute DVD that is a condensed version of the 2-hour group session. It is culturally sensitive and has yielded knowledge and self-efficacy levels comparable with those we found immediately after the group session.

The next logical step is to compare the outcomes of the DVD format of the bladder health class with those of the efficacious face-to-face format. If levels of knowledge, self-efficacy, adherence, and, most importantly, a salutatory effect on incontinence prevention are demonstrated, it will be appropriate to disseminate this information widely. The DVD addresses some of the key concerns of the face-to-face format in that the DVD could be expeditiously incorporated into a woman's annual examination. A brief positive provider comment about the high prevention capacity of the self-management practices, in conjunction with a copy of the DVD and provider encouragement to the woman to view it, could yield results similar to those seen in brief provider interventions related to smoking cessation. With further development of the bladder health content into an interactive computer-based program, the self-management information could be readily incorporated into downloadable podcasts.

POLICY IMPLICATIONS FOR PRIMARY AND SECONDARY PREVENTION

Like many other chronic conditions, UI is quite treatable in the early stages and may be preventable (or at least mutable, with onset deferred and progression impeded) in many cases. A two-pronged approach is most likely to be effective, with the first strategy emphasizing the point of service and the second focusing on the public health arena.

Point of Service

Using the models available for other high-prevalence conditions that have benefited from early detection, such as hypertension and diabetes, targeting the healthcare provider will be valuable in order to encourage routine screening and assure up-to-date knowledge about available treatment and prevention strategies. Evidence-based information made available to women's health providers via such projects as the Continence for Women project sponsored by the Association for Women's Health Obstetric and Neonatal Nurses has yielded significant benefits for women's bladder health (Sampselle et al., 1997; Sampselle et al., 2000). More recently, practice journals have published papers that summarize the evidence base and provide materials that can be readily incorporated into primary care (Wyman, Burgio, & Newman, 2009).

With so many conditions competing for priority in the brief period of contact between provider and patient that characterizes current healthcare, it is essential that the needed knowledge be available in a format that does not impose undue time demands. Hence, a DVD or other computer-based format such as that described earlier may increase the likelihood that the provider will screen for incontinence, since the requisite information can be provided efficiently.

Targeting highest-risk populations can yield high cost–benefit ratios. For example, women in the childbearing years who often experience incontinence for the first time may present a "teachable moment" that can be used to maximum benefit for the institution of lifelong self-management practices that will benefit bladder health. Some women know about pelvic floor muscle training but elect not to practice it. These individuals might be motivated by the linkage of this practice to benefits beyond continence prevention. For example, the knowledge that recent research has shown that increased pelvic muscle strength resulting from adherence to pelvic floor muscle training enhances sexual function (Zahariou, Karamouti, & Papaioannou, 2008) might have a greater impact on women being encouraged to adopt the practice than does information about the potential for avoiding incontinence later in life.

In addition to making the self-management information readily available to women, system-level change is needed to assure that providers are compensated for the training they provide. Considering the estimated numbers of any and severe incontinence cases that could be avoided with intensive conservative management information delivered to childbearing women, third-party payers should consider reimbursement a logical investment in prevention over a woman's life course. This is particularly germane when the treatment requires the expense of electromyographic biofeedback or intensive group therapy led by a skilled therapist. Impeccable cost-benefit studies will be needed to provide the necessary evidence for such a policy change.

Public Health Initiative

Given the high prevalence of UI, it is useful to consider prevention efforts as a widespread public health initiative using the PRECEDE-PROCEED model. This model, developed by Greene and Kreuter (1991) and extended by Gielen and McDonald (2002), is based upon the disciplines of epidemiology; the social, behavioral, and educational sciences; and health administration. It advances health promotion efforts with the recognition that health and health risks are determined by multiple factors. Thus, it is not sufficient to only provide the patient with the information that is needed, such as diet change or an exercise prescription. Rather, because of multiple determinants, efforts to effect the widespread adoption of protective self-management practices for bladder health must be multisectorial, involving providers, media, and innovative partnerships.

Partnerships with businesses, such as Jenny Craig or Weight Watchers, could disseminate health education materials and encourage their use. This approach could not only link weight loss to improved continence but also could provide simple instruction and encouragement to practice the self-management strategies that are effective in its prevention and control. An obvious point of dissemination for incontinence self-management information is in absorbent products developed to conceal incontinence. The educational materials, of course, need to be developed in collaboration with communication and media experts who are skilled in capturing attention and in planting sustainable messages.

The accomplishment of a widespread translational effort entails interdisciplinary collaboration. This call was sounded by Steven Woolf (2008), who recommended partnering with experts in communication theory, system redesign, informatics, and public policy, among others, in the service of effectively translating discoveries that benefit human health into widespread practice. It is essential that we follow this path, and nurses, with their longstanding tradition of interdisciplinarity, are well positioned to outline best practices for successful partnerships. Such leadership will better enable us to achieve the charge extended by the NIH Clinical and Translational Science Award Initiative to accelerate the translation of scientific discoveries into widespread use to make tangible differences in human health.

REFERENCES

Agency for Healthcare Quality Research. (2007). *Prevention of Fecal and Urinary Incontinence in Adults.* (2007). Publication No. 8-E003.

Aggazzotti, G., Pesce, F., Grassi, D., Fantuzzi, G., Righi, E., De Vita, D., . . . Artibani, W. (2000). Prevalence of urinary incontinence among institutionalized patients: A cross-sectional epidemiologic study in a midsized city in northern Italy. *Urology, 56,* 245.

Aksac, B., Aki, S., Karan, A., Yalcin, O., Isikoglu, M., & Eskiyurt, N. (2003). Biofeedback and pelvic floor exercises for the rehabilitation of stress urinary incontinence. *Gynecologic Obstetric Investigation, 56*(1), 23–27.

Antonakos, C. L., Miller, J. M., & Sampselle, C. M. (2003). Indices for studying urinary incontinence and levator ani function in primiparous women. *Journal of Clinical Nursing, 12,* 554–561.

Betts, C. D., D'Mellow, M. T., & Fowler, C. J. (1993). Urinary symptoms and the neurological features of bladder dysfunction in multiple sclerosis. *Journal of Neurology, Neurosurgery, and Psychiatry, 56,* 245–50.

Bo, K., Talseth, T., & Holme, I. (1999). Single blind, randomized controlled trial of pelvic floor exercises, electrical stimulation, vaginal cones, and no treatment in management of genuine stress incontinence in women. *British Medical Journal, 318,* 487–493.

Brown, J. S., Nyberg, L. M., Kusek, J. W., Burgio, K. L., Diokno, A. C., Foldspang, A., et al. (2003). Proceedings of the National Institute of Diabetes and Digestive and Kidney Diseases. International Symposium on Epidemiologic Issues in Urinary Incontinence in Women. *American Journal of Obstetrics and Gynecology, 188,* S77–S88.

Brown, J. S., Vittinghoff, E., Wyman, J. F., Stone, K. L., Nevitt, M. C., Ensrud, K. E., et al. (2000). Urinary incontinence: Does it increase risk for falls and fractures? *Journal of the American Geriatrics Society, 487,* 721–725.

Burgio, K. L., Zyczynski, H., Locher, J. L., Richter, H. E., Redden, D. T., & Wright, K. C. (2003). Urinary incontinence in the 12-month postpartum period. *Obstetrics & Gynecology, 102*(6),1291–1298.

Coyne, K. S., Sexton, C. C., Irwin, D. E., Kopp, Z. S., Kelleher. C. J., & Milsom, I. (2008). The impact of overactive bladder, incontinence and other lower urinary tract symptoms on quality of life, work productivity, sexuality and emotional well-being in men and women: Results from the EPIC study. *BJU International, 101,* 1388–1395.

Davis, G., Sherman, R., Wong, M. F., McClure, G., Perez, R., & Hibbert, M. (1999). Urinary incontinence among female soldiers. *Military Medicine, 164*(3), 182–187.

DeLancey, J. O., Morgan, D. M., Fenner, D. E., Kearney, R., Guire, K., Miller, J. M., et al. (2007). Comparison of levator ani muscle defects and function in women with and without pelvic organ prolapsed. *Obstetrics & Gynecology, 109,* 295–302.

Diokno, A. C., Sampselle, C. M., Herzog, A. G., Raghunathan, T. E., Hines, S., Messer, K. L., et al. (2004). Prevention of urinary incontinence by behavioral modification program: A randomized controlled trial among older women in the community. *The Journal of Urology, 171,* 1165–1171.

Dougherty, M. C., Dwyer, J. W., Pendergast, J. F., Boyington, A. R., Tomlinson, B. U., Coward, R. T., . . . Rooks, L. G. (2002). A randomized trial of behavioral management for continence with older rural women. *Research in Nursing and Health, 1,* 3–13.

Fantl, J. A., Wyman, J. F., McClish, D. K., Harkins, S., Elswick, R. K., Taylor, J. K., & Hadley, E. C. (1991). Efficacy of bladder training in older women with urinary incontinence. *Journal of the American Medical Association, 265*(5), 609–613.

Faudes, A., Guarisi, T., & Pinto-Neto, A. M. (2001). The risk of urinary incontinence of parous women who delivered only by cesarean section. *International Journal of Gynecology & Obstetrics, 72,* 41–46.

Fitzgerald, S. T., Palmer, M. H., Kirkland, V. L., & Robinson, L. (2002). The impact of urinary incontinence in working women: A study in a production facility. *Women & Health, 35*(1), 1–16.

Gielen, A., & McDonald, E. (2002). Using the PRECEDE-PROCEED planning model to apply health behavior theories. In L. W. Green & M. W. Kreuter (1991). *Health promotion planning: An educational and environmental approach* (2nd ed.). Mountain View, CA: Mayfield.

Goode, P. S., Burgio, K. L., Locher, J. L., Roth, D., Umlauf, M. G., Richter, H. E., . . . Lloyd, L. K. (2003). Effect of behavioral training with or without pelvic floor electrical stimulation on stress incontinence in women: A randomized controlled trial, *Journal of the American Medical Association, 290*(3), 345–352.

Green, L. & Kreuter, M. (1991). *Health Promotion Planning: An Educational and Environmental Approach* (2nd ed.). Mountain View, CA: Mayfield Publishing.

Hay Smith, J., Berghmans, B., Burgio, K. et al. (2009). Adult Conservative Management. In P. Abrams, L. Cardozo, S. Khouri, & A. Wein (Eds). *Proceedings from the 4th International Consultation on Incontinence.* Plymouth, UK: Health Publication.

Hines, S. H., Seng, J. S., Messer, K. L., Raghunathan, T. E., Diokno, A. C., & Sampselle, C. M. (2007). Adherence to a behavioral program to prevent incontinence. *Western Journal of Nursing Research, 29*(1), 36–56.

Hu, T. W., Wagner, T. H., Bentkover, J. D., Leblanc, K., Zhou, S. Z., & Hunt, T. (2004). Costs of urinary incontinence and overactive bladder in the United States: A comparative study. *Urology, 63*(3), 461–465.

Hunskaar, S., Burgio, K., Clark, A., Lapitan, M., Nelson, R., Sillen, U., et al. (2005). Epidemiology of urinary incontinence (UI) and faecal incontinence (FI) and pelvic organ prolapsed (POP). *Incontinence,* 255.

Jakobsson, U., & Hallberg, I. R. (2002). Pain and quality of life among older people with rheumatoid arthritis and/or osteoarthritis: A literature review. *Journal of Clinical Nursing, 11,* 430–443.

Jumadilova, Z., Zyczynski, T., Paul, B., & Narayanan, S. (2005). Urinary incontinence in the nursing home: Resident characteristics and prevalence of drug treatment. *American Journal of Managed Care, 11,* S112.

Kirschstein, R. (2000). National Institutes of Health, disease specific estimates of direct and indirect costs of illness and NIH Support.

Lagro-Janssen, A. L., Debruyne, F. M., Smits, A. J., & Van Weel, C. (1992). The effects of treatment of urinary incontinence in general practice. *Family Practice,* (3), 284–289.

Landefeld, C. S., Bowers, B. J., Feld, A. D., Hartmann, K. E., Hoffman, E., Ingber, M. J., et al. (2008). National Institutes of Health State-of-the-Science conference statement: Prevention of fecal and urinary incontinence in adults. *Annals of Internal Medicine, 148*(6), 449–458.

Lien, K. C., Mooney, B., DeLancey, J. O., & Ashton-Miller, J. A. (2004). Levator ani muscle stretch induced by simulated vaginal birth. *Obstetrics & Gynecology, 103*(1), 31–40.

Longworth, J., Davila, Y., & Sampselle, C. M. (2003). La perdida de orina: Hispanic women's experience of urinary incontinence. *Hispanic Health Care International: The Official Journal of the National Association of Hispanic Nurses, 2*(1), 13–21.

MacLennan, A. H., Taylor, A. W., Wilson, D. H., & Wilson, D. (2001). The prevalence of pelvic floor disorders and their relationship to gender, age, parity and mode of delivery. *Obstetrical & Gynecological Survey, 56*(6), 335–336.

McGrother, C. W., Donaldson, M. M., Shaw, C., Matthews, R. J., Hayward, T. A., Dallosso, H. M., . . . MRC Incontinence Study Team, University of Leicester. (2004). Storage symptoms of the bladder: Prevalence, incidence and need for services in the UK. *BJU International, 93*(6), 763–769.

Melville, J. L., Katon, W., Delaney, K., & Newton, K. (2005). Urinary incontinence in US women: A population-based study. *Archives of Internal Medicine, 165,* 537.

Miller, J. M., Ashton-Miller, J. A., & DeLancey, J. L. (1998). A pelvic muscle precontraction can reduce cough-related urine loss in selected women with mild SUI. *Journal of the American Geriatrics Society, 46*(7), 870–874.

Miller, J., Sampselle, C. M., Ashton-Miller, J., Hong, G. R., & DeLancey, J. (2008). Clarification and confirmation of the knack maneuver: The effect of volitional pelvic floor muscle contraction to preempt expected stress incontinence. *The International Journal of Urogynecology, 19*(6), 773–782.

Monz, B., Chartier-Kastler, E., Hampel, C., Samsioe, G., Hunskaar, S., Espuna-Pons, M., . . . Chinn, C. (2007). Patient characteristics associated with quality of life in European women seeking treatment for urinary incontinence: Results from PURE. *European Urology, 5,* 1073–1082.

Morkved, S., Bo, K., Schei, B., & Salvesen, K. A. (2003). Pelvic floor muscle training during pregnancy to prevent urinary incontinence: A single-blind randomized control trial. *Obstetrics & Gynecology, 101,* 313–319.

Nygaard, I. E., & Linder, M. (1997). Thirst at work—An occupational hazard? *International Urogynecology Journal and Pelvic Floor Dysfunction, 8,* 340–343.

Ouslander, J. G., Kane, R. L., & Abrass, I. B. (1982). Urinary incontinence in elderly nursing home patients. *Journal of the American Medical Association, 248,* 1194.

Rortveit, G., Daltveit, A. K., Hannestad, Y. S., & Hunskaar, S. (2003). Urinary incontinence after vaginal delivery or cesarean section. *The New England Journal of Medicine, 348,* 900–907.

Sampselle, C. M., Burns, P., Dougherty, M., Kelly-Thomas, K., Newman, D. K., & Wyman, J. (1997). Continence for women: Evidence-based practice. *Journal of Obstetric, Gynecologic, and Neonatal Nursing, 26*(4), 375–385.

Sampselle, C. M., Harlow, S. D., Skurnick, J., Brubaker, L., & Bondarenko, I. (2002). Urinary incontinence predictors and life impact in ethnically diverse perimenopausal women. *Obstetrics and Gynecology, 100,* 1230.

Sampselle, C. M., Messer, K. L., Seng, J. S., Raghunathan, T. E., Hines, S. H., & Diokno, A. C. (2005). Learning outcomes of a group behavioral modification program to prevent urinary incontinence. *International Urogynecology Journal, 16,* 441–446.

Sampselle, C. M., Miller, J. M., Mims, B. M., DeLancey, J. O., Ashton-Miller, J. A., & Antonakos, C. L. (1998). Effect of pelvic muscle exercise on transient incontinence during pregnancy and after birth. *Obstetrics and Gynecology, 91*, 406–412.

Sampselle, C. M., Wyman, J. F., Thomas, K. K., Newman, D. K., Gray, M., Dougherty, M., et al. (2000). Continence for women: A test of AWHONN's evidence-based protocol in clinical practice. *Journal of Obstetric, Gynecologic, and Neonatal Nursing, 29*(1), 18–26.

Schnelle, J. F., Cadogan, M. P., Grbic, D., Bates-Jensen, B. M., Osterweil, D., Yoshii, J., et al. (2003). A standardized quality assessment system to evaluate incontinence care in the nursing home. *Journal of the American Geriatrics Society, 51*, 1754–1761.

Sherman, R. A., Davis, G. D., & Wong, M. F. (1997). Behavioral treatment of exercise-induced urinary incontinence among female soldiers. *Military Medicine, 162*, 690–694.

Subak, L. L., Wing, R., West, D. S., Franklin, F., Vittinghoff, E., Creasman, J. M., et al. (2009). Weight loss to treat urinary incontinence in overweight and obese women. *New England Journal of Medicine, 360*(5), 481–490.

Tennstedt, S. L., Fitzgerald, M. P., Nager, C. W., Xu, Y., Zimmern, P., Kraus, S., et al. (2007). Quality of life in women with stress urinary incontinence. *International Urogynecology Journal, 18*, 543–549.

Thom, D. H., Haan, M. N., & Van Den Eeden, S. K. (1997). Medically recognized urinary incontinence and risks of hospitalization, nursing home admission and mortality. *Age and Ageing, 26*, 367–368.

Watson, N. M., Brink, C. A., Zimmer, J. G., & Mayer, R. D. (2003). Use of the Agency for Health Care Policy and Research Urinary Incontinence Guideline in nursing homes. *Journal of the American Geriatrics Society, 51*, 1779–1786.

Wilson, L., Brown J. S., Shin, G. P., Luc, K. O., & Subak, L. L. (2001). Annual direct cost of urinary incontinence. *Obstetrics and Gynecology, 98*, 398–406.

Woolf, S. H. (2008). The meaning of translational research and why it matters. *Journal of the American Medical Association, 299*(2), 211–213.

Wymann, J., Burgio, K., & Newman, D. (2009). Practical aspects of lifestyle modifications and behavioral interventions in the treatment of overactive bladder and urgency urinary incontinence. *The International Journal of Clinical Practice, 63*(8), 1177–1191.

Zahariou, A. G., Karamouti, M. V., & Papaioannou, P. D. (2008). Pelvic floor muscle training improves sexual function of women with stress urinary incontinence. *International Urogynecology Journal and Pelvic Floor Dysfunction, 19*, 401–406.

9

Shaping HIV/AIDS Prevention Policy for Minority Youth

Antonia M. Villarruel and Loretta S. Jemmott

It has been a little over 25 years since the beginning of the HIV/AIDS epidemic in the United States—one of the major public health challenges in the 20th century. The dramatic decline in the incidence of HIV/AIDS is due, in part, to advances in the prevention and detection of HIV. These advances include the availability of diagnostic screening and testing for blood donors, pregnant women, and the general population; the use of AZT prophylaxis during pregnancy and in infants after birth; and the development of effective behavioral interventions for at-risk populations (Centers for Disease Control & Prevention [CDC], 2006b). In addition to science advances, decreases in the HIV epidemic have been supported by advocacy efforts of affected communities. These efforts have included involvement in the design of effective programs, the development of prevention and treatment services, and mobilization of policy efforts at local, state, and federal levels (Stall & Mills, 2006).

Despite declines in the rates of overall infection, HIV remains a significant health threat, with about 40,000 new cases of HIV diagnosed each year (CDC, 2006c). Furthermore, there has been a shift in the populations affected by HIV. In the early years of the epidemic, HIV and AIDS were thought to be primarily a gay, White man's disease. In 2000, the rate of HIV/AIDS in Black and Hispanic men overtook that of Whites. Racial and ethnic minorities, particularly African Americans and Hispanics/Latinos, are still disproportionately impacted by HIV/AIDS (CDC, 2008b). Youth, especially minority youth, are also disproportionately affected by HIV/AIDS. In 2004, 13% of all new HIV diagnoses were among young people aged 13–24 years (CDC, 2008a). In the absence of a vaccine, prevention is the best and only defense against HIV/AIDS.

Health policies that support the uptake and dissemination of effective HIV/AIDS primary and secondary prevention programs and strategies are essential. However, as was true since the beginning of the epidemic, HIV/AIDS research and policy are challenging due to the racism, discrimination, stigma, and homophobia associated with the disease (CDC, 2007a). Despite these challenges, however, HIV/AIDS prevention efforts have successfully contributed to the reduction of new HIV/AIDS cases. The effectiveness of HIV/AIDS prevention has been consistently demonstrated in rigorous randomized clinical trials, implemented in practice, and supported through effective policies (CDC, 2006b).

In this chapter, we highlight how prevention research has been used to support policy in preventing HIV in communities of color. We discuss how the development of evidence-based programs has been disseminated to schools, communities, and practitioners through the development of effective national and local policy. We also discuss the importance of advocacy organizations in promoting effective programs and policies. We focus primarily on research conducted with African American and Latino adolescents.

DEVELOPMENT OF EFFECTIVE INTERVENTIONS FOR MINORITY YOUTH

Since the early 1990s, the Jemmott team has responded to the increasing epidemic of HIV/AIDS in African American communities, especially youth, by developing a program of research to develop theoretically based interventions to decrease sexual risk behaviors. The many intervention studies developed as part of this program of research include efforts to (1) elucidate the social psychological factors that underlie HIV/STD and risk-associated sexual behavior; (2) identify the conceptual variables that are most important to achieving sexual behavior change; (3) identify theory-based, culture-sensitive, developmentally appropriate strategies to reduce HIV/STD and risk-associated sexual behaviors; (4) test the effectiveness of interventions using scientifically rigorous methodologies; and (5) tailor and disseminate effective research-based behavioral interventions to end users (e.g., communities and providers).

Interventions to reduce sexual risk behavior were based on social cognitive theory (Bandura, 1986, 1994), the Theory of Reasoned Action (Ajzen & Fishbein, 1980; Fishbein & Ajzen, 1975), and the Theory of Planned behavior (Ajzen, 1991). Formative research with adolescents and parents and extensive collaboration with school and community members and leaders informed the content and format of the program and study approaches. Programs were designed to be culturally and developmentally appropriate for urban youth.

Using these approaches, the results of two randomized controlled trials (RCTs; Jemmott, Jemmott, & Fong, 1992; Jemmott, Jemmott, Fong, & McCaffree, 1999) indicated that a 5-hour cognitive behavioral intervention, "Be Proud! Be Responsible!" (Jemmott, Jemmott, & McCaffree, 1995), developed for African American youth aged 13 to 17 years reduced HIV/STD and risk-associated sexual behavior, reduced frequency of sexual intercourse, reduced unprotected sexual intercourse, and reduced the number of sexual partners. Furthermore, results of the intervention were sustained at 3- and 6-month follow-ups.

The rapid increase in the epidemic in the African American community, coupled with the need for effective interventions to reach affected communities, also directed the team to consider practical questions about the most effective way to implement HIV/STD risk-reduction interventions. For example, one important question addressed in this program of research was to determine if the effectiveness of the intervention was altered by the small group composition (e.g., same- or mixed-gender groups) or facilitator characteristics such as gender, race, and age (e.g., adult vs. peer facilitator). Despite widely held beliefs about the effects of facilitator characteristics and group composition on program effectiveness, there were no differences in intervention effects by age, race, or gender or group composition (Jemmott et al., 1992; Jemmott, Jemmott, & Fong, 1998; Jemmott et al., 1999).

Another study in this program of research addressed the important question as to whether a safer-sex approach or an abstinence-based approach would be effective with younger adolescents (Jemmott et al., 1998). In this randomized controlled study, African American adolescents (mean age = 11.8 years) were randomly assigned to a safer-sex intervention ("Making a Difference"; Jemmott, Jemmott, & McCaffree, 2001), an abstinence-based intervention ("Making Proud Choices"; Jemmott, Jemmott, & McCaffree, 2001), or a health promotion control condition. Results indicated that the abstinence intervention reduced the frequency of intercourse, and for those adolescents who were not sexually active, the intervention delayed the initiation of sexual intercourse, but only at the 3-month follow-up. The abstinence intervention is the only effective intervention to date that has shown behavior changes at 3 months. The safer-sex intervention reduced the frequency of unprotected intercourse and increased condom use at the 3-, 6-, and 12-month follow-up.

The effectiveness of different types of behavioral interventions (e.g., skill based and information based) on reducing sexual behavior and STD incidence was examined in a clinic-based RCT with sexually active female adolescents (Jemmott, Jemmott, Braverman, & Fong, 2005). The interventions were composed of a single session (250 minutes) and were group based. At 12-month follow-up, participants in the skill-based HIV/STD risk-reduction ("Sisters Saving Sisters") intervention reported less unprotected sexual intercourse and fewer sexual partners and were also less likely to have a new STD infection than did adolescents in the health control intervention. There were no significant differences in sexual risk behavior or STD incidence between the skill-based intervention and the information intervention.

Finally, an important research and practice question addressed by the Jemmott team was to determine if similar theoretical approaches could be used to design effective interventions for other minority communities, specifically, Latinos. The intervention "Be Proud! Be Responsible" was first culturally adapted to incorporate Latino cultural beliefs and values (Villarruel, Jemmott, & Jemmott, 2005). Then, in another RCT, conducted with both English- and Spanish-speaking Latino youth, adolescents 13 to 18 years of age were randomly assigned to the *¡Cuídate!* (take care of yourself) intervention or a health-promotion control condition (Villarruel, Jemmott, & Jemmott, 2006). Results indicated that compared with youth in the health-promotion intervention, youth in *¡Cuídate!* reported fewer incidents of sexual intercourse, fewer sex partners, fewer days of unprotected intercourse, and an increase in consistent condom use as a result of the program. Each of these effects continued 12 months after the program ended.

In summary, the program of research by the Jemmott team since the beginning of the AIDS epidemic has advanced the science of prevention for minority youth. Findings from these studies have been used to develop and support effective ways of reducing sexual risk behavior and STD incidence with minorities and youth. Specifically, reviews and meta-analysis of effective interventions from several sources (e.g., Caucus for Evidence Based Prevention, 2006; Kalichman, Carey, & Johnson, 1996; Kirby, 2007; Lyles, Crepaz, Herbst, & Kay, 2006; Marín, 1995; Pedlow & Carey, 2003) indicate that interventions for youth should be guided by a theoretical framework, address theoretical determinants of risk behavior, elicit research, and be tailored to the culture of the target group.

MOVING EFFICACIOUS RESEARCH INTO PRACTICE—FACILITATING POLICIES

An important component of the Jemmott program of research has been the ability to move research into practice. This has been facilitated both by the rigor of the science, working with affected communities in the development and conduct of the intervention, and the infrastructure or dissemination provided predominantly by the CDC. In addition, there have been several national and local policies that have facilitated the use of efficacious interventions.

Mandated by the Congress, in 1992, the CDC initiated "Programs That Work" (PTW) to identify health education programs with credible evidence of effectiveness and, if programs met criteria for scientific rigor, to disseminate programs to education and youth agencies (Collins et al., 2002). Criteria to be met in order to be considered in the PTW included the following: (1) The intervention is a complete program and is more than a single component; (2) the intervention has been tested in a classroom or other group setting with school-aged youth; (3) the intervention has produced a significant positive effect on the basis of self-report behavior or biologic markers such as delay of initiation of first sexual intercourse, reduced frequency of intercourse, reduced number of sexual partners, increased use of condoms or other contraceptives, and decreased pregnancy or STD rates; (4) the intervention does not cause increases in risk behavior; (5) the research design includes a control or comparison group and collection of follow-up data for at least 4 weeks, for sexual risk-reduction outcomes after the end of the intervention; and (6) results from the study have been published, or accepted for publication, in a peer-reviewed journal (CDC, 2001). Of the eight programs selected in the area of HIV/STD and pregnancy prevention, three of the programs were developed by the Jemmott team (i.e. "Be Proud! Be Responsible" [Jemmott et al., 1995], "Making a Difference" [Jemmott et al., 2001], and "Making Proud Choices" [Jemmott et al., 2001]).

In addition to meeting specific criterion, programs selected for PTW also were reviewed by an external evaluation panel and by a program panel. The evaluation panel reviewed the intervention and supporting studies to ensure the scientific rigor by determining if the sample size was adequate, the comparison and intervention groups were comparable, attrition was controlled, measures were adequate and robust, in general, and findings were valid (CDC, 2001). The program panel reviewed the curriculum to ensure that the curriculum was factually correct, the program could be reasonably implemented by a teacher or other adult in a real-world setting, the intensity of training or additional materials required were reasonable, and the curriculum would be applicable to groups other than those targeted in the original study and to determine how barriers encountered might be overcome.

The CDC supported national dissemination efforts in several ways. The CDC provided curriculum and evaluation fact sheets and facilitated distribution through government and other public and professional venues. Several national trainings of the PTW were conducted in select states across the country and the CDC provided trainers and materials for CDC grantees. Although the reach was wide and the interest in the PTW was great, the program was discontinued in 2001, for reasons that will be subsequently discussed.

A venue to support the dissemination of effective HIV prevention interventions has been developed by the CDC's Division of HIV/AIDS Prevention. The first initiative was the development in 1999 of the "Compendium of HIV Prevention Interventions With Evidence of Effectiveness" (CDC, 1999). This compendium, with subsequent updates in 2005 and 2009, is the identification of interventions that have met rigorous standards for evaluating which behavioral interventions have been shown to reduce sex and drug injection risk behaviors. Criteria for being considered an intervention with "best evidence" include a random assignment to study arms, at least a 3-month postintervention follow-up assessment for each study arm, a positive and statistically significant ($p = .05$) intervention effect for one or more relevant outcome measures, and no other statistically significant harmful intervention effect. Three interventions, Be Proud! Be Responsible! (Jemmott et al., 1995), Sisters Saving Sisters (Jemmott & Jemmott, 2008), and ¡Cuídate! (Villarruel, Jemmott, & Jemmott, 2009), were evaluated as having met the criteria for a best evidence intervention.

Another component of the CDC's Division of HIV/AIDS Prevention strategy is the diffusion of effective interventions through Replicating Effective Programs (REP) Project and the Diffusion of Evidence Based Interventions (DEBI; CDC, 2007b). The REP focuses on packaging effective evidence-based interventions so they can be used in community-based, nonacademic settings. Since 1996, over 17 intervention packages have been developed, and ¡Cuídate! is one of the most recent REP packages. The goal of the DEBI is to enhance the capacity to implement effective interventions at the state and local levels. Through a variety of networks, training and technical assistance are provided to health departments and CDC grantees to support local efforts to effectively utilize HIV prevention programs. While both the PTW and DEBI Program are not mandated in order to use evidence-based programs, many health departments and other agencies require the use of selected interventions in state and local funding.

The use of evidence-based programs for HIV prevention, including those for youth, is also facilitated by the development of CDC-required state and local HIV prevention community planning groups (CPG). Beginning in 1994, state, territorial, and local health departments receiving federal prevention funds through the CDC were asked to develop a comprehensive HIV prevention plan with community members, including those who were affected by HIV (CDC, 2006a). The major goal of the CPG is to recommend a comprehensive HIV prevention plan, based on scientific evidence and community needs, with strategies for adapting and tailoring evidenced-based programs for their communities (Academy for Educational Development, 2005). The plan serves as a guide to direct the use of federal and nonfederal funds for the implementation and evaluation of these evidenced-based programs and training of community-based organizations to use these programs. Many of the programs that were part of the PTW and now the DEBI program are important components of prevention plans that are incorporated by many CPGs.

MOVING EFFICACIOUS RESEARCH INTO PRACTICE— POLICIES AS BARRIERS

Two predominant policy approaches have been utilized for the prevention of HIV/AIDS among youth: (1) comprehensive sexuality education and (2) abstinence-only programs. The evidence of the effectiveness of comprehensive sexuality education is evident in the work of the Jemmott team and also recognized as effective in synthesis of similar behavioral interventions (Kirby, 2007). However, despite evidence of effectiveness, comprehensive sexuality education was not a major policy priority in the early 2000. Many advocacy groups argue that pressure from the conservative groups caused a discontinuation of the PTW by the CDC in addition to challenging information about the efficacy of condoms.

In turn, abstinence-only programs have been a predominant approach to preventing pregnancy, STDs, and HIV. Since 1982, more than $1.5 billion has been spent on abstinence-only-until-marriage programs (Howell, 2007). Section 510 of the 1996 Welfare Reform Act provided major funding for abstinence education. This law provided a federal matching grant to states of $25 million for over 5 years, which was later increased to $50 million per year in 2004. In this legislation, detailed guidelines and restrictions were provided for abstinence education. In the Personal Responsibility and Work Opportunity Reconciliation Act of 1996, abstinence education refers to programs that:

- Have as its exclusive purpose teaching the social, psychological, and health gains to be realized by abstaining from sexual activity
- Teach abstinence from sexual activity outside marriage as the expected standard for all school-age children
- Teach that abstinence from sexual activity is the only certain way to avoid out-of-wedlock pregnancy, STDs, and other associated health problems
- Teach that a mutually faithful monogamous relationship in the context of marriage is the expected standard of human sexual activity
- Teach that sexual activity out of the context of marriage is likely to have harmful psychological and physical effects
- Teach that bearing children out of wedlock is likely to have harmful consequences for the child, the child's parents, and the society
- Teach young people how to reject sexual advances and how alcohol and drug use increases vulnerability to sexual advances; and
- Teach the importance of attaining self-sufficiency before engaging in sexual activity.

The Special Projects of Regional and National Significance (SPRANS) created even more stringent policies regarding sex education for youth. Whereas state approval was required for Section 510 funding, SPRANS funding could be accepted directly by community-based organizations, thus bypassing the need for consent at the state level. Organizations funded by SPRANS were prohibited to educate youth, even with their own nonfederal funds, about contraception, sexual orientation, gender identity, or safer sex. The majority of abstinence-only funding since 2001 came from the SPRANS program.

The science to support an abstinence-only policy is not strong. Some argue that criteria for determining effective interventions were changed from data demonstrating behavior change or a reduction in pregnancy or STD incidence to more of a process evaluation (e.g., proportion of program participants who successfully complete or remain enrolled in an abstinence-only education program and proportion of youth who commit to abstain from sexual activity until marriage). Few abstinence programs have been developed and rigorously tested. Those that have been tested do not indicate that these curricula delay the onset of sexual behavior (Santelli et al., 2006). A major issue with this approach is that once adolescents become sexually active, they are at risk because they do not use contraceptives or condoms.

With a new administration comes new policy approaches. In the president's fiscal year 2009 budget, a request was included for increases in comprehensive sexuality education, and in the 2010 budget proposal, requests were allocated for evidence-based teenage pregnancy and prevention programs. Funding will be designated not only for programs that replicate the characteristics of proven programs but also for research and development of new preventive strategies and programs to delay sexual activity and increase contraceptive and condom use (Planned Parenthood, 2009).

APPROACHES TO SHAPING HIV POLICY FOR MINORITY YOUTH

The shifts in policies for sexual risk reduction among youth indicate the precariousness of the relationship between science and policy. Just as we know knowledge is necessary but not sufficient to create behavior change, we know that science is necessary but not sufficient to create policy change. Nurse scientists play an important role in supporting these policy approaches.

There are several strategies and roles we have used in shaping HIV policy for minority youth. Much of what we do can be viewed in the context of connecting communities to science and to policy. Our success in developing effective interventions, moving them into practice, and influencing policy is grounded in our work with and integration with the communities with whom we work. Although we utilize focus groups and community advisory boards in our research as part of the research process, community members and leaders are an important part of the implementation of the research and in dissemination activities. Members of the community who are involved with us also have ownership of the program as they can see that their ideas and suggestions are incorporated into our research. Many community members become involved in advocacy efforts in their communities to sustain our programs.

Importantly, our role as researchers and knowledge of the community give us credibility as effective advocates at the national, state, and local levels. Efforts at the national level have focused on creating and supporting prevention and science policies. At the national level, we have met with congressional staffers and provided testimony at Senate hearings on needs and funding priorities for HIV prevention. Both of us were appointed by the Secretary of Health and Human Services to the CDC/HRSA Advisory Committee on HIV and STD Prevention and Treatment. As members, we provided direction for the development of priorities and activities related to the prevention and control of HIV/AIDS and other STDs, the support of healthcare services to persons living with HIV/AIDS, and education of health professionals and the public about HIV/AIDS and other STDs. We have each led and served on numerous NIH (e.g., National Institute of Mental Health (NIMH) Annual International Research Conference on the Role of Families in Preventing and Adapting to HIV/AIDS, NIH Consensus Conference: Interventions to Prevent HIV Risk Behaviors, Cultural dynamics in HIV/AIDS prevention research among young people) and CDC (e.g., Developing a Strategic Plan to Address HIV Among Latinos, Developing a Strategic Plan for Adolescent Reproductive Health Initiatives) related task forces and initiatives. These initiatives have facilitated the development of health and science policy related to HIV prevention among minority youth.

In addition to work with policy makers and government agencies, an important component of policy work is leadership in advocacy efforts with professional and advocacy organizations. We have participated in numerous task forces and initiatives and key-noted at conferences of major professional (e.g., American Academy of Nursing, Association of Nurses in AIDS Care, American Psychological Association, and Physicians for Social Responsibility) and advocacy and policy organizations (National Campaign to Prevent Teen Pregnancy and Brookings Institute), including two separate Institute of Medicine (1997, 2001) studies on HIV and STDs. Importantly, our work in minority organizations (e.g., National Council of La Raza, National Black Nurses Association, and National Association of Hispanic Nurses) strengthens the voice of affected communities in policy efforts.

In addition, we have also been active in different ways at the state and local levels. We have spoken to school boards, parent groups, church ministers, community leaders, and family planning clinics about the need for comprehensive sexuality and the use of evidence-based programs. We have written editorials supporting approaches for comprehensive sexuality education. We have been involved with the Philadelphia CPG in providing consultation regarding the assessment of local needs, the identification of effective programs, and the development of an evaluation plan. Finally, we have worked with community members in how to work with school boards and other local policy makers to support the use of evidence-based programs. These collective strategies have resulted in the creation of policies at multiple levels to facilitate the national dissemination and use of efficacious evidence-based programs such as the ones we have developed. Furthermore, we have used similar research and policy strategies in our work internationally in Mexico and South Africa.

SUMMARY

In summary, the HIV/AIDS prevention research is critical to the ultimate development and institution of effective policies. Policy recommendations should be based on evidence-based research to create supportive legislation to ensure confidentiality, reduce discrimination and stigma to prevention and treatment, and increase access to preventive and treatment healthcare services. In regard to future policy, some suggestions include advocating for evidence-based comprehensive sexuality education in schools across the country, supporting funding that is earmarked for comprehensive sexuality education, providing public health expertise to school boards and state education departments, and providing study findings and concerns with community and political leaders (Trigg, 2008).

In addition, future policies, as well as their interconnected funding and research, must support strategies that promote (1) dialogues between researchers, practitioners, and communities; (2) preparation of nurse scientists to lead complex research efforts; (3) partnerships among people, communities, agencies, and the private sector; and (4) improved collaboration across disciplines and governmental agencies. Advances have been made in the prevention and treatment of HIV/AIDS; however, much more remains to be done. Nurse scientists have played a critical role to date and will undoubtedly continue to lead advances in science, practice, and policy.

REFERENCES

Academy for Educational Development (AED). (2005). *HIV prevention: Community planning: An orientation guide.* Retrieved September 28, 2009, from http://www.cdc.gov/hiv/topics/cba/resources/guidelines/Orientation_Final.pdf

Ajzen, I. (1991). The theory of planned behavior. *Organizational Behavior and Human Decision Processes, 50,* 179–211.

Ajzen, I., & Fishbein, M. (1980). *Understanding attitudes and predicting social behavior.* Englewood Cliffs, NJ: Prentice-Hall.

Bandura, A. (1986). *Social foundations of thought and action: A social cognitive theory.* Englewood Cliffs, NJ: Prentice-Hall.

Bandura, A. (1994). Health promotion by social cognitive means. *Health Education Behavior, 31*(2), 143–164.

Caucus for Evidence-Based Prevention. (2006). HIV prevention for and with youth people. Retrieved September 28, 2009, from http://www.hiv-prevention.org/docs/topics/Youth-HIV_FactSheet.pdf

Centers for Disease Control and Prevention (CDC). (1999). Compendium of HIV prevention interventions with evidence of effectiveness. Retrieved September 29, 2009 from http://minority-health.pitt.edu/archive/00001008/01/HIVcompendium.pdf

Centers for Disease Control and Prevention (CDC). (2001). Programs that work. Retrieved September 28, 2009, from http://web.archive.org/web/20010606142729/www.cdc.gov/nccdphp/dash/rtc/index.htm

Centers for Disease Control and Prevention (CDC). (2006a). HIV prevention community planning guidance. Retrieved September 28, 2009, from http://www.cdc.gov/hiv/topics/cba/resources/guidelines/hiv-cp/section1.htm

Centers for Disease Control and Prevention. (CDC). (2006b). The past 2 decades: How far have we come? Retrieved May 17, 2009 from http://www.cdc.gov/hiv/resources/reports/hiv3rddecade/chapter1.htm

Centers for Disease Control and Prevention (CDC). (2006c). Twenty-five years of HIV/AIDS—United States, 1981–2006. *Morbidity and Mortality Weekly Report, 55*(21), 585–589.

Centers for Disease Control and Prevention. (CDC). (2007a). CDC HIV prevention strategic plan: Extended through 2010. Retrieved May 15, 2009, from http://www.cdc.gov/hiv/resources/reports/psp/

Centers for Disease Control and Prevention (CDC). (2007b). PRS, REP, and DEBI. Retrieved September 28, 2009, from http://www.cdc.gov/hiv/topics/research/prs/prs_rep_debi.htm

Centers for Disease Control and Prevention (CDC). (2008a). HIV/AIDS among youth. Retrieved May 18, 2009, from http://www.cdc.gov/hiv/resources/factsheets/youth.htm

Centers for Disease Control and Prevention (CDC). (2008b). New estimates of U.S. HIV prevalence, 2006. Retrieved May 18, 2009, from http://www.cdc.gov/hiv/topics/surveillance/resources/factsheets/prevalence.htm

Collins, J., Robin, L., Wooley, S., Fenley, D., Hunt, P., Taylor, J., et al. (2002). Programs-that-work: CDC's guide to effective programs that reduce health-risk behavior of youth. *The Journal of School Health, 72*(3), 93–99.

Fishbein, M., & Ajzen, I. (1975). *Belief, attitude, intention and behavior.* Boston: Addison-Wesley.

Howell, M. (2007). Advocates for youth: The history of federal abstinence-only funding. Retrieved September 30, 2009, from http://advfy.nonprofitsoapbox.com/storage/advfy/documents/fshistoryabonly.pdf

Institute of Medicine (IOM). (1997). In T. R. Eng & W. T. Butler (Eds.), *The hidden epidemic: Confronting sexually transmitted disease.* Washington: National Academies Press.

Institute of Medicine (IOM). (2001). In M. S. Ruiz, A. R. Gable, E. H. Kaplan, M. A. Soto, H. V. Fineberg, & J. Trussell (Eds.), *No time to lose: Getting more from HIV prevention.* Washington: National Academies Press.

Jemmott, L. S., & Jemmott J. B. (2008). *Sisters Saving Sisters: A three hour group intervention for teenage women.* New York, NY: Select Media Publications.

Jemmott, J. B., Jemmott, L. S., Braverman, P. K., & Fong, G. T. (2005). HIV/STD risk reduction interventions for African American and Latino adolescent girls at an adolescent medicine clinic: A randomized control trial. *Archives of Pediatric and Adolescent Medicine, 159*, 440–449.

Jemmott, J. B., Jemmott, L. S., & Fong, G. T. (1992). Reductions in HIV risk-associated sexual behaviors among black male adolescents: Effects of an AIDS prevention intervention. *American Journal of Public Health, 82*(3), 372–377.

Jemmott, J. B., Jemmott, L. S., & Fong, G. T. (1998). Abstinence and safer sex HIV risk-reduction interventions for African American adolescents: A randomized controlled trial. *Journal of the American Medical Association, 279*(19), 1529–1536.

Jemmott, J. B., Jemmott, L. S., Fong, G. T., & McCaffree, K. (1999). Reducing HIV risk-associated sexual behavior among African American adolescents: Testing the generality of intervention effects. *American Journal of Community Psychology, 27*(2), 161–187.

Jemmott, L. S., Jemmott J. B., & McCaffree, K. (1995). *Be proud! Be responsible! Strategies to empower youth to reduce their risk for AIDS.* New York, NY: Select Media Publications.

Jemmott, L. S., Jemmott, J. B., & McCaffree, K. (2001). *Making a difference: An abstinence based approach to STDs, teen pregnancy and HIV/AIDS.* New York, NY: Select Media Publications.

Jemmott, L. S., Jemmott, J. B., & McCaffree, K. (2001). *Making proud choices: A safer sex approach to STDs, teen pregnancy and HIV/AIDS.* New York, NY: Select Media Publications.

Kalichman, S. C., Carey, M. P., & Johnson, B. T. (1996). Prevention of sexually transmitted HIV infection: A meta-analytic review of the behavioral outcome literature. *Annals of Behavioral Medicine, 18*(1), 6–15.

Kirby, D. (2007). *Emerging answers 2007: Research findings on programs to reduce teen pregnancy and sexually transmitted diseases.* Washington, DC: The National Campaign to Prevent Teen Pregnancy.

Lyles, C. M., Crepaz, N., Herbst, J. H., & Kay, L. S. (2006). Evidence-based HIV behavioral prevention from the perspective of the CDC's HIV/AIDS Prevention Research Synthesis Team. *AIDS Education and Prevention, 18*(Suppl. A), 21–31.

Marín, B. V. (1995). *Analysis of AIDS prevention among African Americans and Latinos in the United States.* Report prepared for the Office of Technology Assessment, US Congress. Washington DC: Office of Technology Assessment.

Pedlow, C., & Carey, M. P. (2003). HIV sexual risk-reduction interventions for youth: A review and methodological critique of randomized controlled trials. *Behavior Modification, 27*(2), 135–190.

Personal Responsibility and Work Opportunity Reconciliation Act of 1996. (1996). Public Law 104–193, 104th Cong.

Planned Parenthood. (2009). Planned parenthood statement on President Obama's 2010 budget. Retrieved May 18, 2009, from http://www.plannedparenthood.org/about-us/newsroom/press-releases/planned-parenthood-statement-president-obamas-2010-budget-26882.htm

Santelli, J., Ott, M. A., Lyon, M., Rogers, J., Summer, D., & Schleifer, R. (2006). Abstinence and abstinence-only education: A review of U.S. policies and programs. *Journal of Adolescent Health, 38,* 72–81.

Stall, R., & Mills, T. C. (2006). A quarter century of AIDS. *American Journal of Public Health, 96*(6), 959–961.

Trigg, B. (2008). What we have learned from 25 years of federally funded abstinence-only-until-marriage programs? Retrieved May 18, 2009, from http://cdc.confex.com/recording/cdc/std2008/ppt/free/4db77adf5df9fff0d3caf5cafe28f496/paper15253_5.ppt

Villarruel, A. M., Jemmott, L. S., & Jemmott, J. B., III. (2005). Designing a culturally based intervention to reduce HIV sexual risk for Latino adolescents. *Journal of the Association of Nurses in AIDS Care, 16*(2), 23–31. doi:/10.1016/j.jana.2005.01.001

Villarruel, A. M., Jemmott, J. B., & Jemmott, L. S. (2006). A randomized controlled trial testing an HIV prevention intervention for Latino youth. *Archives of Pediatrics & Adolescent Medicine, 160*(8), 772–777.

Villarruel, A. M., Jemmott, L. S., & Jemmott, J. B. (2009). *¡Cuídate!: A program to reduce HIV sexual risk behavior among Latino youth.* New York, NY: Select Media Publications.

10

Health Promotion and Prevention in Early Childhood: The Role of Nursing Research in Shaping Policy and Practice

Deborah Gross and Angela Crowley

The future of our nation's health begins with the health of its youngest citizens. Children's health and well-being in the first 5 years of life are particularly important because it is during this period that health behaviors and the basic building blocks for learning, social relationships, and internal regulation of one's emotions are first formed (Shonkoff & Phillips, 2000). Healthy habits, such as consumption of nutritious foods and daily physical activity, established in the early years are critical in reducing morbidity and mortality (Guo & Chumlea, 1999; Whitlock, Williams, Gold, Smith, & Shipman, 2005). Similarly, if children do not acquire the most basic skills for managing their behavior and emotions in early childhood, they will have difficulty functioning well in school, developing healthy peer relationships, and becoming a contributing member of the adult workforce (Heckman, 2006). For this reason, scientists and economists have concluded that the most cost-effective investments we can make as a society is to invest in the first 5 years of life. Skills acquired early in life lead to the formation of new, more sophisticated skills that are essential for healthy development. In addition, when investments are targeted to the very young, children have a longer time in which to fully benefit from those investments and ultimately give back to society. As Nobel Laureate James Heckman (2002) has argued, "The returns to human capital investments are greatest for the young" (p. 5).

The difficult task facing policy makers is deciding which programs or strategies warrant public investments. The purpose of policy research is to provide policy makers clear guidance in identifying practical, cost-effective solutions for making those decisions. To that end, nursing research has never been more important. In fact, the American Academy of Nursing recently initiated the "Raise the Voice" campaign to highlight the important role of nursing research for guiding policy. Led by Donna Shalala, former secretary of the Department of Health and Human Services (DHHS), the "Raise the Voice" campaign is designed to offer policy makers practical, evidence-based solutions for solving complex healthcare problems. The purpose of this chapter is to describe the importance of nursing research in early childhood and how one evidence-based solution, the Chicago Parent

Program, is improving the lives of young children enrolled in early-childcare programs serving families from low-income communities.

The Chicago Parent Program is a 12-session program designed to promote positive parenting and child mental health by addressing the challenges of raising young children in urban environments. Developed in collaboration with ethnic minority parents of young children, the Chicago Parent Program was originally designed to be used in childcare centers to support parenting and enhance the quality of existing early-childhood programs (Gross, Garvey, Julion, & Fogg, 2007). Based on the growing body of evidence showing the negative effects of poverty on young children's development (Engle & Black, 2008), the Chicago Parent Program specifically targeted early-childcare centers serving young children from low-income communities (Breitenstein et al., 2007).

This chapter will first describe the important role that early-childhood programs[1] can play in the promotion of physical and mental health and the management of chronic conditions in the lives of young children and their families. We will then present three key conditions illustrating how nursing research in early-childhood programs could advance the health and well-being of young children: asthma screening and management, obesity prevention, and child mental health. We will also describe collaborations with the Chicago Department of Children and Youth Services to disseminate the Chicago Parent Program in Head Start centers as one example of how nursing research is changing practice and informing policy. Finally, important considerations for ensuring that nursing research can inform health policy will be highlighted.

THE DEMOGRAPHICS OF EARLY CHILDCARE

In 2005, 62.5% of mothers with children under 6 years old and 59% of mothers with children under 3 years old were employed. Among single mothers, those rates were 70.4% and 65%, respectively (U.S. Department of Labor, 2005). As a result of these high maternal employment rates, most children under 6 years old who are not yet in kindergarten are enrolled in nonparental care (Child Trends Data Bank, 2005). Recent data show that approximately 11 million children between birth and 4 years of age in the United States are enrolled in childcare programs, and two-thirds of these children are in center-based care, including licensed childcare centers, Early Head Start, and Head Start (National Association of Child Care Resource and Referral Agencies, 2009). Mothers employed full-time (48%), mothers who are college graduates (46%), working families living in poverty (42% are most likely to utilize center-based care), and children with guardians (44% are most likely to utilize center-based care). Center-based care also attracts an ethnically diverse population of families. For example, national Head Start statistics show that 30% of enrolled children are African American and 35% are Hispanic (U.S. DHHS, Administration for Children & Families, 2008).

On average, young children in center-based care spend about 36 hours per week in that care. That so many children spend that many hours per week in early-childcare programs is an important demographic change, placing early-childcare programs at the center of young children's lives. According to Shonkoff and Phillips (2000), "Second only to the immediate family, childcare is the context in which early childhood unfolds" (p. 297). Unlike in elemen-

---

[1] For the purposes of this chapter, early childhood refers to birth through 5 years of age. Early-childhood programs include center-based and family child care as well as more comprehensive early childhood programs focusing on school readiness, such as Early Head Start, Head Start, and pre-Kindergarten.

tary and high school, most parents participate to some degree in their children's childcare center, if only to drop off and pick up their children. As a result, early-childhood programs have enormous potential to reach large numbers of young children and their parents to improve health outcomes through health promotion and prevention interventions.

Early-childhood programs also offer important opportunities for improving the health of young children with chronic illnesses. According to the National Survey of Children With Special Health Care Needs (2005–2006), 14% of children have special healthcare needs that require medications (86%), specialty medical care (52%), and mental health-care (25%) (U.S. Department of Health and Human Services, Health Resources and Services Administration, Maternal and Child Health Bureau, 2008). Data on the number of children enrolled in childcare with special healthcare needs are not available. However, Head Start reports that at least 10% of enrolled children have a special healthcare need (U.S. DHHS, Administration for Children and Families, Office of Head Start, 2008). Among the parents surveyed, 18% reported that their child's chronic illness contributed to financial problems, and 24% reported that it led to a reduced number of working days. Although most parents reported having health insurance coverage, one third of insured respondents described insurance limitations including inadequate coverage, unreasonable charges, and lack of access to appropriate healthcare providers, all of which influence quality of care and health outcomes.

THE ROLE OF HIGH-QUALITY EARLY CHILDCARE PROGRAMS IN THE WELL-BEING OF YOUNG CHILDREN AND THEIR FAMILIES

Research shows that high-quality early-childhood education is associated with positive outcomes in children, particularly for children from low-income families (Campbell, Ramey, Pungello, Sparling, & Miller-Johnson, 2002; Schweinart et al., 2005) Economic evaluations indicate that for every $1 spent on high-quality early-childhood education, there is a $3–$17 return on investment secondary to reduced special education costs, less grade retention, higher adult earnings, more tax revenues, and reduced crime (Lucas, 2008). As a result, states and local governments are looking to support new initiatives for improving the quality of early care and education (Duncan, Ludwig, & Magnuson, 2007; Johnson & Knitzer, 2005).

Harms, Clifford, and Cryer (1998) identified three domains of high-quality early care and education:

1. Physical: health, safety, and abuse prevention,
2. Social/Emotional: supporting relationships with children, families, and community,
3. Cognitive: supporting opportunities for development and learning.

In addition, the characteristics of the childcare workforce are also associated with high-quality care in early childhood. Specifically, these include high staff-to-child ratios, higher levels of teacher preparation, better teacher wages, and lower staff turnover (Helburn et al., 1995; Phillips, Howes, & Whitebrook, 1991). Better provider-to-child ratios and small group size are especially important for infants and toddlers and are linked to higher quality, more sensitive caregiving (NICHD Early Child Care Research Network, 1996; Phillipsen, Burchinal, Howes, & Cryer, 1997).

Center-based childcare continues to be an important resource for working poor families. Almost one out of five children in the United States is living in poverty, and African

American and Hispanic children are more than twice as likely to live in poverty as non-Hispanic White and Asian children (Moore, Redd, Burkhauser, Mbwana, & Collins, 2009). Child poverty is linked to poorer outcomes across a number of physical and emotional health indicators (Engle & Black, 2008). Parents living below the poverty line are also at substantially higher risk for physical and emotional problems, including chronic stress, depression, and substance abuse (Beeber, Perreira, & Schwartz, 2008), all of which affect their ability to parent. For this reason, early-childhood programs serving children from low-income families also need to include services for assisting those families with accessing health, mental health, and social services (Schumacher, Hamm, & Ewen, 2007).

Even better, providing those services *within* early-childhood programs as part of a comprehensive care menu would represent a significant advance toward promoting the health of young children and their families. Despite 12 primary care visits in the first 3 years of life, pediatric clinicians have limited time to address health promotion topics in addition to conducting a history, examination, and screening and delivering immunizations. In a survey of parents of young children enrolled in Medicaid (Bethell et al., 2002), 40% of parents reported at least one concern about their child's social, emotional, behavioral, or cognitive development during well child visits; however, only 23% received preventive and developmental services. Furthermore, 40% of the parents reported that their pediatric healthcare provider did not routinely inquire about concerns regarding their children's development or well-being and only 46% reported receiving sufficient information to address their concerns.

One strategy that has been evaluated for providing health promotion services within childcare centers is the use of health consultants, most of whom are nurses (Alkon, Farrer, & Bernzweig, 2004; Crowley, 1990, 2000; Dellert, Gasalberti, Sternas, Lucarelli, & Hall, 2006; Ulione, 1997). Nurses have provided health consultation to early-childhood programs for over 30 years in Head Start and as a regulatory requirement in some states (Crowley, 1988, 2001). In a comprehensive literature review, Ramler, Nakatsukasa-Ono, Loe, and Harris (2006) reported that the use of childcare health consultants was associated with stronger health and safety childcare policies and practices and with increased numbers of children with access to healthcare and current immunizations and was beneficial in promoting mental health, nutrition, physical activity, and oral health. Crowley's (2001) Ecological Model of Child Care Health Consultation provides a family-centered model based on Bronfenbrenner's ecological theory of human development. Within a family-centered perspective, the health consultant promotes child health as well as health and safety within the early-childhood education program and encourages constructive interactions and care coordination among families, childcare teachers, primary health care providers, and other health providers and services, thus influencing not only program health and safety but also child and family health and development.

SOCIAL, EMOTIONAL, AND PHYSICAL NEEDS OF YOUNG CHILDREN IN EARLY CHILDCARE PROGRAMS: KEY AREAS FOR NURSING RESEARCH

Early-childhood programs are important settings for nursing intervention research that can inform health policy. Screening and management of chronic health conditions, early intervention, and health promotion and prevention are key areas where nursing research could make important contributions. Specific examples within each of these areas are described in the following sections.

Screening and Management of Chronic Conditions: Pediatric Asthma

Asthma is the most common chronic illness among children, and its prevalence has increased steadily since 1960 (Cope, Ungar, & Glazier, 2008). According to the Centers for Disease Control and Prevention (Akinbami, 2006), asthma affects approximately 9 million children in the United States. Children who are of ethnic minority, less than 5 years old, and living in low-income urban environments suffer at disproportionate rates. Low-income children with asthma are also more likely to be undermedicated or to receive the wrong medication. In one study of preschool children hospitalized for asthma, Finkelstein et al. (1995) found that only 7% of African American and 2% of Hispanic children were prescribed routine medication at discharge that would prevent future asthma exacerbations. Evidence suggests that poor medication adherence is a significant problem leading to higher rates of emergency department visits, hospitalization, and death (Horne, 2006).

Childcare participation presents additional opportunities and barriers to medication adherence. Many childcare providers are reluctant to administer medications for fear of liability. Despite the Americans With Disabilities Act of 1990, most state childcare regulations do not require medication training, and providers report lack of accessible and affordable training (Catenzaro, 1999). While nurses in several states are leading efforts to design and implement medication administration training programs for childcare providers (Crowley, 2010), nurses in some states are reluctant to train providers because of delegation issues (Heschel, Crowley, & Cohen, 2005). Because of the importance of medication adherence for asthma symptom management in early childhood, effective models for collaboration between nurses and childcare providers is an important area of study.

The annual healthcare cost for pediatric asthma has been estimated to be approximately $3 billion (Mellon & Parasuraman, 2004). Children with asthma incur 80% higher medical expenses than do children without asthma. Clearly, a reduction in asthma-related illness would represent significant cost savings. Not surprisingly, reducing asthma morbidity has been a national healthcare objective of Healthy People 2010.

Prevention guidelines highlight the importance of identifying and avoiding asthma triggers and using asthma medications that control symptoms (National Heart, Lung, and Blood Institute, 2007). One nursing study of young children with asthma living in an inner city community found that families who used asthma care routines had better preventive medication adherence and less exposure to environmental triggers than did those with no asthma care routine (Peterson-Sweeney, Halterman, Conn, & Yoos, in press). However, more research is needed. For example, could nurse childcare health consultants who screen and manage children's asthma in coordination with childcare providers, parents, and primary care providers lead to improved child health status, reductions in child absences from care, and increased parent productivity? Of particular interest are studies evaluating the cost-effectiveness of asthma screening and management education programs in early-childhood programs conducted in coordination with primary care providers.

Early Intervention: Reducing Preschool Obesity Rates

Over the past 30 years, the obesity prevalence rate in the United States has increased almost threefold. Recent data suggest that 14% of preschool children (Ogden et al., 2006) and 11.4% of infants and toddlers (Kim, Peterson, Scanlon et al., 2006) are overweight (defined by weight ≥85th percentile). Higher rates are found among low-income and ethnic minority children. For example, in one study of Mississippi Head Start preschoolers (Harbaugh, Jordan, Johnson, Hovan, & Nugent, 2009), overweight and obesity rates exceeded 38% of children. Rising obesity rates are occurring simultaneously with decreasing physical activity levels. The Children's Activity and Movement in Preschools Study collected detailed observations of physical activity among preschool children in 24 South Carolina childcare centers (Brown et al., 2009). They found that 89% of children's daily activities were characterized as sedentary; only 3% of their activities were defined as moderate to vigorous physical activity.

Overweight preschool children are more than five times as likely to be overweight at age 12 years (Nader et al., 2006), and most overweight children remain overweight into adulthood (U.S. Preventive Services Task Force, 2005). These statistics are concerning given the high morbidity and mortality risks associated with obesity and the annual costs, which are estimated to exceed $100 billion (Simpson & Cooper, 2009).

Interventions to increase physical activity and reduce obesity in preschool children are needed. A recent review of interventions to prevent or treat obesity in preschool children (Bluford, Sherry, & Scanlon, 2007) found very few controlled studies targeting young children, and only three of seven studies reviewed documented sustained reductions in weight status or body fat. A promising randomized control study that is examining the effect of a training curriculum to improve nutrition and increase physical activity for 600 preschool children in childcare centers across three states is in progress (Kotch, Crowley, Alkon, & Benjamin, 2007–2010). Nurse childcare health consultants are delivering the curriculum to childcare providers and providing support through onsite and offsite consultation. Studying cost-effective interventions for reducing preschool obesity and increasing physical activity in early-childhood programs is a priority area for nursing research (Bluford, Sherry, & Scanlon, 2007).

Health Promotion and Prevention: Promoting Early Childhood Mental Health

In 2000, U.S. Surgeon General Dr. David Satcher noted that "the burden of suffering experienced by children with mental health needs and their families has created a health crisis in this country" (U.S. DHHS, 2000). It has been estimated that from 6% to 30% of children under 6 years of age have significant behavior problems (Anthony, Anthony, Morrel, & Acosta, 2005; Gross, Sambrook, & Fogg, 1999; Razzino, New, Lewin, & Joseph, 2004), and most children who need mental health services do not receive them (U.S. DHHS, 2000). Although the causes of early-onset behavior problems are multifactorial, these children are at higher risk for poorer social, emotional, and academic outcomes in later childhood. Moreover, mental health problems in children are often accompanied by mental health problems in their parents. In one study of Head Start parents (Razzino et al., 2004), 43% of parents reported high rates of mental health problems, including depression and anxiety.

Without intervention, chronic behavior problems in children become costly social problems. In early childhood, children with high rates of behavior problems face a higher likelihood of being expelled from childcare (Gilliam, 2005), leading to lost wages and reduced productivity for parents. Over time, public costs for untreated childhood behavior problems have been estimated to range from almost $24,000 per child to over $61,000 per child for mental health services, grade retention, special education, and juvenile justice involvement (Foster & Jones, 2005).

Among the most promising interventions for preventing behavior problems in young children are those that directly target parents (Breismeister & Schaefer, 2007). These parenting programs focus on improving knowledge and parenting skills, raising parenting self-efficacy, and reducing child behavior problems.

One program designed to be delivered as a universal prevention intervention in early-childcare centers is the Chicago Parent Program (Gross, Garvey, Julion, & Fogg, 2007). The goal of the Chicago Parent Program is to help parents clarify their childrearing goals and values and apply positive parenting strategies for reaching those goals. Most importantly, the program is designed to build on parents' strengths and provide information in a nonstigmatizing way. Tested in a randomized trial of seven childcare centers serving low-income families in Chicago, the Chicago Parent Program was shown to reduce parents' use of corporal punishment, improve parenting behavior, and reduce child behavior problems (Gross et al., 2009). In addition, some parents who completed the program sought additional mental health services, including individual and marital therapy, in part because of the nonjudgmental and supportive environment created within the parent groups (Breitenstein et al., 2007). The following section describes efforts to disseminate the Chicago Parent Program in Chicago-area Head Start to improve young children's mental health and inform health policy.

Case Example: A Practical, Cost-Effective Program for Promoting Mental Health in Early Childhood

In 2005, the Chicago Parent Program Team[2] was approached by the commissioner of the Chicago Department of Children and Youth Services approached the Chicago Parent Program team[2] about the potential to disseminate the Chicago Parent Program in Head Start sites in Chicago. At this time, the team had just completed a randomized trial testing the efficacy of the program in seven childcare centers serving low-income families in Chicago, of whom 59% were African American and 33% were Latino. Results showed that the Chicago Parent Program led to significant reductions in child behavior problems in the childcare classroom (Gross et al., 2007) and improvements in parenting behavior and observed parent–child interactions (Gross et al., 2009). In addition, parent satisfaction was high; all of the participating parents reported that they would "highly recommend" (88%) or "recommend" (12%) the program to other parents.

The team agreed to work with the Department of Children and Youth Services to develop a feasible plan for training Head Start staff to deliver the program at reasonable cost while retaining high quality. This involved developing a business plan that included costs for training, coordination, technical assistance, and program delivery at the site level. However, we first wanted to pilot test the dissemination plan to better understand issues related to site-level readiness and organizational capacity for implementing the Chicago Parent Program. Of particular concern was that in our clinical trials, Chicago Parent Program group leaders were mostly graduate-prepared

---

[2] The Chicago Parent Program team includes the program's authors, Deborah Gross, Wrenetha Julion, Christine Garvey, and Susan Breitenstein, and the project coordinator Alison Ridge.

nurses and social workers; we had not tested the effectiveness of the program when delivered by paraprofessionals. We therefore recommended that we conduct a small pilot test with staff from five Head Start sites and evaluate their ability to deliver the Chicago Parent Program within their sites. The $50,000 budget for this pilot project was used to cover the cost of training and intervention materials, project coordination, and conducting five 12-session parent groups with approximately 12 parents per group.

Six staff from five Head Start sites attended a 2-day training workshop in 2006. By the end of 2006, three of the five sites had developed and implemented a plan for conducted parent groups at their site. In one site, the group leader decided to practice using the Chicago Parent Program by first leading a group with Head Start teachers who were also parents of young children. At the end of the pilot, graduate students working with the Chicago Parent Program team conducted interviews with site directors, teachers, parents, and group leaders to examine feasibility, acceptability, and perceived utility. To understand barriers to implementation, they also interviewed the site directors and Head Start staff who attended the training workshop but did not conduct parent groups. The team analyzed the written abridged transcripts of these interviews for themes relating to strengths and challenges along the dimensions of program feasibility, acceptability, and perceived utility by the different constituencies interviewed.

Overall, the parents found the program very beneficial. All described stories about the benefits of sharing experiences with other parents and of feeling less isolated. Many parents said that they felt that they communicated more with teachers and with their children since completing the program. In terms of improvements in parenting, parents reported that they "yelled" less, used more consistent discipline, and established more routines at home. All reported that their children's behavior was better than before they started the program. One 20-year-old mother of a 4-year-old boy explained it this way:

> "It started helping me calm myself down, be more patient, and it basically showed me different ways to do things besides spanking. . . . When you sum it all up, it's about building better communication with your child . . . and that's basically my number one problem, communicating. He's opening up to me more, I'm giving him more of my time, and so I'm getting more positive feedback."

Teachers also reported observing better behavior in the children and acknowledged more interaction with the parents who participated in the program. Teachers who had gone through the program were particularly enthusiastic and, according to one site director, became "the biggest cheerleaders for the program." The three group leaders who completed parent groups were also enthusiastic. They were particularly pleased by the positive changes they perceived in the parents who attended the groups and felt good about their ability to make a difference with parents.

However, there were significant challenges, particularly with regard to the limited resources available for implementation. Although costs associated with conducting the parent groups were reimbursed (such as food and childcare during parent groups), all of the sites struggled with covering those costs until the reimbursement checks arrived. Other events, such as preparing for accreditation site visits, parent meetings, and staff vacations, competed for limited human resources. Buy-in from teachers and site directors was necessary for getting sufficient support for recruiting parents and getting childcare staff to work overtime to supervise the children during parent group meetings. In one site that did not implement the program, insufficient buy-in from the site administrator was offered as the primary reason. In the other site, too many demands on staff time and not having enough other staff to cover overtime childcare were identified as the primary barriers to implementation. Head Start staff who did implement parent groups felt that although they had support from the agency, they wanted more technical assistance from the Chicago Parent Program team for ongoing consultation and support once parent groups were started.

Based on these pilot data, a report was presented to the Chicago Department of Children and Youth Services with recommendations for the next dissemination stage. These recommendations included increased financial support for Chicago Parent Program staff to provide (1) an initial assessment of each site's organizational capacity, readiness, and administrative buy-in prior to initiating parent groups, (2) more support for coordinating reimbursements to Head Start sites, and (3) technical assistance to group leaders conducting parent groups. Recommendations also included an expanded and improved group leader training to better prepare staff for facilitating parent groups. As part of this training, all novice group leaders would initially be paired with an experienced group leader until they become comfortable and competent leading parent groups. Finally, to more closely evaluate implementation fidelity, all parent groups would need to be audiotaped and submitted weekly to the Chicago Parent Program office to be assessed for adherence and competence by independent raters.

The administrators in the Chicago Department of Children and Youth Services were pleased by the outcomes and supported the recommendations. Over the following years, the project has continued to be funded to expand training and implementation. In addition, a Chicago Parent Program Head Start advisory board was formed to advise the team on innovative ways to address site-level barriers and expand the program without loss to quality or affordability.

In its first 3 years, over 300 children and their parents were served, with up to a 30% reduction in child behavior problems. The Chicago Parent Program is now one of the evidence-based programs listed on the menu of recommended interventions for Head Start in Chicago. In addition, the cost for implementing the 12-session program has been low—approximately $22 per child per week to deliver.[3]

FRAMING RESULTS TO GUIDE POLICY

The goal of nursing research is to develop and test interventions that improve health and well-being, reduce suffering and disability associated with chronic illness, and promote quality of life. Nursing research studies emphasize rigorous designs, strategies to control error, and statistical significance. However, there are many more considerations for making research useful for guiding policy. Although programs need strong evidence, policy makers want to know whether those programs can function at the same high quality at

---

[3] Estimate based on 12 parents per group, each with an average of two children, and includes direct costs for food and childcare during parent groups, group leader stipends, and fidelity monitoring in 2008 dollars.

reasonable cost in the real world (Huston, 2005). To that end, the following is a brief list of some key considerations for nurse researchers.

1. *Estimate the cost-effectiveness of interventions.* Estimating the cost of implementing interventions is essential for research to inform policy. However, this does not mean that programs have to be inexpensive to be useful. In fact, expensive programs can be very cost-effective when the health outcome being treated or prevented is a costly problem (Foster, Jones, & the Conduct Problems Prevention Research Group, 2006). As described earlier, early-childhood obesity, mental health problems, and chronic illnesses that are poorly managed are costly to families and society. Therefore, these are significant areas for nursing research where cost-effective interventions can make important contributions to policy. However, nurse researchers must include plans for estimating cost-effectiveness or cost-benefit in their research plans.

2. *Attend to implementation in the real world.* Clinical trials do not mimic real life (Fogg & Gross, 2000). One reason why interventions that worked well in clinical trials do not produce similar outcomes outside the clinical trial is poor attention to fidelity (Bellg et al., 2004; Breitenstein, Gross, Garvey, Hill, Fogg, & Resnick, 2010a). When the Chicago Parent Program team first reflected on how to disseminate the program in Head Start, our attention immediately focused on how we could monitor and ensure quality, safety, and fidelity with paraprofessional group leaders on a large scale. This led to a revision of our protocols to include more training and supervision of group leaders and independent ratings of their adherence and competence while conducting parent groups. We also evaluated the effectiveness of this revised protocol, the outcomes of which were then used to improve our training (Breitenstein, Fogg, Garvey, Hill, Resnick, & Gross, 2010b). Thus, researchers need to think through the feasibility of enacting interventions not only within the careful conditions of a clinical trial but also how it can be implemented with quality at an affordable price in real life.

3. *Understand context and local adaptation.* Although early-childhood programs share a common mission to support the well-being of young children and their families, each is affected by a unique context by virtue of its location, history, and leadership; the cultural values of its constituents; and the resources available to it. For this reason, Shorr (1998) found that the programs most likely to function well in the community were those that had not only a strong theory delineating its core components but also an understanding of which components could be flexed to meet the needs of local context. This means that nurse researchers need to understand what are the essential ingredients of the intervention that make it work and what components can be adapted at the local level. Clarifying this balance between strict adherence and local adaptation increases the likelihood that programs can be scaled up and still function successfully, an important consideration for policy makers. However, it also suggests that more research is needed on how to work with local agencies in tailoring evidence-based programs to fit with local context and the extent to which adaptations will affect targeted outcomes.

4. *Effect size is important, but so is a good story.* It is important to communicate results in ways that are easily understood. A 0.25 effect size between the intervention and the comparison group has little meaning to nonresearchers. However, a 30% reduc-

tion in behavior problems or a $52,000 savings in healthcare cost makes an impact. Even better, tell a story about a child whose behavior dramatically changed after his mother participated in the parent group or a child whose asthma once triggered regular visits to the emergency room and three hospitalizations is now well controlled. According to Goodman (2006), "[Good stories] not only make facts more memorable, [they] arouse the emotions and engage the audience in ways numbers do not" (p. 25).

Most researchers have not learned how to communicate their data in ways that engage the public and policy makers. More times than not, research presentations are lengthy, detailed, technical, and mind numbing. In contrast, short, nontechnical executive summaries and research briefs make the data easier to digest while stories give the data life. Although researchers should not overinterpret their data, it is important to make the results meaningful and usable to those in positions to change the health landscape.

CONCLUSIONS

There continues to be a significant gap between what we know about the importance of early childhood and our willingness to invest in young children in a comprehensive and sustained way. The public reticence is understandable; the upfront investments and required infrastructure changes are substantial, and the gains may not be apparent for years to come. Arguing for change is complicated by the fact that the problems we seek to change are complex and the "usual care" control groups against which we compare the new treatments are usually exposed to a range of alternative interventions. As a result, even small program effects are difficult to demonstrate on a large scale (Ludwig & Phillips, 2008). Further obscuring program effects, childhood obesity, mental health problems, and chronic illness all occur at higher rates in low-income populations already at heightened risk for poor health outcomes. Yet these three health problems constitute significant burdens on the health of our nation's children and on society and further contribute to widening racial and ethnic health disparities.

One answer may lie in concentrating evidence-based health promotion and early interventions in natural settings where economically disadvantaged families with young children are most likely to be found. What if, for example, childcare centers became health promotion centers? As argued in this paper, early-childhood programs serve a large number of poor families and, as such, represent an underutilized opportunity for providing innovative, cost-effective health promotion and early intervention services. From a policy perspective, nursing research focused on the behavioral and physical health of young children has great potential to improve the overall health of individuals and families from the most vulnerable populations.

ACKNOWLEDGMENT

We acknowledge the funding from the National Institute for Nursing Research (grant #R01 NR004085).

REFERENCES

Akinbami, L. J. (2006). The state of childhood asthma, United States 1980–2005. Advance data from Vital Health Statistics, no. 381. Hyattsville, MD: National Center for Health Statistics.

Alkon, A., Farrer, J., & Bernzweig, J. (2004). Child care health consultants' roles and responsibilities: Focus group findings. *Pediatric Nursing, 30*(4), 315–321.

Americans with Disabilities Act of 1990, 42 U.S.C.A. § 12101 *et seq.*

Anthony, B. J., Anthony, L. G., Morrel, R. M., & Acosta, M. (2005). Evidence for social and behavior problems in low-income urban preschoolers: Effects of site, classroom, and teacher. *Journal of Youth and Adolescence, 34,* 31–39.

Beeber, L., Perreira, K. M., & Schwartz, T. (2008). Supporting the mental health of mothers raising children in poverty: How do we target them for intervention studies? *Annals of the New York Academy of Sciences, 1136,* 86–100.

Bellg, A. J., Borrelli, B., Resnick, B., Hecht, J., Minicucci, D. S., Ory, M., . . . the Treatment Fidelity Workshop of the NIH Behavioral Change Consortium. (2004). Enhancing treatment fidelity in health behavior change studies: Best practices and recommendations from the NIH behavior change consortium. *Health Psychology, 23,* 443–451.

Bethell, C., Peck, C., Abrams, M., Halfon, N., Sareen, H., & Scott, K. S. (2002). Partnering with parents to promote the healthy development of young children enrolled in Medicaid: Results from a survey assessing the quality of preventive and developmental services for young children enrolled in Medicaid in three states. Retrieved on May 4, 2009, from: http://www.commonwealthfund.org/content/publications/fund-reports/2002/sep/partnering-with-parents-to-promote-the-healthy-development-of-young-children-enrolled-in-Medicaid.aspx#citation

Bluford, D. A. A., Sherry, B., & Scanlon, K. S. (2007). Interventions to prevent or treat obesity in preschool children: A review of evaluated programs. *Obesity, 15,* 1356–1372.

Breismeister, J. M., & Schaefer, C. E. (2007). *Handbook of parent training: Helping parents prevent and solve problem behaviors* (3rd ed). Hoboken, NJ: Wiley.

Breitenstein, S., Gross, D., Garvey, C., Hill, C., Fogg, L., & Resnick, B. (2010a). Implementation fidelity in community-based interventions. *Research in Nursing & Health, 33,* 164–173.

Breitenstein, S., Fogg, L., Garvey, C., Hill, C., Resnick, B., & Gross, D. (2010b). Measuring implementation fidelity in a community-based parenting intervention. *Nursing Research, 59,* 158–165.

Breitenstein, S. M., Gross, D., Ordaz, I., Julion, W., Garvey, C., & Ridge, A. (2007). Promoting mental health in early childhood programs serving families from low-income neighborhoods. *Journal of the American Psychiatric Nurses Association, 13,* 313–320.

Brown, W. H., Pfeiffer, K. A., McIver, K. L., Dowda, M., Addy, C. L., & Pate, R. R. (2009). Social and environmental factors associated with preschoolers' nonsedentary physical activity. *Child Development, 80,* 45–58.

Campbell, F. A., Ramey, C. T., Pungello, E., Sparling, J. J., & Miller-Johnson, S. (2002). Early childhood education: Young adult outcomes from the Abecedarian Project. *Applied Developmental Science, 6,* 42–57.

Catenzaro, S. (1999). *Issues and barriers to medication administration in child care programs.* Unpublished thesis, Yale University School of Nursing, New Haven, CT.

Center for Law and Social Policy, Early Head Start Participants, Programs, Families and Staff in 2005 (2006). Retrieved on May 3, 2009, from www.clasp.org/publications/hs_brief8_2005data.pdf

Child Trends Data Bank. (2005). Child care. Retrieved March 26, 2009, from www.childtrendsdatabank.org/tables21_table_1.htm

Cope, S. F., Ungar, W. J., & Glazier, R. H. (2008). Socioeconomic factors and asthma control in children. *Pediatric Pulmonology, 43,* 745–752.

Crowley, A. A. (1988). The child care dilemma: Expanding nurse practitioner involvement. *Journal of Pediatric Health Care, 2,* 128–134.

Crowley, A. A. (1990). Health services in child day care centers: A survey. *Journal of Pediatric Health Care, 4*(5), 252–259.

Crowley, A. A. (2000). Child care health consultation: The Connecticut experience. *Maternal and Child Health Journal, 4,* 67–75.

Crowley, A. A. (2001). Child care health consultation: An ecological model. *Journal of the Society of Pediatric Nurses, 6* (4), 170–181 (erratum: *JSPN,* 2002, 7(1): 41).

Crowley, A. A. (2010). Medication administration. In E. A. Donoghue & C. A. Kraft (Eds.), *Managing chronic health needs in child care and schools.* American Academy of Pediatrics: Elk Grove Village. IL.

Dellert, J. C., Gasalberti, D., Sternas, K., Lucarelli, P., & Hall, J. (2006). Outcomes of child care health consultation services for child care providers in New Jersey: A pilot study. *Pediatric Nursing, 32,* 530–535.

Duncan, G., Ludwig, J., & Magnuson, K. A. (2007). Reducing poverty through preschool interventions. *The Future of Children, 17*(2), 143–160.

Engle, P. L., & Black, M. M. (2008). The effect of poverty on child development and educational outcomes. *Annals of the New York Academy of Sciences, 1136,* 243–245.

Finkelstein, J. A., Brown, R. W., Schneider, L. C., Weiss, S. T., Quintana, J. M., Goldman, D. A., & Homer, C. J. (1995). Quality of care for preschool children with asthma: The role of social factors and practice setting. *Pediatrics, 95,* 389–394.

Fogg, L., & Gross, D. (2000). Threats to validity in randomized clinical trials. *Research in Nursing & Health, 23,* 79–87.

Foster, E. M., & Jones, D. E. (2005). The high costs of aggression: Public expenditures resulting from conduct disorder. *American Journal of Public Health, 95,* 1767–1772.

Foster, E. M., Jones, D., and the Conduct Problems Prevention Research Group. (2006). Can a costly intervention be cost-effective? An analysis of violence prevention. *Archives of General Psychiatry, 63,* 1284–1291.

Gilliam, W. S. (2005). *Pre-kindergarteners left behind: Expulsion rates in state prekindergarten systems.* Retrieved January 3, 2007, from http://www.fed-us.org/PDFs/NationalPreKExpulsionPaper03.02_new.pdf

Goodman, A. (2006). *Storytelling as best practice: How stories strengthen your organization, engage your audience, and advance your mission.* Available from the author at www.agoodmanonline.com

Gross, D., Garvey, C., Julion, W., & Fogg, L., (2007). Preventive parent training with low-income, ethnic minority families of preschoolers. In J. M. Briesmeister & C. E. Schaefer (Eds.), *Handbook of parent training: Helping parents prevent and solve problem behaviors* (3rd ed., pp. 5–25). Hoboken, NJ: Wiley.

Gross, D., Garvey, C., Julion, W., Fogg, L, Tucker, S., & Mokros, H. (2009). Efficacy of the Chicago Parent Program with low-income African American and Latino parents of young children. *Prevention Science, 10,* 54–65.

Gross, D., Sambrook, A., & Fogg, L. (1999). Behavior problems among young children in low-income urban day care centers. *Research in Nursing & Health, 22,* 15–25.

Guo, S. S. & Chumlea, W. C. (1999). Tracking of body mass index in children in relation to overweight in adulthood. *American Journal of Clinical Nutrition, 70*(1), 145S–148S.

Harbaugh, B. L., Jordan, M., Johnson, K., Hovan, M., & Nugent, K. (2009, February). *A comparative study of weight trends in Head Start preschoolers.* Poster presented at the annual meeting of the Southern Nursing Research Society, Baltimore, MD.

Harms, T., Clifford, R. M., & Cryer, D. (1998). *The early childhood environment rating scale* (Rev. ed.). New York: Teachers College Press.

Heckman, J. J. (2002). *Invest in the very young.* Chicago, IL: Ounce of Prevention Fund and the University of Chicago Harris School of Public Policy Studies.

Heckman, J. J. (2006). Skill formation and the economics of investing in disadvantaged children. *Science, 312,* 1900–1902.

Helburn, S., Culkin, M., Morris, J., Mocan, N., Howes, C., Phillipsen, L., . . . Rustici, J. (1995). *Cost, quality, and child outcomes in child care centers: Public report.* Denver: Economics Department, University of Colorado at Denver.

Heschel, R. T., Crowley, A. A., & Cohen, S. S. (2005). State policies regarding nursing delegation and medication administration in child care settings: A case study. *Policy, Politics and Nursing Practice, 6*(2), 86–98.

Horne, R. (2006). Compliance, adherence, and concordance: Implications for asthma treatment. *Chest, 130,* 655–725.

Huston, A. C. (2005). Connecting the science of child development to public policy. *Social Policy Report, 14*(4), 3–7, 10–18.

Johnson, K., & Knitzer, J. (2005). *Spending smarter: A funding guide for policymakers and advocates to promote social and emotional health and school readiness.* New York: National Center for Children in Poverty.

Kim, J., Peterson, K. E., Scanlon, K. S., Fitzmaurice, G. M., Must, A., & Oken, E., . . . Gillman, M. W. (2006). Trends in overweight from 1980 through 2001 among preschool-aged children enrolled in a health maintenance organization. *Obesity*, 14, 1107–1112.

Kotch, J., Crowley, A., Alkon, A., & Benjamin, S. (2007–2010). *Promoting nutrition and physical activity in child care centers*. HRSA/DHHS/Maternal and Child Health Research Program.

Lucas, K. (2008). Investing in infants and toddlers: The economics of early childhood. Zero to three policy center. Originally published September 6, 2006, updated August 26, 2008. Retrieved from www.zerotothree.org/policy

Ludwig, J., & Phillips, D. A. (2008). Long-term effects of head start on low-income children. *Annals of the New York Academy of Sciences, 1136*, 257–268.

Mellon, M., & Parasuraman, B. (2004). Pediatric asthma: Improving management to reduce cost of care. *Journal of Managed Care Pharmacy, 10*, 130–141.

Moore, K. A., Redd, Z., Burkhauser, M., Mbwana, K., & Collins, A. (2009). Children in poverty: Trends, consequences, and policy options. *Child Trends Research Brief*, Publication #2009–11. Retrieved from www.childtrends.org

Nader, P. R., O'Brien, M., Houts, R., Bradley, R., Belsky, J., Crosnoe, R., . . . Susman, E. (2006). Identifying risk for obesity in early childhood. *Pediatrics, 118*, e594–e601.

National Heart, Lung, and Blood Institute. (2007). Expert Panel Report 3 (EPR 3): Guidelines for the diagnosis and management of asthma. Retrieved on June 3, 2009, from http://www.nhlbi.nih.gov/guidelines/asthma

NICHD Early Child Care Research Network. (1996). Characteristics of infant child care: Factors contributing to positive care giving. *Early Childhood Research Quarterly, 11*(3): 269–306.

Ogden, C. L., Carroll, M. D., Curtin, L. R., McDowell, M. A., Tabak, C. J., & Flegal, K. M. (2006). Prevalence of overweight and obesity in the United States, 1999–2004. *Journal of the American Medical Association, 295*(13), 1549–1555.

Peterson-Sweeney, K., Halterman, J. S., Conn, K., & Yoos, L. (in press). The effect of family routines on care for inner city children with asthma. *Journal of Pediatric Nursing*.

Phillips, D., Howes, C., & Whitebrook, M. (1991). Child care as an adult work environment. *Journal of Social Issues, 47*(2), 49–70.

Phillipsen, L. C., Burchinal, M., Howes, C., & Cryer, D. (1997). The prediction of process quality from structural features of child care. *Early Childhood Research Quarterly, 12*(3), 281–303.

Ramler, M., Nakatsukasa-Ono, W., Loe, C. & Harris, K. (2006). The influence of child care health consultants in promoting children's health and well-being: A report on selected resources. Retrieved on May 5, 2009, from: http://hcccnsc.edc.org

Razzino, B. E., New, M., Lewin, A., & Joseph, J. (2004). Need for and use of mental health services among parents of children in the Head Start program. *Psychiatric Services, 55*, 583–586.

Schumacher, R., Hamm, K., & Ewen, D. (2007). Making pre-kindergarten work for low income families. *Center for Law and Social Policy Child Care and Early Education Series*. Retrieved from http://clasp.org/admin/site/publications/files/0366.pdf

Schweinart, L. J., Montie, J., Xiang, X., Barnett, W. S., Belfield, C. R., & Nores, M. (2005). *Lifetime effects: The High/Scope Perry Preschool Study through age 40*. Monographs of the High/Scope Educational Research Foundation, 14. Ypsilanti, MI: High/Scope Press.

Shonkoff, J. P., & Phillips, D. A. (2000). *Neurons to neighborhoods: The science of early childhood development*. National Research Council and Institute of Medicine. Committee on Integrating the Science of Early Childhood Development. Washington, D.C.: National Academy Press.

Simpson, L. A., & Cooper, J. (2009). Paying for obesity: A changing landscape. *Pediatrics, 123*(Suppl 5), s301–s307.

Ulione, M. S. (1997). Health promotion and injury prevention in a child development center. *Journal of Pediatric Nursing, 12*(3), 148–154.

U.S. DHHS, ACF, Office of Head Start. (2008). Program performance standards and other regulations. Retrieved on May 28, 2009, from http://www.acf.hhs.gov/programs

U.S. Department of Health and Human Services, Health Resources and Services Administration, Maternal and Child Health Bureau (2008). *The national survey of children with special health care needs chartbook 2005–2006*. Rockville, MD: U.S. Department of Health and Human Services.

U.S. Department of Health and Human Services. (DHHS). (2000). US Public Health Service report of the Surgeon General's Conference on Children's Mental Health: A national action agenda. Washington, DC: Author.

U.S. Department of Labor, Bureau of Labor Statistics and Bureau of the Census. (2005). Annual social and economic supplement: Current population survey. Retrieved on March 31, 2009, from http://www.bls.census.gov/cps/asec/adsmain.htm

U.S. DHHS, Head Start Bureau. (2008). Statistical fact sheet. Retrieved on May 4, 2000, from http://www.acf.hhs.gov/program/ohs/about/indes.html#mission

U.S. Preventive Services Task Force. Screening and Interventions for Overweight in Children and Adolescent: Recommendation Statement. AHRQ Publication No. 05-0574-A, July 2005. Agency for Healthcare Research and Quality, Rockville, MD. http://www.ahrq.gov/clinic/uspstf05/choverwt/choverrs.htm

Whitlock, E. P., Williams, S. B., Gold, R., Smith, P. R., & Shipman, S. A. (2005). Screening and interventions for childhood overweight: A summary of evidence for the US Preventive Services Task Force. *Pediatrics, 116*(1), e125–e144.

11

Influencing Policy for Improving End-of-Life Care

Virginia P. Tilden

Few areas of clinical care in the United States have been as politically tumultuous in the last 30 years as care of dying patients. Until the mid-1950s, dying was largely a private affair that typically followed infections, accidents, or cardiac events within short time frames. With the advent of medically more sophisticated life-sustaining treatments that allowed the prolongation of life, controversies arose regarding clinical care standards and stakeholders' decision-making authority. This led to policy changes at multiple levels—institutional, state, and federal—and to numerous legal disputes, both in individual patient cases and in public policy.

In the past 25 years, findings from studies on caring for patients at the end of life have frequently contributed to policy improvement. For example, findings from the SUPPORT investigation (1995), a study of almost 10,000 gravely ill patients hospitalized in five major acute care hospitals, indicated that a large proportion of patients received prolonged aggressive treatments even when patients and families had indicated a preference for palliative care rather than life extension. In addition, one half of all conscious patients reported moderate to severe pain to family members in the final days of life. Thus, the study showed serious inattention to patients' concerns in major hospitals. The findings contributed to gradual improvements across the country in hospital policies related to advance planning and symptom management. The purpose of this chapter is to describe another interprofessional research program that focused on improving end-of-life care and to highlight its influence on the media and policy.

BACKGROUND

Policy issues related to dying in America often have been publicly contentious, beginning in the mid-1970s with the legal battle between the family of Karen Ann Quinlan, a young woman in a persistent vegetative state, and the New Jersey hospital that cared for her (re Quinlan, 355 A2d 647, NJ 1976). The Quinlan case was surrounded by public, medical, and theological debate and was considered to have contributed to the advent of formal ethics committees in hospitals and the development of advance directives. This case also led to efforts to distinguish ordinary and extraordinary means of sustaining life, particularly the administration of artificial food and fluids.

A second high-profile case in the late 1980s concerned a Missouri woman, Nancy Beth Cruzan, who also was in a persistent vegetative state in a long-term care facility (Cruzan *v.* Director, 1990). Cruzan's case ended with a Supreme Court decision that supported a hospital's or other care facility's right to require "clear and convincing evidence" with regard to the patient's wishes before removing life-sustaining treatments. The ruling subsequently led to the passage by Congress of the Patient Self-Determination Act in 1991 (101 PL 508). This act created a federal law that requires hospitals receiving Medicare and Medicaid dollars to routinely notify all newly admitted patients about advance directives so as to encourage patients to complete them.

The most recent highly contentious and very public case was that of a Florida woman, Terri Schiavo, who, like Quinlan and Cruzan before her, lived in a long-term care facility in a persistent vegetative state maintained by minimally aggressive life-sustaining treatments (Quill, 2005). A bitter family feud over Schiavo's prognosis polarized her husband from her parents and brother. A legal battle over the question of removing her feeding tube stretched over 7 years and included numerous rulings and appeals in state court, the Federal District Court, and, eventually, the Supreme Court, ultimately involving the state governor, some members of the Congress, and the president of the United States.

Throughout the approximately 30-year time span of these and other court cases on the question of patient preferences, family rights, clinician responsibilities, and decisional conflicts over life-sustaining treatments, there has been steady improvement in care of the dying throughout the country. Indicators of better care include higher advance directive completion rates by the public, and of citizens' appointment of a personal healthcare power of attorney to represent the patient's wishes in the event of incapacity. In addition, hospice utilization has steadily increased, and formal palliative care teams and pain management services for terminally ill patients have emerged. Nonetheless, policy reform has been slow, generally hampered by widely divergent political and religious views about the best approach to medical care at the end of life and by entrenched healthcare financing laws, such as those associated with hospice care and the required rehabilitative focus of nursing home care.

One State's Environment

Because healthcare and health policy in the United States are generally influenced and directed more at the state than the federal level, considerations about the influence of research investigations on policy typically start with a look at a state's environment. Our program of research was located in western Oregon, where the cultural and social climate tends toward liberal philosophies rooted in progressive citizen activism and respect for natural resources, rugged individualism, and communitarian values. These values are evident in an emphasis on patient autonomy and respect for patient preferences in treatment decisions. These liberal tendencies manifested themselves in the 1990s with the passage of the first physician-assisted suicide law in the country. Although not the first state in the Union to vote on legalizing physician-assisted suicide (Michigan, California, and Washington all had failed referenda on the issue), Oregon was the first in which a citizens' initiative, called the Death With Dignity Act, passed. The initial passing vote was in 1994; however, the act was not legally implemented until 1997 (Gonzales *v.* Oregon, 2006). Surviving numerous legal injunctions against it, the act was upheld again in 2006 by the U.S. Supreme Court. The law allows mentally competent, terminally ill, adult patients under narrow terms pertaining to mental capacity, prognosis, and symptom control to receive after specific waiting periods a prescription for a lethal dose of medication from a licensed physician.

Unrelated to the specific law itself, legalization of physician-assisted suicide created a major window of opportunity for improving care for dying patients. Upon passage of the law, no care agency wished to be associated with insufficient palliative care or to appear unconcerned about the physical and psychological suffering of terminally ill patients. No one in a public policy arena could risk seeming inattentive to the issues and burdens of dying citizens. This made the environment particularly attuned and responsive to the goal of improving clinical care to dying patients. The Center for Ethics in Healthcare at Oregon Health & Science University, directed by Susan Tolle, MD, had earlier embraced this goal. Part of the work toward that goal consisted of a series of research investigations codirected by myself and Dr. Tolle into aspects of terminally ill patient care.

During the debates about physician-assisted suicide, the leading newspaper of the state, *The Oregonian*, began front-page coverage of care of the dying using end-of-life stories that showed compassionate care by clinicians intermixed with true shortcomings in healthcare delivery, financing, symptom management, and practical help for families caring for dying loved ones (e.g., *The Oregonian*, April 1997 and September 1997). The public interest in such information and the paper's willingness to give this in-depth coverage heightened the usefulness of our research findings and the media's appetite for them. The national scope of debate about better quality care and the urgency for research that would improve care led to coverage of our research program by the Robert Wood Johnson Foundation in a publication, *State Initiatives in End-of-life Care*, prepared by the Community-State Partnerships to Improve End-of-life Care of the Foundation's Last Acts Campaign (State Initiatives in End-of-Life Care, 1998). This publication, entitled "Using Qualitative and Quantitative Data to Shape Policy Change," featured the role of the research program's data, both numeric and narrative, in highlighting such critical issues as the different lengths of hospice stay for uninsured versus insured citizens, raising concerns about access to palliative care for the neediest populations.

A second window of opportunity was created in 1990 by a call for applications from the National Institute of Nursing Research (NINR) on "Bioethics and Clinical Decision Making." This Research for Application opened the path for federal funding for studies on end-of-life decision making and launched our series of studies with federal and foundation funding to improve care of the dying. In the years that followed, the NINR became the lead institute for federally supported research on improving end-of-life care and subsequently issued such successive program announcements as "Management of Symptoms at the End-of-Life" (1997), "Research on Care at the End-of-Life" (1999), "Quality of Life for Individuals at the End-of-Life" (2000), "Research to Improve Care for Dying Children and Their Families" (2002), "Reducing Barriers to Symptom Management and Palliative Care" (2004), "Interventions to Improve Palliative Care at the End of Life" (2006), and "Methods to Enhance Palliative Care and End-of-Life Research" (2008).

RESEARCH OVERVIEW

Family Communication and Treatment Decision Making

In the first NINR study (Tilden, principal investigator [PI], 1991–1993), 32 family members were interviewed shortly after their relative died in the hospital after withdrawal of life-sustaining treatment. The purpose of the study was to learn what families thought and felt about the decision and what had helped or made things worse during the decision making time, particularly related to clinician behaviors and communication. All patients were unresponsive at the time treatment decisions were required, and we sampled only patients without advance directives. Families viewed clinician behaviors and communications as either inclusive (timely, honest, unhurried, respectful, or collaborative) or distancing. Distancing behaviors greatly added to family stress, e.g., clinicians talking over the patient's bed about treatment withdrawal or phrasing the question of withdrawing treatments to imply that the decision was solely the family's to make, and clinician avoidance of family members when hope for the patient's recovery ebbed. We found that clinicians tended to seek a single spokesperson for the family, whereas families resisted this designation out of reluctance to put a disproportionate share of responsibility on one family member, i.e., over "life and death decisions," as often phrased by families.

These findings became a primer of "Directions to Clinicians," which we published in the *Archives of Internal Medicine* (Tilden, Tolle, Garland, & Nelson, 1995) because we especially wanted to enhance physician insight about what families need. Two unusual features of this publication were that the first author was a nurse, and second, the data reported were qualitative. While both numeric and narrative data are powerful tools for influencing change, the particular topic of this study and the nuanced lessons from families for clinician behaviors made the piece compelling.

Building on these findings, a second NINR-funded study (Tilden, PI, 1995–1998) allowed the continuation of this work. Using data from hospital records of decedents with and without advance directives whose deaths followed withdrawal of life-sustaining treatments, we collected data about family members' experience of participating in the withdrawal decisions. Data were collected twice from family members and clinicians who had cared for the patients—shortly after patient death and again 6 months later. Family stress associated with the decision, indexed by two well-established measures of stress (Horowitz, Wilner, & Alvarez, 1979; Ware & Sherbourne, 1992), was high immediately after the death and, although it decreased over time, remained high half a year later. Compared with published reports of stress levels using these measures, families in the study were more stressed even 6 months after the death than were other high-stress samples, such as survivors of the 1994 Oakland-Berkeley firestorm (Koopman, Classen, & Spiegel, 1994).

Study families reported high rates of intrusive psychological symptoms, indicated by disturbed sleep and waves of strong feelings. Many said that it was the hardest thing a family will ever do (Tilden, Tolle, Nelson, Thompson, & Eggman, 1999). Several factors significantly affected stress, most notably when the patient had no advance directive. About a quarter of families reported conflict with clinicians. Typically, this included their frustration at the inadequacy of information from clinicians (e.g., wanting more timely information, more candid information, and explanations in lay terms), anger at clinicians for mixed or inconsistent information from different specialists or different nurse shifts, or distress at feeling unheard or disregarded (Norton, Tilden, Tolle, Nelson, & Eggman,

2003). This study was the first to give a quantitative picture of the high level of family stress in the absence of a patient's advance directive, and was evidence for the power of advance directives to reduce the burden on families who face this decision (Tilden, Tolle, Nelson, & Fields, 2001).

Because of the public's already high awareness of issues related to dying, there was significant media interest in the study findings that advance directives have a measureable impact on family stress. Although no specific changes to state laws on advance directives or healthcare power of attorney resulted from these findings, the findings helped raise awareness. Oregon's advance planning laws were already among the most progressive in the nation, and importantly, respect by citizens and healthcare providers for advance planning documents was already high. But the family implications were new information and were featured in NINR reports to the Congress and the scientific community.

A parallel arm of the research program's effort to improve the use of advance directives centered on residents of long-term care facilities, a population at risk for medical events that require decisions about life-sustaining treatments. Under the direction of Patrick Dunn, MD, chair of the National POLST Paradigm Task Force, and with foundation funding (Tolle, PI, 1993–1995, 1995–1997, Greenwall Foundation), the Center for Ethics in Health Care developed a medical cover sheet called the POLST (Physician Orders for Life-Sustaining Treatment), a durable, bright-pink, one-page order form that puts the patient's preferences for medical treatment in the event of serious illness into a *medical order*, thereby enhancing its legal authority. The advantages of the POLST over advance directives are that it is briefer, better standardized, and, most importantly, signed by a physician or nurse practitioner, thus empowering nursing home staff and emergency medical services personnel to honor a patient's wishes.

To assess the POLST's utility, we conducted a 1-year prospective study of POLST outcomes in helping people receive only the aggressive treatments they wanted. We followed 180 residents from eight nursing homes in Oregon. All subjects had a POLST in their record documenting their wishes not to receive cardiopulmonary resuscitation and not to be transferred to a hospital unless necessary to control suffering. During the study year, a third of subjects experienced a life-threatening illness (a rate typical of this population), but none received cardiopulmonary resuscitation. About half were transferred to the hospital, but for most, the transfer occurred because the nursing home could not manage distressing symptoms such as pain or dyspnea. No subject in the hospitalized group was admitted to an intensive care unit or received ventilatory support. About a third of subjects died during the study year, but only two died in the hospital. These rates of aggressive treatment are low, indicating that the POLST likely enhanced an already progressive state's environment in achieving high levels of respect for patients' wishes (Tolle, Tilden, Nelson, & Dunn, 1998; Tilden, Nelson, Dunn, Donius, & Tolle, 2000).

After much work by many POLST champions, a majority of nursing homes and hospices in Oregon now use the POLST. Nationally, regions of the country in approximately 30 states have adopted a POLST, typically adapted to accommodate different state laws or agency regulations. This work over many years progressed through numerous policy forums, such as the delivery of testimony to legislative committees and state licensing boards. The success of the POLST as policy is a credit to the Center for Ethics in Health Care at Oregon Health & Science University. The Center for Ethics has continued its development and promotion of the POLST, which can be found at www.polst.org. This exemplifies the advancement of research-guided policy at the delivery-systems level rather than at the legislation level.

Patient Distress

This period in Oregon's healthcare policy history was particularly tumultuous because of its unique legal option of physician-assisted suicide. Coalitions opposed to physician-assisted suicide typically took a moral and religious stand but also voiced such secular concerns as the legal scope of medical practice, the off-label use of sedating medications, the risks for pharmacists, and concerns for the rights of the disabled. Coalitions in favor of physician-assisted suicide did so typically on grounds of citizens' right to choose and a person's autonomy in medical and health decisions.

Oregon's Death With Dignity Act requires physicians who write the prescription to report information to the state health department, which then summarizes and releases aggregate data each year (as an example, see the most recent year at www.oregon.gov/DHS/ph/pas/docs/year11.pdf). We were more interested in dying patients whose distress led them to *consider* suicide and who asked for a prescription but died of their own disease before using the prescription—in other words, patients *not* represented in the health department data. We conducted telephone interviews in a sample of 1,384 family caregivers of recent decedents. Decedents were 18 years or older, had died from natural causes, and were identified through a random sample of Oregon death certificates. Families reported that 236 (17%) of dying patients had considered physician-assisted suicide seriously enough to talk with their families about it. Those considering it were more likely to be younger, to be white, and to have cancer. Greater symptom distress independently predicted personal consideration, with pain and sadness being most predictive. Of those who considered assisted suicide, 25 (2%) had formally requested a lethal prescription. Of that group, only one patient completed the required waiting period and obtained a prescription but did not use it and died of his or her disease. Thus, patients were nearly 200 times more likely to consider assisted suicide than to obtain a lethal prescription.

These findings, published in *The Journal of Clinical Ethics* (Tolle, Tilden, Drach, Fromme, Perrin, & Hedberg, 2004) and cited by the Oregon Department of Human Services (2006), underscore that symptom distress does lead to considerations and requests for physician-assisted suicide but that, as often reported, completion rates are extremely low. This study and those by others about the Oregon law's effect on the state's rates and causes of death have contributed to the general consensus over 11 years of "one state's experiment," as it was called by former Attorney General Janet Reno, that legalizing physician-assisted suicide does not result in a large number of deaths under the law or open the floodgates to abuse. Such findings likely have contributed to the durability of the law, despite its controversial nature and continued opposition by conservative groups.

Pain and Symptom Management

Although improvements to care of the dying generally occurred in this time frame, the area of symptom management for patients in pain or suffering from other burdensome symptoms was slow to improve. In a study of pain funded by the Open Society Institute's Project on Death in America (Tolle, PI, 1996–1998), we noted an upward trend of moderate to severe pain in the last week of life of 134 hospitalized patients as reported by their family members (Tolle, Tilden, Rosenfeld, & Hickman, 2000). Specifically, 33% of family members reported moderate to severe pain during 11 months of 1996–1997; this proportion climbed to 59% during the last 3 months of 1997 and was approximately that high at 54% in the last 3 months of 1998. This change occurred during the politically volatile time in Oregon in the wake of the passage of the physician-assisted suicide law. Ironically, although the law's ripple effect had been an overall improvement in palliative care, one untoward effect in hospitals appeared to be reduced opioids for terminally ill patients in hospitals.

As a follow-up study, with funding from the Greenwall Foundation (Tolle, PI, 2001–2002), we mail surveyed a stratified random sample of hospital physicians and nurses about their views of the trend in family reports of pain and of factors that may have contributed to the increase. With a response rate of 57%, data from 411 respondents indicated two factors as most explanatory of the change: (1) increased family awareness of pain management, i.e., more reporting, and (2) concern over anticipated scrutiny by the Medical Board of Examiners and the U.S. Drug Enforcement Administration (Hickman, Tolle, & Tilden, 2000). This was at the time when then U.S. Attorney General John Ashcroft attempted to give federal drug agents the go-ahead to take action against physicians in Oregon who assisted terminally ill patients under the law. Although, obviously, a cause-and-effect relationship between Ashcroft's avowed positions and pain management by hospital clinicians cannot be concluded, the association was dramatic. Study findings were widely reported in the media and suggest the trickle-down effect on patient care that policy disputes can have.

In a subsequent NINR-funded study (Tilden, PI, 2000–2003), we broadened the focus of symptom burden to other patient symptoms and issues for family caregivers. Using state death certificates and conducting random sampling for decedents 65 years or older who died of natural causes in community settings (home, nursing home, assisted living facility, and inpatient hospice), we conducted telephone interviews with over 1,000 family caregivers using a standardized 69-item telephone interview that indexed a range of quality-of-life variables in end-of-life care, particularly the patient's symptom experience in the last week of life, as well as caregiver strain and family finances. Significant findings, reported in the *Journal of the American Geriatric Society* (Tilden, Tolle, Drach, & Perrin, 2004), were in three areas: (1) Certain symptoms, such as pain, dyspnea, and constipation, were highly distressing for approximately half of decedents who experienced them; (2) caregivers reported high rates of strain, as manifested in sleep disturbance and physical and emotional exhaustion; and (3) a third of families experienced significant financial loss as a result of the patient's illness. Although we found other favorable quality care indicators such as a high advance directives rate and a high hospice use rate, patient suffering and family burden were unacceptably high. In addition, in a subsample of 423 family respondents, 54% reported that the patient had used some form of complementary and alternative treatment such as herbs, megavitamins, or acupuncture for symptom relief (Tilden, Drach, & Tolle, 2004). Findings from this study lent urgency to the national dialogue about the inadequacies of symptom management for patients and insufficient recognition of family caregiver burden.

THE URGENCY OF POLICY REFORM FOR CARE OF THE DYING

There is urgent need for policy reform in the management and care for citizens at the end of life. With the benefits of better public health and improved medical treatments in both acute and chronic disease, people live much longer, as evidenced by the aging demographics of the population. However, rescue medicine is the default mode in American hospitals, even though, currently, 7 out of 10 deaths result from life-limiting chronic illnesses that follow a slow and often predictable decline. But poorly managed symptoms, overtreatment, clinicians' inattention to preferences, and family stress and financial devastation are all too common.

Compounding these problems is the issue of high and poorly justified resource utilization in the last few months of life in many regions of the country. Medicare claims data reported in the Dartmouth Atlas of Health Care show staggering variation in how hospitals care for patients in the last 6 months of life (Wennberg, Fisher, Goodman, & Skinner, 2008). Such care-intensity indicators as intensive care unit stays, hospice use, and referral to medical specialists vary many-fold across the country. For example, Medicare expenses for this population in Manhattan and Miami vastly exceed those in Minneapolis and Portland, Oregon, with death the outcome in all locations. Treatment decisions appear based more on the prevalence of medical specialists and hospital beds than on realistic appraisals of patients' quality of remaining life or families' and patients' wishes for their care. This "supply side" (Wennberg & Wennberg, 2003) driver of care decisions results in hugely expensive but ultimately futile interventions. Most troubling is the fact that regions of the country where more life-extending services are given and more Medicare dollars are spent show worse patient outcomes (Fisher et al., 2003a, 2003b).

Furthermore, dying in high-utilization regions is not associated with higher family satisfaction or more frequent perceptions of high-quality care. In fact, family respondents in high-intensity regions, where patients were much more likely to have had more frequent physician visits and be treated in a hospital by medical specialists, more often reported inadequate emotional support for the decedent, poor shared decision making, and failure to treat the decedent with respect (Teno et al., 2005). Thus, although Medicare costs for the last year of life have been proportionately stable for decades, at about 25% to 30% of the program budget, the bigger issue is what those dollars are buying if quality of care is not associated with higher spending.

Well-organized data, such as those reported in the Dartmouth Atlas, send a powerful message, but even so, reform is slow. Goldstein and Lynn (2002) reported that the 107th Congress enacted only 1 bill out of 22 introduced during the 2001–2002 legislative period that improved care of dying patients. Undoubtedly, the deep religious and philosophical differences that exist in the American citizenry also characterize members of the Congress. The authors conclude, "At this time, only a few bills have come before Congress attempting to improve care at the end of life; those do not have substantial action, and they do not reflect any coherent view of needed reforms. This is a prescription for inertia in public policy" (pp. 825–826). Thus, despite many gains since the publication of the landmark research by the SUPPORT investigators, which so clearly revealed the range and extent of problems in hospital care of gravely ill patients, and the pivotal 1997 report by the Institute of Medicine (Field & Cassel, 1997) that called for reform, years later, the view by most experts is that gains have been modest at best.

LESSONS LEARNED

For research to influence policy, several factors need to be aligned in the right direction. These include the timing of studies to coincide with visible societal problems; relationship building and communication with the media, the public, and other stakeholders; and the presentation of study findings so as to make a compelling case for change.

As described in this chapter, a major window of opportunity allowed investigators at the Oregon Health & Science University Center for Ethics in Health Care to launch a program of research intended to improve in various ways the care received by patients and their families in the final months of life. In this time frame, the nation had been sensitized to issues of the terminally ill by events such as the Nancy Cruzan decision by the Supreme Court and the notorious activities of Jack Kevorkian in hastening death in Michigan, all of which led to calls for improvement in practice and policy across the country. The NINR's timely announcement of a funding stream for ethical decision making, which later specifically focused on improving care at the end of life, made it possible to study patients, families, and clinicians as they navigated patient care in this time period. Thus, a lesson for investigators is that research is most likely to be funded and research findings are most likely to be influential when the timing is in sync with urgent societal questions.

Various research data characteristics increase their potential for impact. Data must be current, not dated, and preferably locally based rather than extrapolated from elsewhere. Research studies are most credible when conducted by scientists from multiple professions, who bring various perspectives and vantage points, particularly if the research topic is broad in scope. Mechanic and Reinhard (2002) point out that "health policy is by its very nature an interdisciplinary activity, building on networks of people from various professions and disciplines who come together around common interests and shared expertise" (p. 9). In this case, policies that influence care at the end of life, and team-based care itself, are transdisciplinary and of value to each of the health professions involved, including medicine, nursing, clinical pharmacy, social work, the ministry, and public health, not to mention lay caregivers, home health aides, and other concerned and involved citizens.

Timely and broad dissemination of research findings are essential for findings to influence policy. In addition to conference presentations, scientific publications in well-respected journals are essential, and again, the data must be recent to maximize impact. Selecting journals in which to publish is a challenge for interprofessional research teams because each of the members understandably knows his or her own journals best. Furthermore, each likely sees career benefits associated with publishing in his or her own discipline's journals. However, it is important to also publish across disciplinary boundaries. Findings that sit isolated within the journals of any one discipline are more easily overlooked. For many reasons, this problem is especially acute in nursing, including its young history as a true science as opposed to a calling or an art rooted in the religious traditions of selfless service. The reality is that most health policy researchers, physicians, the press, or other power groups typically do not read nursing journals and are seldom aware of nursing research unless specific action is taken to relay the message, such as the NINR's Web site and publications and the American Academy of Nursing's Raise the Voice campaign. Fortunate for our research program, excellent journals in the field of end-of-life care are interprofessional, such as the *Journal of Palliative Medicine*, *The Journal of Clinical Ethics*, *Journal of Palliative Care*, *Journal of Pain and Symptom Management*, *Journal of the American Geriatric Society*, and *The Gerontologist*.

Although publishing scientific findings in top-tier journals is crucial, equally important is working with the lay press and other media to deliver understandable research findings and their implications into the public eye. The local media is the initial target, since "all politics is local, even if the issue is national" (McBride, Coburn, MacKinney,

Mueller, Slifkin, & Wakefield, 2008, p. 152). Release of findings to the media must be strategic and coordinated with journal embargos because premature release of findings violates journal requirements, and leaks are likely to dampen the media's interest in full coverage of a story. A sophisticated public affairs department from the investigators' organization should know how to effectively manage press releases.

With the support of such personnel, it is the investigators' job to prepare the announcement so as to provide the data with clear displays, highlight important findings, emphasize the key implications from the data, and make take-away messages short and to the point. Even policy brief titles are important. McBride et al. (2008) point out that many potential users will overlook information if the title does not entice them to read further. To make findings easily usable for policy makers, we self-published *The Oregon Report Card: Improving Care of the Dying*, a glossy booklet of data and their implications for change (Tolle, Tilden, Hickman, Rosenfeld, & Halvor, 1999).

Simple descriptive statistics can be very revealing. For example, our data displays of length of hospice stays quickly revealed the very short time between admission and death for the majority of patients, illustrating the problem of the greatly truncated benefits of hospice. The descriptive data alone do not tell the "why" story, but they raise the question—in this case, answered by other data that implicate the Centers for Medicare & Medicaid Services hospice requirement that aggressive treatments must be stopped or foregone. This requirement often leads both physicians and patients to delay hospice until very late.

Data are most compelling to policy makers when they quickly paint a full yet precise picture. Quantitative data are powerful for snapshots and big pictures. For example, end-of-life care researchers consider the Dartmouth Atlas data to be among the most effective ongoing data sets to show the high cost of ineffective care on a national level. As a companion to quantitative data, qualitative data put human story detail onto the canvas and more powerfully capture the attention and, sometimes, the hearts of policy makers.

Policy makers often complain that research data are too slow in coming and miss the optimal point in time for being relevant. This problem links back to the need for investigators to seize windows of opportunity and to disseminate findings quickly. A feature of our program of research was that several investigations with different PIs and various funders progressed simultaneously in an overlapping fashion. Thus, at any point in time, proposals for funding were in review, funded studies were underway, and completed studies were in press or published. This was made possible by a relatively large team that included several excellent project managers and a group of dedicated research assistants, typically numbering four to five at a time.

To enhance research's policy impact, the design and methods of a study are important. For example, the study of family stress after withdrawal of life-sustaining treatments specifically sampled patient cases with and without advance directives, allowing a comparison of family stress levels between conditions and leading to the finding of high stress in the absence of advanced directives. As another example, findings from the study of patient symptoms and caregiver burden were particularly credible because of the large sample size of over 1,000 subjects and the random selection of patient cases from all eligible state death certificates. As researchers in a study's design phase become better at anticipating whether a study may have future influence on policy, they may want to speculate on what aspects of the design could be of particular interest to external audiences. Others have suggested engaging end users when framing the study, thus better anticipating the likelihood that study findings, if significant, will be used (McBride et al., 2008). Finally, a lesson from this program of research was the key feature of relationship building, especially by Dr. Tolle, throughout state community agencies interested in improving palliative care.

With the expansion of health services research through funding by the Agency for Healthcare Research and Quality and other funding agencies, investigators are increasingly concerned that study findings lead to systems improvement. Approaches to this, such as those suggested in this chapter, are increasingly in the literature (e.g., McBride et al., 2008) and in editorials (e.g., Berkowitz & Gebbie, 2009) and serve as a focus for some journals (e.g., *Health Affairs*).

Few researchers are policy makers, but all researchers should be policy advocates. The same burning knowledge gaps that drive the need for research can, at the conclusion of studies, drive the agenda for policy reform. In this research program's case study findings were particularly salient because of the confluence of many factors, including a national interest in improving end-of-life care along with national and state-level policy events, such as the passage of the federal Patient Self-determination Act and the Oregon Death With Dignity Act.

With the promise of coming national healthcare reform, much is unclear about what effects changes to access and financing might have on care at the end of life. More certain is that timely, well-designed research that quickly produces credible data for policy makers' consideration will be important in helping steer toward a preferred future in managing life's end.

REFERENCES

Berkowitz, B., & Gebbie, K. M. (2009). Nurses and policy: What more is there to say? *Nursing Outlook, 57*(2), 69.

Cruzan *v.* Director (1990). Missouri Department of Health, 497 US 261.

Field, M. J., & Cassel, C. K. (1997). *Approaching death: Improving care at the end of life.* Washington, D.C.: Institute of Medicine Committee on Care at the End of Life, National Academy Press.

Fisher, E. S., Wennberg, D. E., Stukel, T. A., Gottlieb, D. J., Lucas, F. L., & Pinder, E. L. (2003a). The implications of regional variations in Medicare spending. Part 1: The content, quality, and accessibility of care. *Annals of Internal Medicine, 138,* 273–287.

Fisher, E. S., Wennberg, D. E., Stukey, T. A., Gottlieb, D. J., Lucas, F. L., & Pinder, E. L. (2003b). The implications of regional variations in Medicare spending. Part 2: Health outcomes and satisfaction with care. *Annals of Internal Medicine, 138,* 288–298.

Goldstein, N. E., & Lynn, J. (2002). The 107th Congress' legislative proposals concerning end-of-life care. *Journal of Palliative Medicine, 5*(6), 819–827.

Gonzales *v.* Oregon (2006). 546 US 243.

Hickman, S. E., Tolle, S .W., & Tilden, V.P. (2000). Physicians' and nurses' perspectives on increased family reports of pain in dying hospitalized patients. *Journal of Palliative Medicine, 3*(4), 413–418.

Horowitz, M. J., Wilner, N., & Alvarez, W. (1979). Impact of Event Scale: A measure of subjective stress. *Psychosomatic Medicine, 41*(3), 209–218.

Koopman, C., Classen, C., & Spiegel, D. (1994). Predictors of posttraumatic stress symptoms among survivors of the Oakland/Berkeley, California firestorm. *American Journal of Psychiatry, 151,* 888–894.

McBride, T., Coburn, A., MacKinney, C., Mueller, K., Slifkin, R., & Wakefield, M. (2008). Bridging health research and policy: Effective dissemination strategies. *Journal of Public Health Management and Practice, 14*(2), 150–154.

Mechanic, D., & Reinhard, S. C. (2002). Contributions of nurses to health policy: Challenges and opportunities. *Nursing and Health Policy Review, 1*(1), 7–15.

Norton, S. A., Tilden, V. P., Tolle, S. W., Nelson, C. A., & Eggman, S. T. (2003). Life support withdrawal: Communication and conflict. *American Journal of Critical Care, 12*(6), 548–555.

Oregon Department of Human Services. (2006). Eighth Annual Report on Oregon's Death With Dignity Act. http://egov.oregon.gov/DHS/ph/pas/docs/year8.pdf

Patient Self Determination Act, 101 PL 508 (1991).

Quill, T. E. (2005). Terri Schiavo—A tragedy compounded. *The New England Journal of Medicine, 352*(16), 1630–1633.

Quinlan, 355 A2d 647 (NJ 1976).

SUPPORT Principal Investigators. (1995). A controlled trial to improve care for seriously ill hospitalized patients. *Journal of the American Medical Association, 274*, 1591–1598.

State Initiatives in End-of-Life Care. *Focus Oregon: Using qualitative and quantitative data to shape policy change. Community-state partnerships to improve end-of-life care*, Last Acts Campaign. The Robert Wood Johnson Foundation, Issue 1, June, 1998.

The Oregonian. A Good Death. April 20, 1997.

The Oregonian. Hospice: Dying well. September 29, 1997.

Teno, J. M., Mor, V., Ward, N., Roy, J., Clarridge, B., Wennberg, J., et al. (2005). Bereaved family member perceptions of quality of end-of-life care in U.S. regions with high and low usage of intensive care unit care. *Journal of the American Geriatrics Society, 53*, 1905–1911.

Tilden, V. P., Drach, L. L., & Tolle, S. W. (2004). Complementary and alternative therapy use at end-of-life in community settings. *The Journal of Alternative and Complementary Medicine, 10*(5), 811–817.

Tilden, V. P., Drach, L. L., Tolle, S. W., & Hickman, S. E. (2002). Measurement of quality of care and quality of life at end-of-life (paper commissioned by the National Institutes of Health). *The Gerontologist, 42* (Special Issue III), 71–80.

Tilden, V. P., Nelson, C. A., Dunn, P. M., Donius, M., & Tolle, S. W. (2000). Nursing's perspective on improving communication about nursing home residents' preferences for medical treatments at end of life. *Nursing Outlook, 48*(3), 109–115.

Tilden, V. P., Tolle, S. W., Drach, L. L., & Perrin, N. A. (2004). Out of hospital death: Advance care planning, patient symptoms, and caregiver burden. *Journal of the American Geriatric Society,* (52), 532–539.

Tilden, V. P., Tolle, S. W., Garland, M. J., & Nelson, C. A. (1995). Decisions about life sustaining treatment: Impact of physicians' behaviors on families. *Archives of Internal Medicine, 155*, 633–638.

Tilden, V. P., Tolle, S. W., Nelson, C. A. & Fields, J. (2001). Family decision-making to withdraw life-sustaining treatments from hospitalized patients. *Nursing Research, 50*(2), 105–115.

Tilden, V. P., Tolle, S. W., Nelson, C. A., Thompson, M., & Eggman, S. C. (1999). Family decision making in foregoing life-extending treatments. *Journal of Family Nursing, 5*(4), 426–442.

Tolle, S. W., Tilden, V. P., Drach, L. L., Fromme, E. K., Perrin, N. A., & Hedberg, K. (2004). Characteristics and proportion of dying Oregonians who personally consider physician-assisted suicide. *The Journal of Clinical Ethics, 15*(2), 111–118.

Tolle, S. W., Tilden, V. P., Hickman, S. E., Rosenfeld, A. G., & Halvor, C. B. (1999). *The Oregon report card: Improving care of the dying.* Center for Ethics in Health Care, Oregon Health & Science University.

Tolle, S. W., Tilden, V. P., Nelson, C. A., & Dunn, P. M. (1998). Prospective study of the efficacy of the physician order form for life-sustaining treatment. *Journal of the American Geriatric Society, 46*, 1097–1102.

Tolle, S. W., Tilden, V. P., Rosenfeld, A. G., & Hickman, S. E. (2000). Family reports of barriers to optimal care of the dying. *Nursing Research, 49*(6), 310–317.

Ware, J. E., & Sherbourne, C. D. (1992). The MOS 36-Item Short-Form Health Survey (SF-36). I. Conceptual framework and item selection. *Medical Care, 30*, 473–483.

Wennberg, D. E., & Wennberg, J. E. (2003). Addressing variations: Is there hope for the future? *Health Affairs (Web Exclusive),* W3, 614–617.

Wennberg, J. E., Fisher, E. S., Goodman, D. C., & Skinner, J. S. (2008). *Tracking the care of patients with severe chronic illness.* The Dartmouth Institute for Health Policy & Clinical Practice. www.dartmouthatlas.org.

12

Two Decades of Research on Physical Restraint: Impact on Practice and Policy

Lois K. Evans and Neville E. Strumpf

All myths seem implausible in retrospect, but it is truly audacious to challenge them while we are still in their thrall. —Carol Lindemann

This chapter describes, within historical and sociopolitical contexts, a program of research on restraint use with older adults and traces the complex circumstances by which evidence derived from research helped inform policy and change an embedded practice.

HOW IT STARTED

In 1985, Doris Schwartz sent a clarion call through the world of geriatrics with her "Call for Help" in *Geriatric Nursing*, asking for information on what she considered to be an all-too-prevalent and increasingly recalcitrant clinical problem, the routine use of physical restraints in the care of frail older adults in hospitals and nursing homes (Schwartz, 1985a). Schwartz's query elicited 126 relevant references to published literature on the use of restraints (Schwartz, 1985b). The results of her initial plea set us on a two-decade journey of discovery, dissemination, and advocacy to uncover the reasons for such practices, to provide a scientific rationale for change, and to promulgate a model of individualized, restraint-free care.

Simultaneous with the publication of Schwartz's call, and with her assistance, we were able to interview three residents of a continuing-care retirement community, each of whom had been restrained during a recent hospitalization. Among the residents' recollections were these (Strumpf, Evans, & Schwartz, 1991):

"Sometimes I feel my wrists still hurt. I told the nurse I would write a story if I could, but it would scare people. Usually I meet life by trying to forget the bad things, but this was such a vivid experience. I haven't forgotten the pain and the indignity of being tied" (p. 330).

"I was not exactly out of contact; I realized what was going on. Both of my feet were restrained, making it impossible to turn over or even to pull myself up. If anyone tried to explain, I don't remember, but I can still hear myself saying, 'Please, oh, please undo my feet.' Queer things happened to me. They say it was dreams, but I think I had hallucinations" (p. 330).

Quickly, we recognized how little research existed demonstrating any efficacy whatsoever for the widespread use of physical restraints. We thus began in earnest to systematically examine the literature, gather preliminary data through interviews, and engage in pilot research. In brief, these efforts yielded important insights and several critical papers during the early years of our work.

Our comprehensive review of the literature on physical restraint appeared in the *Journal of the American Geriatrics Society* in 1989, with the opening line, "Everyday in the United States over 500,000 older people in hospitals and nursing homes are tied to their beds and chairs" (Evans & Strumpf, 1989). Later that same year, Tamar Lewin, in a lead article in the *New York Times*, began her story with nearly identical words (but no citation): "Every day more than 500,000 elderly Americans in nursing homes and hospitals, most of them frail and demented, are tied to their beds or wheelchairs. But institutions across the country are re-examining their use of restraints" (Lewin, 1989). At the time our review paper was published, 10 studies had been completed on physical restraint (2 of these were ours), indicating a prevalence rate in various settings from 6% to 86%, a high risk of restraint for persons with cognitive impairment, and no evidence that restraints safeguarded patients from injury. The paper, which laid out an agenda for research, has been cited 176 times (ISI Web of Science).

In a similar vein, we also examined the myths associated with restraint use, which was published as a State-of-the-Science paper in *IMAGE: Journal of Nursing Scholarship* (now the *Journal of Nursing Scholarship*) in 1990 (Evans & Strumpf, 1990); it has been cited some 31 times. Using what was then the extant body of literature, we refuted six myths surrounding the use of physical restraints: (1) The old should be restrained because they are more likely to fall and seriously injure themselves; (2) it is a moral duty to use physical restraints because they protect patients from harm; (3) failure to restrain puts individuals and facilities at risk for legal liability; (4) restraint does not really bother older people; (5) restraint is necessary because of inadequate staffing; and (6) alternatives to physical restraint are unavailable. On the basis of existing evidence, we concluded that not one of these statements was true at the time, nor are they true today, although the evidence is far more compelling now than 20 years ago.

Having critically analyzed what literature did exist, and building on those early interviews with discharged older women, our first study determined (a) the subjective impact of physical restraints on hospitalized patients and (b) their nurses' beliefs about use of restraints (Strumpf & Evans, 1988). We shared their poignant stories in this widely cited (95 times) paper; the findings confirmed the deep emotional impact of restraint on patients, who described anger, discomfort, resistance, and fear in response to the experience of restraint. It was clear as well that the decision to restrain posed for the nursing staff a conflict between protection of the patient and beliefs about professional behavior. In addition, lack of interdisciplinary collaboration in decisions to use a physical restraint was apparent from progress notes written by nurses and physicians in the healthcare record, especially in the case of one patient who was continuously restrained for 121 days! Our conclusions, which have been echoed over and over in many succeeding and more sophisticated studies, with little change, was the following: "When physical restraints are used, they need to be considered a special treatment requiring further assessment, intensive monitoring, and change in management in consultation with other members of the healthcare team. Most urgent is the need for testing alternative interventions and the possible elimination of restraining devices except under the most extreme short-term circumstances" (p. 137).

Two pilot studies (both with intramural funding) followed, focusing on the nursing home setting. In the first, we compared restraint use between residents in a skilled and an intermediate care unit in one facility and described perceptions of residents and nurses and environmental factors that may contribute to behavior resulting in restraint (Strumpf & Evans, 1987). In the second, we observed 826 older adults in nine Scottish acute and long-term care facilities and confirmed what we had been hearing from others: that restraint use was essentially nonexistent (prevalence of 3.8%, consisting of only one side rail, two seat belts, 10 geriatric chairs, and 19 Buxton chairs, the latter used primarily for positioning; Evans, Strumpf, & Williams, 1991). Attention to needs in a personalized, homelike atmosphere was paramount in all facilities.

Among our early studies, the one with the greatest personal impact was an examination of care practices at the Victoria Geriatric Unit in Glasgow, Scotland, and Grabergets Sjukhem in Goteborg, Sweden, in 1990. With support from The Commonwealth Fund, an interdisciplinary team consisting of two nurses, a social worker, a physician, and an architect conducted intensive observations and interviews and collected data on staffing patterns, staff perceptions of restraint use ($n = 210$), and resident incident, functional, demographic, and health data ($n = 460$). We were astounded to discover that there were no vest, wrist, ankle, or other restraining devices in use, despite the moderate to severe functional impairments of most residents; few serious injuries from falls; minimal use of psychotropic medications; and lack of nurses' belief in the efficacy of restraints. We attributed these findings to (1) a philosophy centered on "individualized care," reasonable risk taking, and quality of life; (2) standards set and maintained by nursing and medical staff with geriatric expertise; (3) an environment emphasizing "normalization," with equipment tailored to personal needs; and (4) care practices for behavioral symptoms based on thorough assessment and evaluation. Application of a physical restraint was deemed "a last resort" (Evans, Strumpf, & Williams, 1991; Strumpf, Evans, Williams, Williams, & Middleton, 1991; Strumpf & Tomes, 1993).

Work completed up to this point led to a study funded by the Alzheimer's Association testing the feasibility of an education/consultation protocol to reduce physical restraints in a nursing home (Evans & Strumpf, 1992), and finally, to funding in 1990 by the National Institute on Aging (NIA) of the first, and still only, United States–based clinical trial to reduce restraints in nursing homes (Evans et al., 1997). To proceed with this story, however, requires attention to the historical context of the period and its influence on policy and practice relevant to the use of physical restraints and to our ongoing program of research.

Historical Context

What over time came to be known as the "restraint-free care movement" was possible because of related social movements that began in the 1950s, including the Civil Rights and the Women's Movements. Their associated strategies and outcomes may have influenced reform ideology about elder care. From a broader perspective, the end of the Cold War, with its social and political themes of "containment and control," perhaps fed into the increasing global calls for freedom, liberty, autonomy, community, and humanism (Fairman & Happ, 1998; Judd, 2010a). By the 1980s, these same ideals were also permeating dialogue about access to healthcare, social care for those with disabilities, and the right to die as examples, all in a period of economic and social conservatism (Judd, 2010b). At the same time, the rapid aging of the population was becoming obvious to all, and concerns over cost and quality in healthcare were growing. Many of the leaders and advocates of the restraint-free care movement were molded by these prior movements of the 1950s and 1960s, embracing strong values and commitments to autonomy and humanism. It is possible that the movement may yet come to represent what Delli Carpini (1989) describes as a "restructuring" generational change, one involving institutional development and support sufficient to maintain and transfer alternate norms, values, and behavior (p. 47). Because change begun during this period is still ongoing, only time will tell its outcome. It is important to note, however, that although the social movement itself was supported by the research base produced by our work and that of others, it was fueled by these much broader cultural, social, economic, and political forces interacting at the time.

In 1986, the Institute of Medicine (IOM) issued its sweeping report on "Improving the Quality of Care in Nursing Homes," which came about when the Health Care Financing Administration (HCFA; now the Centers for Medicare & Medicaid Services [CMS]) asked the IOM to undertake a study that would "serve as a basis for adjusting federal (and state) policies and regulations governing the certification of nursing homes so as to make those policies and regulations as appropriate and effective as possible" (IOM, 1986, p. 2). At the time of the IOM study, federal regulations governing nursing homes under the Medicare and Medicaid programs had been in place, essentially unchanged, since the mid-1970s. There was broad consensus that government regulation of nursing homes was unsatisfactory because it allowed too many marginal or substandard nursing homes to continue in operation; many individuals in nursing homes were "subject to physical abuse," and some received "shockingly deficient" care that hastened "deterioration of their physical, mental, and emotional health" (p. 2). Cited as well was a study of resident attitudes conducted by the National Citizens' Coalition for Nursing Home Reform indicating that residents were "often treated with disrespect, and frequently denied choices of food, of roommates, of the time they rise and go to sleep, of their activities, of the clothes they wear, and of when and where they may visit with family and friends" (p. 2).

In its 432-page report, the IOM concluded that (1) quality of care and quality of life in many nursing homes were not satisfactory, (2) more effective government regulation could substantially improve quality in nursing homes, (3) specific improvements were needed in the regulatory system, (4) improvements in quality of care in nursing homes, in many cases, were independent of changes in Medicaid payment policies or bed supply, (5) regulation was necessary but not sufficient for high-quality care, (6) a system to obtain standardized data on residents was essential, and (7) the regulatory system should be dynamic and evolutionary in outlook. A detailed list of recommended regulatory criteria followed, many of which were ultimately legislated with the passage of the Nursing Home Reform Act, part of the Omnibus Budget Reconciliation Act (OBRA) in 1987. Of note, the act included a set of Resident Rights, including the right to be free from restraints. The act went into effect in October 1990, the same year that we received funding for our clinical trial.

The HCFA's Proposed Rules governing use of physical restraints, which appeared in the *Federal Register* (U.S. Government, 1992), defined a physical restraint as "any manual method or physical or mechanical device, material, or equipment attached or adjacent to the resident's body that the resident cannot remove easily, which restricts freedom of movement or access to his body," noting that such devices could be imposed only "to treat the resident's medical symptoms which include but are not limited to physical, emotional and behavioral problems." Other proposed wording addressed emergency and nonemergency circumstances, use of devices as a last resort, progressive removal and least restrictive means of restraint, explanations to families and residents for restraint use, and record keeping (National Citizens' Coalition for Nursing Home Reform, 1992). In a personal correspondence dated April 1, 1992, we addressed our comments to the HCFA, noting that language in the proposed Conditions of Participation and Requirements inadvertently undermined the law's original intent, which was to move away from a care model aimed at "controlling behavior" to one attuned to "individualized approaches to understanding and responding to the needs being expressed by residents." In succeeding iterations of the Conditions of Participation, language was gradually put in place to address these initial concerns, with an emphasis on assessment for underlying problems and individualized care (Department of Health and Human Services [DHHS], 2007). Fortunately, with this far-reaching legislation, a move toward limiting the use of physical restraints in nursing homes, in sharp contrast to the wholesale prevalence of the past, had finally begun.

During the 1980s and early 1990s, the tireless efforts of advocates at the National Citizens' Coalition for Nursing Home Reform in Washington, DC, and at The Kendall Corporation in Kennett Square, Pennsylvania, brought attention to conditions in nursing homes and to the problem of physical restraint, culminating in a 1989 symposium before the U.S. Senate Special Committee on Aging, chaired by Senator John Heinz (Kendal Corporation, 1999) and to which we contributed. In testimony by advocates, healthcare providers, and consumers, physical restraint, a potent symbol of poor quality care affecting the most vulnerable elders, was made visible to legislators, thus creating an opportunity to change practice forever. More or less simultaneously, many investigative reporters began uncovering the horrors of restraint use, among them, Nohlgren's report on restraint reform for the *St. Petersburg Times* (Florida) in 1987 (Nohlgren, 1987), Freedberg's in the *Wall Street Journal* in 1988 (Freedberg, 1988), and Rigert and Lerner's four-part series in 1990 in the *Minnesota Star Tribune* (Rigert & Lerner, 1990). Rigert and Lerner noted the research of Steven Miles, who, through careful examination of Minnesota death records, determined the frequency of death by strangulation and asphyxiation from physical restraints. Miles' shockingly compelling findings later appeared in *The Gerontologist* (Miles & Irvine, 1991; Miles & Irvine, 1992) and the *Journal of the American Geriatrics Society* (Miles, 1996).

Another powerful voice early on was that of social worker Carter Williams, later one of the founders of the Pioneer Network (in 1997), an organization focused on changing the culture of aging and long-term care. Long an advocate for more homelike environments in nursing homes, Williams (1985) became convinced through her observations in Sweden that America could do better. She described the concept of "individualized care" and challenged us to look beyond the mere removal of restraints to ensure the well-being of the whole person and to restore human rights for choice, sense of control over daily life, respect, and dignity. She gave voice to the person living in a nursing home (Williams, 1989). Other important voices include those of Marshall Kapp (1999), whose sage legal treatment of the issue of restraints in both nursing homes and hospitals helped to assuage the angst of healthcare risk managers, and Bart Collopy (1988), who brought an ethical stance to the issue of autonomy and quality of life in nursing homes among caregivers, consumers, and their advocates.

Remarkable during this period was the amount of personal correspondence (more than 200 letters) that we received, before the age of e-mail. (This material is archived at the Barbara Bates Center for the Study of the History of Nursing at the University of Pennsylvania). Initially, many were requests for more information based on talks we had given, media reports, or the article that appeared in *Nursing Research* in 1988. Investigators wishing to replicate the 1988 study in Dublin, Ireland; Calgary, Canada; Dayton and Columbus, Ohio; and Bundoora, Australia, sought permission to use the Perceptions of Restraint Use Questionnaire and the Subjective Experience of Being Restrained tool. These requests continue by e-mail to this day.

Other letters were from nurses expressing gratitude for exposing the dilemmas of restraint use, for example, this from Terri Gallagher in Monroeville, Pennsylvania: "As a young nurse, I often experience personal conflicts between what I was taught in school and the reality I confront daily as a staff nurse. . . . Your article heightened my awareness to really think about the purpose for restraints prior to using them." A handwritten note (1990) came from Evelyn Cole, a physical therapist in Santa Barbara, California, indicating that she had read an article in her local newspaper; she "found the use of restraints unsatisfactory and demeaning" and wanted to "learn more about ending restraints in nursing homes." A nurse from Boonville, Mississippi, had likewise read an article referencing our work in a newspaper and wanted more information on restraint-free nursing homes and alternatives to restraint. We also heard from those who had experienced success in reducing restraints, like this from Carol Love with the Illinois Department of Public Aid, where 90% of the residents had been restrained in one Illinois nursing home. With the arrival of a "dedicated and dynamic nurse," a totally restraint-free environment was created at Fountain Terrace, where Love reported that "residents who haven't talked in years are talking and residents who haven't walked in years are walking! . . . Staff have more time for resident interactions and while not researched, the staff morale and job satisfaction seem improved."

Others explicitly asked for help in implementing a standard of restraint-free care at their institutions, including the Massachusetts General Hospital in Boston (1990). As an interesting postscript to the latter request, we were the first nurses ever invited to give medical grand rounds at Massachusetts General Hospital in 2003, where we spoke to a packed auditorium of physicians, nurses, and other healthcare providers on restraint-free care for hospitalized elders. Increasingly, requests for information and assistance came from organizations, including the American Red Cross to review their Nurse Assistant Training Program (Bruce Spitz, 1988); the U.S. Senate Special Committee on Aging, to give testimony at Senate hearings (David Pryor, 1989; Philip Boyle [The Hastings Center], 1991); the American Nurses' Association (Pam Mittelstadt, 1990), to review the Resident Assessment Protocols for the Minimum Data Set; the HCFA, to provide guidance on strengthening the standards for restraint use in nursing homes (Sam Kidder, 1990); and the Mental Health Legal Advisors Committee for the Supreme Judicial Court of the Commonwealth of Massachusetts (1991), to supply research findings that would help end "barbaric, harmful, and inhumane modalities of treatment."

Media reports, consumer anguish, and advocacy, however, do not, in and of themselves, create an evidence base for changing practice. As noted above, other than what had been uncovered up until 1990 by our preliminary research and that of several others in the United States and abroad (Appelbaum & Roth, 1984; Cape, 1983; Yarmesch & Sheafor, 1984; Mitchell-Pederson, Edmund, Fingerote et al., 1985; Frengley & Mion, 1986; Morrison, Crinklaw-Wiancko, King, Thibeault, & Wells, 1987; Robbins, Boyko, Lane et al., 1987; Mion, Frengley, Jakovcic & Marion, 1989), the state of the science remained meager, and resistance to change was considerable. In his Kent Lecture at the Annual Meeting of the Gerontological Society of America in 1987, T. Franklin Williams, then Director of the NIA, started by reminding the audience that "good care for older people depends upon what we have learned from research" (Williams, 1988, p. 579). Williams then went on to give numerous examples of the positive impact of research on care, then asked, paradoxically, "why is it that we have trouble accepting modest but clearly valuable advances" when, for example, "we know that restraints are very harmful to people . . . yet we tolerate them in most nursing homes?" (p. 583). He observed further that the evidence from a few nursing homes in the United States and abroad had already "demonstrated that, through truly individualized approaches to care, restraints are never needed" (p. 583). Despite all of the progress in basic science and its importance, Williams concluded that "We need more professionals, more leaders, who have personal experience in both research and care, who through their own experiences can best spot and appreciate the ways that research can gain from the observations made in caring for older people" (p. 585).

It is worth noting as well that the NIA was founded in 1974, only 13 years before Williams' address, to improve the health and well-being of older adults through research and training in aging (National Institutes of Health [NIH], 2009a). By the late 1980s, its portfolio in the three designated research areas—biomedical, social, and behavioral—was well developed and focused not only on biological aging and disease processes in late life but also on other special problems and needs of the aged, including integrated longitudinal studies. At the still nascent National Center for Nursing Research (created by the Congress in 1985, later the National Institute for Nursing Research), consensus on a National Nursing Research Agenda was just beginning to emerge by the end of the 1980s. Seven priority areas were finally identified, one of which was long-term care for older adults (NIH, 2009b). (The NIH has continued to support the development of science relevant to restraint practice and quality of care for older adults. A review of funded research using the CRISP database [fall, 2009] revealed 27 studies directly or indirectly related to restraint use funded primarily by the NIA, NINR, or Agency for Healthcare Research and Quality between 1990 and 2008. These studies include training [F31 and K series] and R series mechanisms that are nearly equally divided in setting, with 12 situated in hospitals and 15 in nursing homes. There were no clinical trials on reducing restraints, but many trials for prevention of falls or agitation included restraint as one covariate or outcome.)

BUILDING A PROGRAM OF RESEARCH ON PHYSICAL RESTRAINT

Against this backdrop, during the early implementation of the Nursing Home Reform Act, we carried out a prospective 12-month NIA-funded clinical trial to reduce restraints in nursing homes from 1990 to 1992 (Evans et al., 1997). Framed within change theory, its purpose was to investigate the relative effects of two experimental interventions on the use of physical restraints. Three voluntary nursing homes in the Philadelphia area were randomly assigned to one of three conditions: restraint education (RE), RE with consultation

(REC), and control (C). A total of 463 of the 643 nursing home residents over the age of 60 years who were enrolled at baseline remained to completion (1 year). Both the RE and REC homes received intensive education by a master's-prepared gerontologic nurse to increase staff awareness of restraint hazards and knowledge about assessing and managing resident behaviors likely to lead to use of restraints. In addition, the REC home received 12 hours per week of unit-based nursing consultation to facilitate restraint reduction in residents with more complex conditions. The intervention lasted for 6 months. Compared with baseline, the REC home had a statistically significant reduction in restraint prevalence, whereas the RE and C homes did not. Relative to baseline, the rates represented an average reduction in restraint use of 23% for the RE, 11% for the C, and 56% for the REC home. The differences in changes over time were consistently significant ($p = .01$), whether considering survivors or those present at each time point and also when controlling for differences between groups at baseline. Furthermore, given any change in restraint use, REC residents were between 25% and 40% more likely than either RE or C residents to experience decreased restraint use. Most importantly, results were achieved without increased staff, psychoactive drugs, or serious fall-related injuries. That this was possible refuted many past arguments for the continued practice of physical restraint.

Accompanying the research report was a collaborative commentary by social worker Carter Williams and basic scientist Caleb Finch, with a definitive conclusion: "physical restraint places highly destructive, measurable stress on people and animals" (Williams & Finch, 1997, p. 773). With publication of the results of the first controlled clinical trial on the removal of restraints (now cited 78 times, and its data recently contributed to a meta-analysis in process for a Cochrane review), Williams and Finch noted a "significant point at which to take stock and chart a new direction," urging "restraint-free care that will promote wellbeing and avoid adding further stress, injury, and disability to older people whose function is already compromised" (p. 774).

In addition to the paper reporting the chief findings of this clinical trial, nine other data-based papers from this trial were published. These further evaluated restraint reduction in relation to psychoactive drugs (Siegler et al., 1997), falls and injuries (Capezuti, Strumpf, Evans, Grisso, & Maislin, 1998; Capezuti, Strumpf, Evans, & Maislin, 1999), behavioral syndromes (Kolanowski, Hurwitz, Taylor, Evans, & Strumpf, 1994), initiation of restraint and predictors of continued use (Sullivan-Marx, Strumpf, Evans, Baumgarten, & Maislin, 1999a; Sullivan-Marx, Strumpf, Evans, Baumgarten, & Maislin, 1999b), side-rail use and bed-related fall outcomes (Capezuti, Maislin, Strumpf, & Evans, 2002), correlates of aggression (Talerico, Evans, & Strumpf, 2002), and depression in dementia (Kurlowicz, Evans, Strumpf, & Maislin, 2002). Taken together, there was now substantive evidence, with regard to physical restraint use in nursing homes, that (1) physical restraints could be safely removed from frail nursing home residents; (2) symptoms such as falls, treatment interference, and behaviors required careful assessment and targeted individualized interventions; (3) physical restraint contributed to falls and serious injuries, as well as aggression and other mental health symptoms; (4) implementation of stringent guidelines and standards did not, by themselves, alter practice behaviors; and (5) maintenance in changes in practice and a culture of caring required ongoing vigilance and professional expertise, preferably guided by advanced practice nurses.

Observing that nursing home residents were frequently restrained when admitted to the hospital, we continued our research with a second R01 to follow nonrestrained nursing home residents as they were transferred to acute care. We employed an advanced practice nurse intervention to reduce the initiation and duration of in-hospital restraint.

Findings from this study included that behavioral symptoms were the only preadmission characteristic that predicted initiation of restraint use by the hospital nurse (Evans, Capezuti, Strumpf, & Maislin, 1999) and that postdischarge physical function was more than three times worse for patients who were restrained, controlling for preadmission and hospital status (Strumpf, Evans, Capezuti, & Maislin, 1997). Elders with the advanced practice registered nurse (APRN) intervention were 6.8 times less likely to be restrained at any time during their hospital stay ($p = .002$; Sullivan-Marx, Strumpf, Evans, Capezuti, & Maislin, 2003). Organizational factors contributing to restraint initiation and continued use were also identified (Bourbonniere, Strumpf, Evans & Maislin, 2003).

In 2000, in the *Annual Review of Nursing Research*, Sue Donaldson undertook a review of breakthroughs in nursing research that have changed thinking about human health within and beyond the discipline of nursing (Donaldson, 2000). She described our work as "pathbreaking" and a contribution to "philosophical debate and research that stimulated a multidisciplinary shift in thinking about the care of elders from a view of usefulness of physical restraints for safe care to acceptance of restraint-free environments as the approach for humane and individualized care" (p. 258). Donaldson acknowledged as well the significance of the timing of our early work "during a period of growing societal rebellion against the then prevalent custodial care of elders in the United States."

In 1995, we were recognized with the Sigma Theta Tau Baxter Foundation Episteme Award, affording us the opportunity to reflect on our research to date. In that acceptance, we noted that "changing practice was not as simple as merely reducing restraints, or removing them altogether, but involved an entire paradigm shift" (and that) "perceptions and habits developed and reinforced over decades would have to be replaced by more individualized approaches to care."

FACTORS RELATED TO THE SHIFT IN PRACTICE

As described previously, the rights of vulnerable people, from adults living with disabilities to frail older people in nursing homes, were embraced during the 1980s–1990s. The Nursing Home Reform Act (OBRA 1987) included most of the points made in the IOM report of 1986 and put into motion a mandated change in the use of physical (and chemical) restraints. As demonstrated by data from our clinical trial, however, regulations alone were ineffective in changing restraint practices, at least in the short run. In our control nursing home, for example, very little occurred in the 12 months after the implementation of OBRA, despite sufficient concern by the facility to seek consultation and to replace many restraints with less restrictive devices (Evans et al., 1997; Evans, Strumpf, Capezuti, Taylor, & Jacobsen, 1992). National Citizen's Coalition for Nursing Home Reform advocates and others continued to urge that behavior be viewed as a symptom of "something gone awry," a problem to be addressed, not "controlled" (Happ, Williams, Strumpf, & Burger, 1996). Providers in nursing homes and hospitals throughout the country struggled to comply with new regulations and standards but found it challenging to change entrenched practice. For a brief period, at least one CMS region published a newsletter on restraints, noting the successes by various states to decrease their rates (Strumpf & Evans, 1993). Other projects, including that of the Jewish Home and Hospital, with support from The Commonwealth Fund (Neufeld et al., 1999), assisted nursing homes on a larger scale to change practice through education, often using train-the-trainer models. In addition, statewide projects, like the Pennsylvania Restraint Reduction Initiative (Blakeslee, 1999) and Untie the

Elderly of the Kendal Corporation (1999), together with training efforts by the National Citizens' Coalition for Nursing Home Reform (NCCNHR) and other groups, achieved positive change in many facilities.

In 1991, the Joint Commission for Accreditation of Healthcare Organizations (JCAHO, 1991) released guidelines for restraint use in hospitals. These focused on medical need for restraint but did not address patient behavior as a symptom or sign of altered health status or communication of an unmet need. The 1996 revisions of the JCAHO acknowledged the risks associated with restraint but not "risky behavior" as a serious reason for assessment and intervention (JCAHO, 1996). Although no national data are available even now, a series of hospital-based research projects, most notably those of Mion and Minnick (Mion et al., 2001; Minnick, Mion, Johnson, Catrambone, & Leipzig, 2007), demonstrated success in hospital medical and surgical units in nearly eliminating restraint, except for intensive care units, which continue to struggle with the challenge of balancing risk and dignity. Despite mounting evidence of restraint-associated deaths, the Food and Drug Administration (FDA), with jurisdiction over such medical devices, was slow to respond. In 1992, after a spate of exposés in the media and professional journals, the FDA issued a Medical Alert on the potential hazards of restraint devices and required better labeling and reporting (U.S. FDA, 1992). As Capezuti and colleagues (2008) describe, however, industry pressure contributed to the FDA's 7-year delay in posting new expert panel recommendations on hazardous hospital bed design, posing another barrier to continued improvements in practice.

In hospitals, especially, but also nursing homes, healthcare risk managers supported routine use of physical restraint and felt that failure to restrain posed a greater legal liability than did injuries or death from restraint (Kapp, 1999). As our work was increasingly published and cited, we were bombarded with requests to serve as expert witnesses on legal cases of restraint and nonrestraint. Unable to take most of these consultations while conducting research, yet recognizing the importance of changing case law as a way to alter practice, we utilized the existing University of Pennsylvania School of Nursing Gerontologic Nursing Consultation Service (now Penn Nursing Consultation Service; Evans, McCausland, Lang, Chiverton, & Strumpf, 2004) and recruited and trained additional geriatric APRNs in the standards of nonrestraint and individualized care. An analysis of requests regarding restraints received between 1994 and 2006 revealed that, of 60 restraint or restraint-related cases reviewed by consultants, 56 were referred between 1997 and 2002 (unreported data from Gerontologic Nursing Consultation Service files), a peak period for litigation on restraint use. By the 2000s, it was generally understood that the standard of practice had become appropriate assessment and intervention, not restraint (Kapp, 2008).

Dialogue and dissemination were also critically important to changes in practice and policy. An interdisciplinary work group on "Risk Taking, Choice and Control: The Case of Physical Restraints" was created within the Gerontological Society of America, which grew to include 50 members over its course (1992–1995). During the late 1980s through the 1990s, papers regarding restraint were highlighted at the annual meetings of nearly every professional and multidisciplinary society related to older adults. These efforts built greater awareness, including the subtleties of language (e.g., *protective device* as a substitute for *physical restraint*), which served to deny the cruel realities of restraint practices. As can be seen in Figure 12.1, during this early period, we presented at grand rounds, national and international keynote addresses, and regional talks. Figure 12.1 further attests to our dissemination efforts, through peer-reviewed papers (research

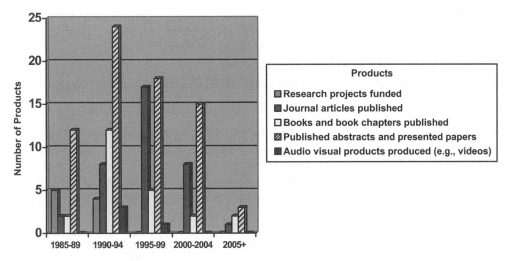

FIGURE 12.1 Research and dissemination activities over time.

and clinical), published abstracts, books, and book chapters. Every new text and encyclopedia included a chapter on restraints; we also produced a practical book (Strumpf, Robinson, Wagner, & Evans, 1998) and two papers (Strumpf, Evans, Wagner & Patterson, 1992; Patterson, Strumpf, & Evans, 1995) based on the educational program tested in our clinical trial, as well as four videotapes, all aimed at end users "at the bedside" and emphasizing a paradigmatic shift in practice. Titles of papers reflect our commitment to research translation and organizational change, e.g., "Creating a Restraint-Free Environment"' and "Framing Difficult Behaviors: Strategies to Reduce Restraints."

Finally, evidence-based clinical practice guidelines related to patient safety or care of persons with dementia or delirium published on www.guidelines.gov now include research-based statements regarding the use of restraints. Currently, only one guideline directly related to physical restraint use is posted (University of Iowa Gerontological Nursing Interventions Research Center, 2005). Focused on changing the practice of restraint use in acute care, it emphasizes understanding and assessing the meaning of behavior versus automatic application of restraint. Current guidelines on delirium and dementia consistently recommend "avoid restraint," "eliminate restraint," and "provide restraint-free care"; the guideline on falls identifies restraint as a risk factor for falling.

EVOLUTION OF A NEW PARADIGM OF PRACTICE

Our program of research provided much needed evidence on the harmful effects of restraint use, the lack of interdisciplinary dialogue and problem solving about complex geriatric care, and the strongly held beliefs about the efficacy of restraints. Indeed, as Kane and colleagues (1993) noted, "it was not until the late 1980s that the articles by Evans and Strumpf raised awareness of American professionals to the possibility that restraining patients was often not only unnecessary, but harmful" (p. 548). After two NIH-funded clinical studies, we concluded that changing an embedded practice is indeed possible, but sustaining change requires ongoing vigilance and organizational commitment. Taken as a whole, the research refined a standard of practice and a concept of individualized care (Evans, 1996) and contributed to a multidisciplinary paradigm shift regarding safe and humane care for frail elders in all settings (Evans & Strumpf, 2004).

The early paper published in *Nursing Research* giving voice to elders' experience of restraint was instrumental in facilitating this change. Once restraints were accurately labeled and removed, it became not only *possible* but also impossible *not* to view nursing home residents as people, existing in an often deficient, noxious environment. Such awareness provided fertile ground for the Pioneer Network (2009) movement, studies of at-homeness (Moloney, McDonald, & Palmisamo-Mills, 2007) "green" and small houses (Kane, Luan, Cutler et al., 2007), and renewed efforts for individualized restraint-free care. Research on side rails and falls prevention (Capezuti, Wagner, Brush et al., 2002), as well as nonpharmacologic management of agitated and aggressive behavior (Kong, Guevera, & Evans, 2009), also contributed to an understanding of resident behavior and ways to provide for normal safety, while not robbing the person of freedom of movement.

CAUTIONARY TALES

Castle and Mor (1998), in a review of the literature describing the impact of the Health Care Reform Act (OBRA 87) on restraint use, found a reduction in the years after its implementation, from 44% in 1989 to 27% in 1991 to 21% in 1996. When we concluded our clinical trial, the restraint rate at the *best* of the three facilities was 14% (down from 32%), whereas the national average was ~27% (Evans et al., 1997). Overall, the restraint rates have continued to decline, such that in 2009, the national average for nursing homes is 4% and 2% in Pennsylvania (CMS, 2009). Lest we think that this means that the problem is solved, however, one must take note that while at least 20% of nursing homes across the country have *no* restraint use, some 10% report between 20% and 40%, and there remains wide regional and state variation (Capezuti, Brush, Won, Wagner, & Lawson, 2008). Furthermore, a recent report substantiates the negative health effects for residents when restraints are initiated in nursing homes (Engberg, Castle, & McCaffrey, 2008). Just a few weeks ago, evoking memories of that flurry of letters in the 1980s, we received an e-mail plea for help from a son for advice about his father's behavior and subsequent restraint. Just last week, the palliative care team in our own institution reported an increase in restraint of elders in the home setting, purportedly by family members. Restraint use in home care is described in a recent paper from The Netherlands published in the *Journal of the American Geriatrics Society* (de Veer, Francke, Buijse, & Friele, 2009). Assisted-living facilities also utilize restraints, as identified in a recent study comparing large and small assisted-living facilities in Maryland (see Leroi et al., 2007), and racial differences in nursing home restraint raise a new concern (Miller, Papandonatos, Fennell, & Mor, 2006).

Indeed, a surprising number of publications regarding restraint prevalence and associated factors are appearing in recent journals from around the world, primarily Australia (Myers, Nikoletti, & Hill, 2001; Moore & Haralambous, 2007; Mott, Poole, & Kenrick, 2005; Retsas, 1998), Canada (Milke, Kendall, Neumann, Wark, & Knopp, 2008), Great Britain (Healey, Cronberg, & Oliver, 2009; Gallinagh, Nevin, McAleese, & Campbell, 2001; Healey, Cronberg, & Oliver, 2009), Germany (Bredthauer, Becker, Eichner, Koczy, & Nikolaus, 2005), Israel (Hendel, Fradkin, & Kidron, 2004), China (Woo, Hui, Chan, Chi, & Sham, 2004), Taiwan (Chuang & Huang, 2007), Norway (Testad, Aasland, & Aasland, 2005), Sweden (Fonad, Wahlin, Winblad, Emami, & Sandmark, 2008), Finland (Pekkarinen, Elovainio, Sinervo, Finne-Soveri, & Noro, 2006), and the Netherlands (de Veer et al.,

2009). One cross-national study in nine European countries reported restraint prevalence rates of from zero to 22% in geriatric hospital departments and from 2% to 19% in nursing homes (de Vries, Ligthart, & Mikolaus, 2004). Most of these papers are focused on describing the practice, its prevalence, and associated factors, including the experience, perceptions, and/or attitudes of nurses, elders, and families (Chuang & Huang, 2007; Hendel, Fradkin, & Kidron, 2004; Hardin, Magee, Vinson, Owen, & Hyatt, 1994; Myers, Nikoletti, & Hill, 2001; Gallinagh, Nevin, McAleese, & Campbell, 2001; Gallinagh, Nevin, Campbell, Mitchell, & Ludwick, 2001; Molassiotis & Newell, 1996). Taken as a whole, these papers are reflective of American publications 20 years ago. They are concerning because they are from many of these same countries that we first learned and were inspired, in the late 1980s, about restraint-free care! To date, only one paper from Norway and two others from one team in the Netherlands report trials to test the effect of staff training on restraint use or initiation in nursing homes (Testad, Aasland, & Aasland, 2005) or psychogeriatric units (Huizing, Hamers, Gulpers, & Berger 2006; Huizing, Hamers, Gulpers, & Berger 2009), the latter two with mixed results.

In the United States, in the early 1990s, it was not uncommon to see reports of research to facilitate the proper application and monitoring of restraints (Schnelle, Simmons, & Ory, 1992); now, in 2007, we have a study to test the comparative safety of the net bed against standard restraint in agitated hospital patients (Nawaz et al., 2007), demonstrating that the paradigm shift is not yet complete. A further, perhaps unplanned, threat is the introduction of a quality initiative to focus attention on potentially preventable iatrogenic hospital events. One of the first events for attention is falls, and advocates have raised concern about the likelihood of a return to restraint as a short-sighted, short-term solution to prevent falls (Inouye, Brown, & Tinetti, 2009). Thus, it appears that, nationally and globally, the work is not yet done.

WHAT CAN WE CONCLUDE AND WHERE DO WE GO FROM HERE?

The story of restraint reduction or elimination is one of exposing, uprooting, and abandoning an embedded, non-evidence-based practice. Among its profound lessons: changing the law is one thing, but changing minds (values, attitudes, and beliefs) and practice is far more difficult. Sometimes, "the stars are aligned" and we find ourselves in a "perfect storm" or, at least, at a "tipping point" (Gladwell, 2000). In the case of physical restraints, a social movement was already afoot in the United States when we began our work. The late 1980s represented a period of ferment about restraints: The IOM report on quality of care in nursing homes was published; newspaper reporters uncovered stories of related deaths; and the NCCNHR campaigned for improved standards of care. A few clinicians demonstrated the possibility of restraint-free care. Policy makers, attorneys, ethicists, researchers, and consumers increasingly were drawn into this discussion and debate. Our program of research and dissemination, strategically planned to include a focus on patients, hospitals, and nursing homes—American and European—and a model to change the practice provided the needed impetus for the movement. The research was timely and, without precedent, then became status quo.

Today, the moral correctness of the restraint-free care movement seems much less strident, yet at the same time, work quietly continues at the CMS to update the interpretive guidelines on an ongoing basis. The most recent set of tags embrace many examples of choice in every aspect of daily life for residents (DHHS, 2009), and the CMS recently published in the *Federal Register* a new rule requiring training for staff to assure appropriateness of treatment (DHHS, 2007). Beryl Goldman (2008), an early leader for the Kendal Corporation's Untie the Elderly program, describes consumer (family) pressure as a continuing barrier to achieving restraint-free care. Her observation is supported by the research of Moore and Haralambous (2007). Targeting families (consumers) may be pivotal in moving the practice of restraint to its next level, even, we hope, to its elimination in our lifetime. Perhaps, it is time again to give voice to elders. Compelling stories of continued elder restraint, together with new science aimed at careful evaluation of the safest and most compassionate means for treating very ill older people, whether in intensive care or any place where frail, confused, and dying older people find themselves, are needed to provide the next "turning point" in this evolution in practice and policy.

REFERENCES

Appelbaum, P. S., & Roth, L. H. (1984). Involuntary treatment in medicine and psychiatry. *American Journal of Psychiatry, 141,* 202.
Blakeslee, J. A. (1999). The first ten years. *Untie the Elderly, 11*(3), 2–3.
Bourbonniere, M., Strumpf, N. E., Evans, L. K., & Maislin, G. (2003). Organizational characteristics and restraint use for hospitalized nursing home residents. *Journal of the American Geriatrics Society, 51,* 1079–1084.
Bredthauer, D., Becker, C., Eichner, B., Koczy, P., & Nikolaus, T. (2005). Factors relating to the use of physical restraints in psychogeriatric care: A paradigm for elder abuse. *Zeitschrift for Gerontology and Geriatrics, 38,* 10–18.
Cape, R. D. T. (1983). Freedom from restraint. *The Gerontologist, 23,* 217.
Capezuti, E., Brush, B. L., Won, R. M., Wagner, L. M. & Lawson, W. T. (2008). Least restrictive or least understood? Waist restraints, provider practices, and risk of harm. *Journal of Aging & Social Policy, 20*(30), 305–322.
Capezuti, E., Maislin, G., Strumpf, N., & Evans, L. (2002). Siderail use and bed-related fall outcomes among nursing home residents. *Journal of the American Geriatrics Society, 50,* 90–96.
Capezuti, E., Strumpf, N., Evans, L., Grisso, J. A., & Maislin, G. (1998). The relationship between physical restraint removal and falls and injuries among nursing home residents. *Journal of Gerontology: Medical Sciences, 53A*(1), M47–M52.
Capezuti, E., Strumpf, N., Evans, L., & Maislin, G. (1999). Outcomes of nighttime physical restraint removal for severely impaired nursing home residents. *American Journal of Alzheimer's Disease, 14*(13), 157–164.
Capezuti, E., Wagner, L. M., Brush, B. L., et al. (2007). Consequences of an intervention to reduce restrictive side rail use in nursing homes. *Journal of the American Geriatrics Society, 55,* 334–341.
Castle, N. G., & Mor, V. (1998). Physical restraints in nursing homes: A review of the literature since the Nursing Home Reform Act of 1987. *Medical Care Research & Review, 55,* 139–170.
Centers for Medicare and Medicaid Services. (2004). Nursing home compare. Available at http://www.medicare.gov/nhcompare/home.asp
Chuang, Y-H., & Huang, H-T. (2007). Nurses' feelings and thoughts about using physical restraints on hospitalized older patients. *Journal of Clinical Nursing, 16,* 486–494.
Collopy, B. (1988). Autonomy in long-term care: Some crucial distinctions. *The Gerontologist, 28*(Supplement), 10–17.
Delli Carpini, M. X. (1989). Age and history: Generations and sociopolitical change. In R. S. Sigel (Ed.), *Political learning in adulthood: A sourcebook of theory and research* (pp. 11–55). Chicago: University of Chicago Press.
de Veer, A. J. E., Francke, A. L., Buijse, R., & Friele, R. D. (2009). The use of physical restraints in home care in the Netherlands. *Journal of the American Geriatrics Society, 57,* 1881–1886.
de Vries, O. J., Ligthart, G. J., Mikolaus, T. (2004). Differences in period prevalence of the use of physical restraints in elderly inpatients of European hospitals and nursing homes. *Journals of Gerontology: Medical Sciences, 59A,* 922–923.

Department of Health and Human Services. (2007). Interpretive guidelines for restraints, §483.13(a). Available at http://www.cms.hhs.gov/CFCsAndCoPs/Downloads/som107ap_pp_guidelines_ltcf.pdf

Department of Health and Human Services. (2009). *CMS manual. System, Pub.100-07 State Operations Provider Certification.* Baltimore: Author.

Donaldson, S. (2000). Breakthroughs in scientific research: The discipline of nursing, 1960-1999. In J. J. Fitzpatrick (Ed.), *Annual Review of Nursing Research* (pp. 247–311). New York: Springer.

Engberg, J., Castle, N. G., & McCaffrey, D. (2008). Physical restraint initiation in nursing homes and subsequent resident health. *The Gerontologist, 48*(4), 442–452.

Evans, L. K. (1996), 'Knowing the patient': The route to individualized care. *Journal of Gerontological Nursing, 22*(3), 15–19.

Evans, L., Capezuti, E., Strumpf, N., & Maislin, G. (1999). Nursing home problem behavior scale: A screening tool to facilitate individualized care planning for older adults. *Proceedings of the 6ᵗʰ Annual Key Aspects Conference: Preventing and Managing Chronic Illness.* Chapel Hill: University of North Carolina.

Evans, L. K., McCausland, M. P., Lang, N. M., Chiverton, P., & Strumpf. N. E. (2004). Making academic nursing practice work in universities: Structure, function and synergy. In L. K. Evans & N. M. Lang (Eds.), *Academic nursing practice: Helping to shape the future of health care* (pp. 92–120). New York: Springer.

Evans, L. K., & Strumpf, N. E. (1989). Tying down the elderly: A review of the literature on physical restraint. *Journal of the American Geriatrics Society, 37*, 65–74.

Evans, L. K., & Strumpf, N. E. (1990). Myths about elder restraint. *IMAGE: Journal of Nursing Scholarship, 22*(2), 124–128.

Evans, L. K., & Strumpf, N. E. (1992). Reducing restraints: One nursing home's story. In S. G. Funk, E. M. Tornquist, M. T. Champagne, & R. A.Weise (Eds.), *Key aspects of elder care* (pp. 118–128). New York: Springer.

Evans, L. K., & Strumpf, N. E. (2004). Changing embedded practice: Lessons from gerontology. *Journal of Psychosocial Nursing, 42*(9), 14–17.

Evans, L. K., Strumpf, N. E., Allen-Taylor, S. L., Capezuti, E., Maislin, G., & Jacobsen, B. (1997). A clinical trial to reduce restraints in nursing homes. *Journal of the American Geriatrics Society, 45*, 675–681.

Evans, L. K., Strumpf, N. E., Capezuti, E., Taylor, L., & Jacobsen, B. (1992). Short-term effects of regulatory change on nursing home practice: The case of physical restraints. *The Gerontologist, 32*(Special Issue II), 60.

Evans, L. K., Strumpf, N. E., & Williams, C. (1991). Redefining a standard of care for frail older people: Alternatives to routine physical restraint. In P. Katz, R. Kane, & M. Mezey (Eds.), *Advances in long term care* (Vol. 1, pp. 81–108). New York: Springer.

Fairman, J., & Happ, M. B. (1998). For their own good? A historical examination of restraint use. *HEC Forum, 10*(3), 290–299.

Fonad, E., Wahlin, T.-B. R., Winblad, B., Emami, A., & Sandmark, H. (2008). Falls and fall risk among nursing home residents. *Journal of Clinical Nursing, 126*–134. doi:10.1111/j.1365-2702.2007.02005.x.

Freedberg, S. (1988, January 29). A week in a Florida nursing home shows a week of sorrow and strain. *The Wall Street Journal.*

Frengley, J. D., & Mion, L. C. (1986). Incidence of physical restraints on acute medical wards. *Journal of the American Geriatrics Society, 34*, 565–568.

Gallinagh, R., Nevin, R., McAleese, L., & Campbell, L. (2001). Perceptions of older people who have experienced physical restraint. *British Journal of Nursing, 10*, 852–859.

Gallinagh, R., Nevin, R., Campbell, L., Mitchell, F., & Ludwick, R. (2001). Relatives' perceptions of siderail use on the older person in hospital. *British Journal of Nursing, 10*(6), 391–399.

Gladwell, N. (2000). *The tipping point.* Boston: Little, Brown & Co.

Goldman, B. D. (2008). Commentary: Barriers to a sustained restraint-free environment. *Journal of Aging & Social Policy, 20*(3), 286–294.

Happ, M. B., Williams, C. C., Strumpf, N. E., & Burger, S. (1996). Individualized care for frail elders: Theory and practice. *Journal of Gerontological Nursing, 22*, 7–14.

Hardin, S. B., Magee, R., Vinson, M. H., Owen, M., & Hyatt, E. C. (1994). Patient and family perceptions of restraints. *Journal of Holistic Nursing, 11*(4), 383–397.

Healey, F. M., Cronberg, A., & Oliver, D. (2009). Bedrail use in English and Welsh hospitals. *Journal of the American Geriatrics Society, 57,* 1887–1891.

Hendel, T., Fradkin, M., & Kidron, D. (2004). Physical restraint use in health care settings: Public attitudes in Israel. *Journal of Gerontological Nursing, 30,* 12–19.

Huizing, A. R., Hamers, J. P. H., Gulpers, M. J. M., & Berger, M. P. F. (2006). Short-term effects of an educational intervention on physical restraint use; A cluster randomized trial. *BMC Geriatrics, 6,* 17. doi:10.1186/147-2318-6-17.

Huizing, A. R., Hamers, J. P. H., Gulpers, M. J. M., & Berger, M. P .F. (2009). Preventing the use of physical restraints on residents newly admitted to psycho-geriatric nursing home wards: A cluster-randomized trial. *International Journal of Nursing Studies, 46,* 459–469.

Inouye, S. K., Brown, C. J., & Tinetti, M. E. (2009). Medicare nonpayment, hospital falls and unintended consequences. *New England Journal of Medicine, 360*(23), 2390–2393.

Institute of Medicine. (1986). *Improving the quality of nursing homes.* Washington, DC: National Academy Press.

Joint Commission on Accreditation of Healthcare Organizations. (1991). Restraint and seclusion scoring guidelines. *Joint Commission Perspectives.* January–February, Insert D1-5.

Joint Commission on Accreditation of Healthcare Organizations. (1996). Restraint and seclusion standards plus scoring: Standards TX.7.1-TX.7.1.3.3. In *1996 Comprehensive accreditation manual for hospitals.* Oakbrook Terrace, IL: Author.

Judd, D. M. (2010a). Nursing in the United States from the 1960s to the early 1980s. In D. Judd, K. Sitzman, & G. M. Davis (Eds.), *A history of American nursing: Trends and eras* (pp. 150–179). Boston: Jones & Bartlett.

Judd, D. M. (2010b). Nursing in the United States from the 1980s to the present. In D. Judd, K. Sitzman, & G. M. Davis (Eds.), *A history of American nursing: Trends and eras* (pp. 180–209). Boston: Jones & Bartlett.

Kane, R. A., Luan, T. Y., Cutler, L. J., et al. (2007). Resident outcomes in small-house nursing homes: A longitudinal evaluation of the initial green house program. *Journal of the American Geriatrics Society, 55*(6), 832–839.

Kane, R. L., Williams, C. C., Williams, T. F., & Kane, R. A. (1993). *Annual Review of Public Health, 14,* 545–584.

Kapp, M. B. (1999). Restraint reduction and legal risk management. *Journal of the American Geriatrics Society, 47,* 375–376.

Kapp, M. B. (2008). Resistance to nursing home restraints reduction revisited: Introduction to a symposium. *Journal of Aging & Social Policy, 20*(3), 279–28.

Kendal Corporation. (1999). Special 10th anniversary issue. *Untie the Elderly, 11* (3), 1–12.

Kong, E. H., Guevera, J., & Evans, L. K. (2009). Non-pharmacologic interventions for agitation in dementia: A systematic review and meta-analysis. *Aging and Mental Health, 13*(4), 512–520.

Kolanowski, A., Hurwitz, S., Taylor, L., Evans, L., & Strumpf, N. (1994). Contextual factors associated with disturbing behaviors in institutionalized elders. *Nursing Research, 43*(2), 73–79.

Kurlowicz, L., Evans, L., Strumpf, N., & Maislin, G. (2002). A psychometric evaluation of the Cornell Scale for depression in dementia in a frail nursing home population. *American Journal of Geriatric Psychiatry, 10,* 600–608.

Leroi, I., Samus, Q. M., Rosenblatt, A., Onyike, C. U., Brandt, J., Baker, A. S., Rabins, P., & Lyketsos, C. (2007). A comparison of small and large assisted living facilities for the diagnosis and care of dementia: The Maryland Assisted Living Study. *International Journal of Geriatric Psychiatry, 22,* 224–232.

Lewin, T. (1989, December 28). Nursing homes rethink merits of tying the aged. *The New York Times.*

Miles, S. H. (1996). A case of death by physical restraint: New lessons from a photograph. *Journal of the American Geriatrics Society, 44,* 291–292.

Miles, S. H., & Irvine, P. (1991). Common features of deaths caused by physical restraints. *The Gerontologist, 31,* 42.

Miles, S. H., & Irvine, P. (1992). Deaths caused by physical restraints. *The Gerontologist, 32,* 762–765.

Milke, D. L., Kendall, T. S., Neumann, I., Wark, C. F., & Knopp, A. (2008). A longitudinal evaluation of restraint reduction within a multi-site, multi-model Canadian Continuing Care Organization. *Canadian Journal on Aging, 27*(1), 35–43.

Miller, S. C., Papandonatos, G., Fennell, M., & Mor, V. (2006). Facility and county effects on racial differences in nursing home quality indicators. *Social Science and Medicine, 63,* 3046–3059.

Minnick, A. F., Mion, L. C., Johnson, M. E., Catrambone, C., & Leipzig, R. (2007). Prevalence and variation of physical restraint use in acute care settings in the US. *Journal of Nursing Scholarship, 39*(1), 30–37.

Mion, L. C., Frengley, J. D., Jakovcic, C., & Marino, J. (1989). A further exploration of the use of physical restraints in hospitalized patients. *Journal of the American Geriatrics Society, 37*, 949–956.

Mion, L. C., Fogel, J., Sendhu, S., Palmer, R. M., Minnick, A. F., et al. (2001). Outcomes following physical restraint reduction programs in two acute care hospitals. *Joint Commission Journal of Quality Improvement, 51*, 1031–1035.

Mitchell-Pederson, L., Edmund, L., Fingerote, E., et al. (1985). Let's untie the elderly. *OAHA Quarterly, 21*, 10.

Molassiotis, A., & Newell, R. (1996). Nurses' awareness of restraint use with elderly people in Greece and the UK: A cross-cultural pilot study. *International Journal of Nursing Studies, 33*(2), 201–211.

Moloney, S. L., McDonald, D. D., & Palmisano-Mills, C. (2007). Psychometric testing of an instrument to measure the experience of home. *Research in Nursing and Health, 30*, 518–530.

Moore, K., & Haralambous, B. (2007). Barriers to reducing the use of restraints in residential elder care facilities. *Journal of Advanced Nursing, 58*(6), 532–540.

Morrison, J., Crinklaw-Wiancko, D., King, D., Thibeault, S., & Wells, D. L. (1987). Formulating a restraint use policy for adults based on the research process. *Journal of Nursing Administration, 17*(3), 39.

Mott, S., Poole, J., & Kenrick, M. (2005). Physical and chemical restraints in acute care: Their potential impact on the rehabilitation of older people. *International Journal of Nursing Practice, 11*, 95–101.

Myers, H., Nikoletti, S., & Hill, A. (2001). Nurses' use of restraints and their attitudes toward restraint use and the elderly in an acute care setting. *Nursing and Health Sciences, 3*, 29–34.

National Citizens' Coalition for Nursing Home Reform. (1992). Preliminary comments on HCFA proposed regulations. Washington, DC: Author.

National Institutes of Health. (2009a). A brief history of NIA. Available at http://www.nih.gov/about/almanac/organization/NIA.htm

National Institutes of Health. (2009b). A brief history of NINR. Available at http://www.nih.gov/about/almanac/organization/index.htm

Nawaz, H., Abbas, A., Sarfraz, A., Slade, M. D., Calvocoressi, L., Wild, D. M. G., & Tessier-Sherman, B. (2007). A randomized clinical trial to compare the use of safety net enclosures with standard restraints in agitated hospitalized patients. *Journal of Hospital Medicine, 2*(6), 385–393.

Neufeld, R. R., Libow, L. S., Foley, W. I., Dunbar, J. M., Cohen, C., & Brewer, B. (1999). Restraint reduction reduces serious injuries among nursing home residents. *Journal of the American Geriatrics Society, 47*(10), 1202–1207.

Nohlgren, S. (1987, December 16). Edging toward restraint reform. *St. Petersburg Times.*

Patterson, J., Strumpf, N. E., & Evans, L. K. (1995). Nursing consultation to reduce restraints in a nursing home. *Clinical Nurse Specialist, 9*(4), 231–235.

Pekkarinen, L., Elovainio, M., Sinervo, T., Finne-Soveri, H., & Noro, A. (2006). Nursing working conditions in relation to restraint practices in long-term care units. *Medical Care, 44*, 1114–1120.

Pioneer Network. Available at http://www.pioneernetwork.net/AboutUs/About/

Retsas, A. P. (1998). Survey findings describing the use of physical restraints in nursing homes in Victoria, Australia. *International Journal of Nursing Studies, 35*, 184–191.

Rigert, J., & Lerner, M. (1990, December 2). For the frail and the elderly, restraints are often deathtraps. *Minnesota Star Tribune.*

Robbins, L. J., Boyko, E., Lane, J., et al. (1987). Binding the elderly: A prospective study of the use of mechanical restraints in an acute care hospital. *Journal of the American Geriatrics Society, 35*, 290.

Schnelle, J. F., Simmons, S. F., & Ory, M. G. (1992). Risk factors that predict staff failure to release nursing home residents from restraints. *The Gerontologist, 32*, 767–770.

Schwartz, D. (1985a). Call for help. *Geriatric Nursing, 6*(1), 4, 9.

Schwartz, D. (1985b). Replies to 'call for help.' *Geriatric Nursing, 6*(6), 250–251.

Siegler, E., Capezuti, E., Maislin, G., Baumgarten, M., Evans, L., & Strumpf, N. (1997). Effects of a restraint reduction intervention and OBRA '87 regulations on psychoactive drug use in nursing homes. *Journal of the American Geriatrics Society, 45*, 791–796.

Strumpf, N. E., & Evans, L. K. (1987). Patterns of restraint use in a nursing home (Abstract). *Nursing Advances in Health.* Proceedings of the American Nurses Association Council of Nurse Researchers Meeting, 410. Washington: ANA.

Strumpf, N. E., & Evans, L. K. (1988). Physical restraint of the hospitalized elderly: Perceptions of patients and nurses. *Nursing Research, 37*(3), 132–137.

Strumpf, N. E., & Evans, L. K. (1993). Making sense of behavior. *HCFA Region III Restraint Reduction Newsletter, 7*(3), 2–3.

Strumpf, N., Evans, L., Capezuti, E., & Maislin, G. (1997). Consequences of hospital restraint use on older nursing home residents. *The Gerontologist, 37*(Special Issue I), 252.

Strumpf, N. E., Evans, L. K., & Schwartz, D. (1991). Physical restraint of the elderly. In C. Chenitz, J. Stone, & S. Salisbury (Eds.), *Clinical Gerontological Nursing* (pp. 329–344). Philadelphia: Saunders.

Strumpf, N. E., Evans, L. K., Wagner, J., & Patterson, J. (1992). Reducing physical restraints: Developing an educational program. *Journal of Gerontological Nursing, 18*(11), 21–27.

Strumpf, N. E., Evans, L. K., Williams, C. C., Williams, T. F., & Middleton, W. G. (1991). Patterns of care in restraint-free facilities: Lessons from abroad. *Search, 14*(2), 5.

Strumpf, N. E., Robinson, J. P., Wagner, J. S., & Evans, L. K. (1998). *Restraint-free care: Individualized approaches for frail elders.* New York: Springer.

Strumpf, N. E., & Tomes, N. (1993). Restraining the troublesome patient: An historical perspective on a contemporary debate. *Nursing History Review, 1*(1), 3–24.

Sullivan-Marx, E., Strumpf, N., Evans, L., Baumgarten, M., & Maislin, G. (1999a). Initiation of physical restraints in nursing home residents following restraint reduction. *Research in Nursing and Health, 22*, 369–379.

Sullivan-Marx, E., Strumpf, N., Evans, L., Baumgarten, M., & Maislin, G. (1999b). Predictors of continued physical restraint use in nursing home residents following restraint reduction efforts. *Journal of the American Geriatrics Society, 47*, 342–348.

Sullivan-Marx, E., Strumpf, N., Evans, L., Capezuti, E., & Maislin, G. (2003). Effects of an advanced practice nursing intervention with physical restraint use among hospitalized nursing home residents. *The Gerontologist, 43*(Special Issue I), 310.

Talerico, K., Evans, L., & Strumpf, N. (2002). Mental health correlates of aggression in nursing home residents with dementia. *The Gerontologist, 42*, 169–177.

Testad, I., Aasland, A. M., & Aasland, D. (2005). The effect of staff training on the use of restraint in dementia: A single-blind randomized controlled trial. *International Journal of Geriatric Psychiatry, 20*, 587–590.

University of Iowa Gerontological Nursing Interventions Research Center. (2005). Changing the practice of physical restraint in acute care. Available at http://www.guidelines.gov/summary/summary.aspx?doc_id=8626&nbr=004806&string=physical+AND+restraints

U.S. Food and Drug Administration. (1992). *FDA safety alert: Potential hazards with restraint devices* (CDRH, HFZ0250). Rockville MD.

U.S. Government. (1992). HCFA proposed regs 483.13 Resident behavior and facility practices. *Federal Register, 57*(24), February 5.

Williams, C. (1985). And *this* is home? In E.L. Schneider (Ed.), *The teaching nursing home: A new approach to geriatric research, education and clinical care* (pp. 137–144). New York: Raven Press.

Williams, C. C. (1989). Liberation: Alternative to physical restraints. *The Gerontologist, 29*(5), 585–586.

Williams, T. F. (1988). Research and care: Essential partners in aging. *The Gerontologist, 28*, 579–585.

Williams, C. C., & Finch, C. E. (1997). Physical restraint: Not fit for woman, man, or beast. *Journal of the American Geriatrics Society, 45*, 773–775.

Woo, J., Hui, E., Chan, F., Chi, I., & Sham, A. (2004). Use of restraints in long term residential care facilities in Hong Kong SAR, China: Predisposing factors and comparison with other countries. *Journal of Gerontology: Medical Sciences, 59A*, 921–923.

Yarmesch, M., & Sheafor, M. (1984). The decision to restrain. *Geriatric Nursing, 5*, 242–244.

13

Research on Human Sleep: Need to Inform Public Policies

David F. Dinges

Understanding the need for sleep in modern humans has been the focus of my scientific studies of sleep deprivation for the past 32 years. The National Institutes of Health National Institute of Nursing Research (NINR) has funded much of my laboratory's research on two of the most fundamental questions in sleep science: How much sleep do healthy adult humans need? What happens to humans when sleep need is not met? These are the scientific questions and data that will be discussed in this chapter relative to the increasing pressure to curtail sleep for lifestyle, economic, and societal reasons. The focus will be substantially on the policy issues relative to the consequences of not satisfying human sleep need. Before discussing these issues, it is important to note that many other scientists have also contributed to this area. It is also noteworthy that this chapter does not deal with sleep disorders and the growing recognition of the burden that they place on public health and the need for effective policies regarding sleep disorder diagnosis and treatment (Walsh, Dement, & Dinges, 2005).

The research that the NINR began supporting in my laboratory in the mid-1990s involved the first well-controlled, sleep-dose-response experiments to establish the neurobehavioral effects of chronic partial sleep deprivation in a representative sample of healthy adults. It came at a critical phase in my decades-long scientific search to understand the consequences of sleep deprivation and the temporal dynamics of changes to the brain and body when sleep need is not fulfilled. Although we have known for some time that normal human sleep need shows a Gaussian distribution at all ages of life, substantial scientific disagreement has persisted over the center of that normal distribution (for example, is it 4, 5, 6, 7, or 8 hours?) and the degree to which humans could reduce their sleep without adverse consequences for safety or health. With the NINR's support, I turned my attention from understanding the effects of total sleep deprivation toward investigations of chronic partial sleep deprivation. I did this in large measure because partial sleep deprivation is vastly more common in humans than acute total sleep deprivation and is therefore much more relevant to a wide range of public policies. However, chronic sleep curtailment studies are also vastly more labor-intensive and experimentally costly than acute sleep deprivation studies, which explains why so few had been well conducted prior to our experiments. It is to the NINR's credit that they recognized the importance of performing tightly controlled experimental studies of the physiological and neurobehavioral effects of chronic partial sleep deprivation. This has allowed us to perform five seminal experiments on sleep restriction in more than 300 healthy adults (50% women; 50% minorities; mean age, 30 years) involving more than 4,000 laboratory days.

The scope of this effort markedly increased the scientific certainty of our seminal findings (see "Consequences of Chronic Sleep Restriction" below). The results triggered a new focus on chronic sleep restriction as a substantial risk factor of relevance to policies in many industries and areas of society, including health policies involving patients and the sleep and work hours of nurses and physicians. The findings and their policy impacts also brought considerable recognition from different organizations.[1] This success notwithstanding, policy changes that emphasize the critical importance of people obtaining sleep have been slower to come due to the pace and priorities of modern culture. Although there is a growing recognition of the importance for health and safety of protected time for adequate sleep, society struggles with how to do it. The solutions most often championed involve the use of behavioral, pharmacological, and technological strategies to keep people "going" in the face of sleep loss or to protect them and others from any incapacitation suffered from sleep loss (Dinges & Rogers, 2008). These efforts to manage sleep loss are reasonable for those segments of society that must operate 24/7 for the greater public good (e.g., military and first responders). However, for the vast majority of people, the most appropriate solution to sleep loss is to obtain the sleep needed to ensure healthy and behaviorally effective functioning.

IN DEFENSE OF SLEEP

Although its biological functions are not yet fully understood, sleep is a fundamental feature of life on Earth and a manifestly obvious biological imperative that must be met daily in humans and many other complex life forms (Cirelli & Tononi, 2008; Meerlo, Mistiberger, Jacobs, Heller, & McGinty, 2009; Siegel, 2008, 2009). However, justifications for the human need for sleep have increasingly been demanded in the past 100 years as industrialization and the technology revolution have swept the planet and brought a higher quality of life to billions of people. As modern human societies began exploiting time 24 hours a day and lit the night with enormous urban areas and incessant transportation systems, sleep began to be viewed as an expendable commodity. Since World War II, policy makers from government to the military, transportation, industrial production, healthcare, and many other public and private sectors have wondered why sleep need could not be eliminated or at least reduced to serve the imperative to have millions

---

[1] Awards I have received after the studies were published on the neurobehavioral and physiological effects of chronic partial sleep deprivation include the following: Senator Mark O. Hatfield Public Policy Award from the American Academy of Sleep Medicine (2001); First Decade of Behavior Research Award from the American Psychological Association (2004); National Aeronautics and Space Administration (NASA) Distinguished Public Service Medal (2007), which is the highest honor that NASA awards to a nongovernment employee—it is granted to individuals whose distinguished accomplishments contributed substantially to the NASA mission; and the Raymond F. Longacre Award for Outstanding Accomplishment in the Psychological and Psychiatric Aspects of Aerospace Medicine, Aerospace Medical Association (2009).

of people awake at any hour of the day or night, as defenders, emergency personnel, healthcare providers, workers, consumers, and others. Tens of millions of people who experience regular night-shift work are perhaps the best example of cultural priority to have people awake at all times to serve the 24/7 economy that now dominates much of the world.

While governments and industries have created the need to have more people awake more of the time, humans have also sought to reduce sleep time for personal benefits. The availability of 24-hour television, satellite communications, transportation, and shopping have made many people wonder why sleep need could not be reduced or made more efficient to increase leisure time or time to get more things accomplished. The cultural dependence on caffeine, the most widely used stimulant in the United States, illustrates people's desire to reduce one of the consequences of not obtaining adequate sleep (i.e., sleepiness). We have shown that caffeine blunts the morning sleep inertia (i.e., grogginess, lethargy, and cognitive slowing) that is a hallmark of people prematurely curtailing their sleep with artificial awakenings (via alarm clocks), resulting in chronic partial sleep deprivation (Van Dongen, Rogers, & Dinges, 2003a). More importantly, we have found that chronic restriction of human sleep duration has cumulative negative effects on neurobehavioral functions and that the theories and claims that humans can behaviorally learn to reduce their sleep time without consequence are not supported by scientific evidence.

CUMULATIVE EFFECTS OF CHRONIC PARTIAL SLEEP DEPRIVATION

For nearly 50 years, the concept of "sleep debt" was used to refer to the effects of chronic partial sleep deprivation (also referred to a chronic sleep restriction). The concept is predicated on the notion of a basal sleep need that must be met to ensure daily recovery of brain and bodily functions. More importantly, the concept of sleep debt implied that a cumulative process was underway—each consecutive day of partial sleep restriction should produce more severe neurobehavioral problems (i.e., greater physiological and subjective sleepiness, more frequent and serious cognitive deficits, and more microsleeps and behavioral lapses).

Despite the heuristic utility of sleep debt as a construct, its theoretical and empirical basis remained very controversial for decades. A prominent scientific theory held that only "core sleep" in the first 4–6 hours of sleep at night—especially that dominated by EEG slow wave activity—was required for adequate daytime functioning to be maintained (Horne, 1988). This view gave hope to those who wanted to shorten their sleep need, and it drew support from some published studies on healthy adults' sleep chronically restricted to 4–6 hours a night for a week, which concluded that there were few, if any, detrimental effects on objective neurobehavioral functions.

Importance of Sound Scientific Methods

Many of the early investigations that found no adverse effects from chronic partial sleep deprivation had serious methodological limitations. Those done before 1965 bordered on the anecdotal and lacked adequate sample sizes and control groups. Most subsequent reports between 1970 and 1995 allowed subjects to go home for practicality sake, thereby failing to ensure that subjects maintained the assigned sleep–wake schedules.[2] Some studies used very infrequent, confounded, and/or insensitive measures of sleep and waking; lacked sophisticated time series analyses of results; and generally drew conclusions not substantiated by their data (for reviews of this work, see Banks & Dinges, 2007; Van Dongen et al., 2003a). This body of flawed science nevertheless resulted in three widely repeated conclusions: (1) that reducing nightly sleep duration to between 4 and 6 hours had little adverse effects on daily functions; (2) that only a "core sleep" duration of 4–6 hours was physiologically essential, and any additional sleep beyond that core duration was "optional sleep" that reflected residual capacity; and (3) that an individual could adapt to a reduced amount of sleep with few neurobehavioral consequences. These three claims were subsequently demonstrated to be categorically *incorrect*.

Not all of the early experiments on the effects of chronic sleep restriction lacked methodological rigor. In particular, a seminal study of a week of 5 hours of sleep a night at Stanford University (Carskadon & Dement, 1981) and a pilot study of 5 hours of sleep a night that we conducted at the University of Pennsylvania (Dinges et al., 1997) both carefully controlled subjects' sleep–wake times and other critical variables (e.g., no caffeine) and found clear evidence for cumulative effects of chronic sleep restriction on objective neurobehavioral functions. Although modest in scope, these two studies demonstrated the proof of principle for cumulative sleep debt, and they formed the basis for our subsequent large-scale experiments supported by the NINR.

Consequences of Chronic Sleep Restriction

To determine if chronic restriction of sleep below 7–8 hours a night results in neurobehavioral and physiological deficits in healthy adults, we conducted three laboratory experiments in which subjects (22–45 years of age) were randomized to 4-, 6-, or 8-hour (control condition) sleep periods each day for up to 10–14 days. The experiments differed only by the time of day (circadian phase) at which sleep was permitted. These large-scale, laboratory-controlled, sleep-dose-response experiments resulted in three important new facts regarding chronic partial sleep deprivation.

1. *Sleep restriction to 6 hours or less adversely affected healthy adults.* Relative to the control condition in which subjects had 8 hours for sleep, restriction of sleep duration between 4 and 6 hours had adverse effects on a range of neurobehavioral outcomes, resulting in decreased physiological alertness, increased lapses of attention, slowed working memory, reduced cognitive throughput, perseveration on wrong responses, and increased sleepiness, fatigue, and negative moods. However, cognitive performance deficits accumulated near linearly over days of sleep restriction, whereas subjective ratings of sleepiness

---

[2] It is problematic when methodologically compromised science is justified by convenience or practicality and even more problematic to find it used in policy development. Science is a method for identifying cause-and-effect relationships in nature. If the method is misapplied, claims of cause and effect as well as claims of no cause and effect are without merit. In such cases, one can only state that the scientific methods used were inadequate to conclude anything reliable.

and fatigue showed an acute response to sleep restriction but only small further increases on subsequent days of restriction (Van Dongen, Maislin, Mullington, & Dinges, 2003b).[3] These findings suggest that as sleep restriction continues, brain-based deficits increase steadily, but subjects may not be fully aware of these decrements. This may explain why people engage in chronic sleep restriction—they may be unaware of the neurobehavioral impairments accumulating in their neurobiology.

2. *Neurobehavioral deficits were accumulated across days of sleep restriction.* The rate of the accumulation in neurobehavioral deficits across days of sleep restriction was inversely proportional to the amount of sleep permitted. Thus, deficits increased faster across days of restriction as the amount of sleep allowed was decreased. Moreover, the accumulation of neurobehavioral deficits from sleep restriction occurred regardless of the circadian phase at which restricted sleep was obtained (Van Dongen et al., 2003b). These findings suggest that the consequences of chronic sleep restriction are not rescued by the time of day sleep is taken or by the circadian phase of wakefulness and that the amount of sleep restriction influences how quickly cognitive deficits develop.

3. *Cumulative deficits were equivalent to those of total sleep deprivation.* All doses (durations) of sleep restricted to between 4 and 6 hours a day produced neurobehavioral deficits equivalent to those found after at least 1 day of acute total sleep deprivation (i.e., 24–40 hours awake). As sleep restriction continued beyond a week, neurobehavioral deficits progressed to levels equivalent to two nights without sleep (i.e., 48–64 hours awake). At 4 hours of sleep per night, attention lapses were equivalent to three nights without sleep (i.e., 72–88 hours awake) by Day 12 of restriction (Van Dongen et al., 2003b).

Our findings (shown in Figure 13.1) were confirmed by another large-scale laboratory-based study of chronic sleep restriction (Belenky et al., 2003) and by our own recent research (Banks, Van Dongen, & Dinges, 2009; Mollicone, Van Dongen, Rogers, & Dinges, 2008). Collectively, these studies indicate that the neurobehavioral effects of chronic sleep restriction are not less serious than those observed with acute total sleep deprivation. If the public would find it unacceptable for a commercial airline pilot, or a school bus driver, or a nurse, or a physician, or a truck driver, or a nuclear power plant operator to be working after being awake for 24 hours, why would it be acceptable for the same individual to be at work after 4 days of 4 hours sleep a day? This is the kind provocative policy inquiry that should elicit serious discussion of how to protect sleep time and ensure that people use that time for sleep and come to work alert and fit to perform. It is perhaps one of the reasons why these findings were highlighted (on p. 141) in the Institute of Medicine (IOM) report on *Sleep Disorders and Sleep Deprivation* (2006) (Colten & Altevogt, 2006).

Our findings on the effects of chronic partial sleep deprivation also leave no doubt that (1) reducing sleep duration to between 4 and 6 hours per day has widespread and serious consequences for neurobehavioral functions in healthy adults; (2) that the concept of 4-hour "core sleep" versus "optional sleep" is emphatically incorrect; and (3) that there was no adaptation to the adverse neurobehavioral (objective) effects of sleep loss,

---

[3] One indication a scientific study's impact on the scientific community is the number of times the work is cited in other peer-review scientific publications. Our seminal study of chronic sleep restriction (Van Dongen et al., 2003b) supported by the NINR has been cited 380 times in the past 7 years. Most science studies are cited less than 50 times.

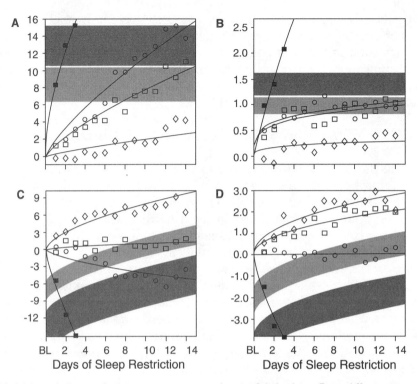

FIGURE 13.1 Neurobehavioral responses to varying doses of daily sleep. Four different neurobehavioral assays served to measure cognitive performance capability and subjective sleepiness. Each panel displays group averages for subjects in the 8 h (◊), 6 h (□), and 4 h (○) chronic sleep period conditions across 14 days, and in the 0 h (■) sleep condition across 3 days. Subjects were tested every 2 h each day; data points represent the daily average (07:30h–23:30h) expressed relative to baseline (BL). Panel A shows the pattern of changes across days for psychomotor vigilance task (PVT) performance lapses; panel B shows the pattern for Stanford Sleepiness Scale (SSS) self-ratings; panel C shows the pattern for digit symbol substitution task (DSST) correct responses; and panel D shows the pattern serial addition/subtraction task (SAST) correct responses (per minute). Upward corresponds to worse performance on the PVT and greater sleepiness on the SSS, and to better performance on the DSST and the SAST. The curves through the data points represent statistical non-linear model-based best-fitting profiles of the response to sleep deprivation for subjects in each of the four experimental conditions. The mean ± s.e. ranges of neurobehavioral functions for 1 and 2 days of 0 h sleep (total sleep deprivation) are shown as light and dark gray bands, respectively, allowing comparison of the 3-day total sleep deprivation condition and the 14-day chronic sleep restriction conditions. For the DSST and SAST, these gray bands are curved parallel to the practice effect displayed by the subjects in the 8 h sleep period condition, to compensate for different amounts of practice on these tasks. Figure reprinted with permission from Van Dongen, H. P. A., Maislin, G., Mullington, J. M., Dinges, D. F. (2003). The cumulative cost of additional wakefulness: Dose-response effects on neurobehavioral functions and sleep physiology from chronic sleep restriction and total sleep deprivation. *SLEEP*, 26 (2):117–126.

although there was subjective adaptation in that people generally did not report greater sleepiness as their cognitive deficits worsened with continuing sleep restriction.

Finally, our studies also reveal that there is substantial individual variability in neurobehavioral responses to sleep restriction, the basis of which remains to be discovered. In addition, while the neurobehavioral effects of chronic sleep restriction are indisputable, the causal role for reduced sleep duration in adverse health outcomes remains less certain. Our laboratory studies of healthy adults subjected to chronic sleep restriction have found adverse effects on certain endocrine and inflammatory responses, which suggests that sleep restriction produces physiological consequences that may be unhealthy. Other investigators have reported metabolic consequences of sleep restriction (Knutson, Spiegel, Penev, & Van Cauter, 2007).

SQUEEZING TIME FOR SLEEP IN A 24/7 WORLD

Having reviewed our results on human sleep need and the consequences of it being unmet, it is important to understand how pervasive and entrenched are the policies that reduce sleep in a world that operates 24 hours a day, 7 days a week, and the risks that these pose to the public and the environment. The IOM report *Sleep Disorders and Sleep Deprivation* (Colten & Altevogt, 2006) highlighted the risks posed to public health by inadequate sleep when they noted:

> The negative public health consequences of sleep loss and sleep-related disorders are enormous. Some of the most devastating human and environmental health disasters have been partially attributed to fatigue-related performance failures, sleep loss, and night shift work-related performance failures, including the tragedy at the Union Carbide chemical plant in Bhopal, India; the nuclear reactor meltdowns at Three Mile Island and Chernobyl; and the grounding of the *Exxon Valdez* oil tanker (Dinges et al., 1989; Moss & Sills, 1981; NCSDR, 1994; United States Senate Committee on Energy and National Resources, 1986; USNRC, 1987). Each of these incidents not only cost millions of dollars but also had a disastrous impact on the environment and the health of local communities. (p. 20).

Reasons for Reduced Sleep Duration

Adequate sleep is vital for healthy neurobehavioral functioning (Cirelli & Tononi, 2008; Goel, Rao, Durmer, & Dinges, 2009; Meerlo et al., 2009). Insufficient sleep occurs in millions of people who have medical conditions that disrupt sleep (e.g., untreated or ineffectively treated sleep apnea; certain types of insomnia, restless legs syndrome, and periodic limb movements; circadian rhythm sleep disorders such as shift work disorder and delayed sleep phase type; and disorders that produce nocturnal pain, nocturia, or otherwise fragmented sleep consolidation or increased premature awakenings). Inadequate sleep duration leading to chronic partial sleep deprivation also occurs in millions of people working night shifts and prolonged shifts (e.g., 24 hours). Population studies reveal that demographic factors, such as being a non-Hispanic African American, and lifestyle factors, such as having children under 2 years of age, job stress, or working long hours are also associated with sleep curtailment (Basner et al., 2007; Basner & Dinges, 2009; Hublin, Kaprio, Partinen, & Koskenvuo, 2001; Krueger & Friedman, 2009).

Reducing sleep time may harbor significant health risks. Although it is unknown whether the association between short sleep and morbidity/mortality is causal, dozens of population-based studies from around the world have found reduced sleep duration (<7 hours) to be a risk factor for obesity, cardiovascular disease and diabetes, depression, and prospective mortality (e.g., Cappuccio et al., 2008; Chaput, Despres, Bouchard, & Tremblay,

2007; Eguchi et al., 2008; Ferrie et al., 2007; Ikehara et al., 2009; King et al., 2008; Shankar, Koh, Yuan, Lee, & Yu, 2008; Vgontzas, Liao, Bixler, Chrousos, &Vela-Bueno, 2009).

It is estimated that 20% to 40% of the adult U.S. population sleep fewer than 7 hours per night (Kripke, Garfinkel, Wingard, Klauber, & Marler, 2002; National Sleep Foundation, 2006), which is the minimum sleep duration that we and others have found was necessary to prevent cumulative deterioration in neurocognitive functions (see Figure 13.1, and Belenky et al., 2003; Dinges et al., 1997; Van Dongen et al., 2003b). The proportion of people curtailing their sleep due to lifestyle appears to be increasing (Centers for Disease Control and Prevention, 2008) and may be even higher than surveys suggest because physiological sleep duration is as much as an hour or more below habitual sleep duration in population studies (Lauderdale, Knutson, Yan, Liu, & Rathouz, 2008).

American Lifestyle and Reduced Time for Sleep

There is increasing evidence that the most common reasons for the reduction in sleep time in the past 50 years may derive from a combination of lifestyle and cultural factors related to both work and leisure. As part of our research for the NINR on the causes and consequences of chronic partial sleep deprivation, my laboratory sought to identify what waking activities were most likely to be reciprocally related to sleep duration in the U.S. population. To answer this question, we used the publicly available American Time Use Survey (ATUS), which is a federally administered, continuous telephone survey sponsored by the Bureau of Labor Statistics and conducted by the U.S. Census Bureau. Using data from 2003 to 2005 on 47,731 Americans over the age of 14 years, we found that among more than 17 ATUS categories, the top three categories reciprocally related to sleep time, in order of importance, were time spent *working*, time spent *traveling* (which included commute time to/from work), and time spent at *leisure*, which includes socializing and relaxing (Basner et al., 2007). More work time and more travel time (for any reason) were particularly associated with less sleep time. These findings suggest that sleep time may be increasingly squeezed by work commutes that are starting earlier in the morning and extending later into the day. My colleague Mathias Basner and I speculate that the reasons commute times are getting longer are associated with such factors as urban sprawl (i.e., people living further from work) and traffic volume growing faster than transport capacity—both of which have occurred steadily over the past 30 years. In other words, the policy area of urban planning (or more accurately, the lack of effective planning) has contributed to reduced sleep in America.

A second study Dr. Basner and I conducted on the ATUS database for the period 2003–2006 identified additional factors that were related to reduced sleep time in people who worked longer hours ($\geq$8 hours on the interview day; $n = 6,116$) versus those who worked <8 hours ($n = 5,589$) and those who did not have compensated work that day ($n = 9,770$; Basner & Dinges, 2009). This study showed precisely why those who worked longer hours obtained less sleep. Long workers ($\geq$8 hours) arose from bed in the morning an average of 41 minutes earlier than did short workers (<8 hours, $p < .0001$) and 1 hour and 19 minutes earlier than did those people not working on the interview day ($p < .001$). Surprisingly, however, bedtime did not differ among the three groups. Watching television was the primary activity people engaged in before going to bed, accounting for 55 minutes (46%) of the 2-hour prebed period (see Figure 13.2). Thus, watching television played a major role in the timing of nocturnal sleep onset for the vast majority of Americans, and work hours plus commute time played a major role in the timing of morning sleep offset

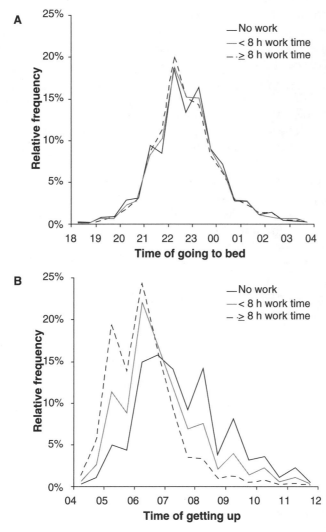

FIGURE 13.2 Panels A and B show distributions of time of going to bed (A) and time of getting up (B) for respondents in the American Time Use Survey (ATUS) who did not work (*black* lines, N = 9,770), who worked less than 8 hours (*gray* lines, N = 5589), and for those who worked 8 hours or more (broken black lines, N = 6,116) on the day of the interview. Figure reprinted with permission from Basner, M., and Dinges, D. F. (2009). Dubious bargain: Trading sleep for Leno and Letterman. *SLEEP* 32(6):747–752.

for a large proportion of Americans. Therefore, watching less television in the evening and postponing work start time in the morning appear to be candidate behavioral changes for efforts to increase sleep in Americans who work long hours.

My colleague in this research, Dr. Mathias Basner, and I concluded that although work and commute times may not be flexible, giving up some television viewing in the evening should be possible to reduce chronic sleep debt and promote adequate sleep in those who need it (Basner & Dinges, 2009). In addition, there are broader health policy issues relevant to these findings. Although it has not been proven that the frequent epidemiological associations between short sleep and medical morbidity/mortality are causal, many investigators believe that the evidence is reliable enough to warrant prospective studies of increased sleep time to improve health. In a published commentary on one of the more comprehensive review articles establishing a reliable association between short sleep duration and obesity (Cappuccio et al., 2008), Professor Terry Young of the Department of Health Sciences at the University of Wisconsin concluded:

> . . .with 700 studies behind us and well summarized by Cappuccio and colleagues, certainty that short sleep is not healthy, that short sleepers are more likely to be obese, (with a good chance that short sleep is the culprit in a meaningful number of children and adults), we *do* have enough to advocate for population-targeted educational initiatives and policies to increase sleep duration as a means of reducing obesity. No, I would not tell an individual that they can sleep away their obesity, but, with a moderate degree of certainty, I expect that if short sleepers increase their sleep time, the population as a whole will be healthier and rank lower in mean BMI. In the words of one renown for his logic, "the needs of the many *outweigh* the needs of the one" (Spock, *Wrath of Khan*, 1982). (p. 594 in Young, 2008)

With regard to our own data on the role of work hours, commute times, and television watching (Basner et al., 2007; Basner & Dinges, 2009), we suggest that if public policies would shift to more aggressively finding ways to reduce commute times, and if commercial primetime television shows would shift to 1 hour earlier in the evening, many Americans may obtain more sleep, which may attenuate the costly epidemics of obesity and diabetes underway in Americans. As importantly, other benefits would include more alert and less accident-prone workers, less stress-related illnesses, and potentially even reduced mortality.

We harbor no delusions that sleep will be prioritized in the near term in major health policy decisions regarding obesity, morbidity, and mortality, although my colleague Dr. Basner has had success in getting public policies in place that balance noise from commercial aircraft traffic at urban airports in Germany with the need to minimize disruption of sleep in the surrounding population (Basner, Samel, & Isermann, 2006). This kind of success may be more difficult in the United States, where economic models dominate virtually every facet of life.

Children, Adolescents, and Young Adults

While increasing sleep time by reducing television viewing and other nonessential activities near bedtime may be very difficult in American society as a whole, it may be far more feasible in children, adolescents, and young adults, who are particularly vulnerable neurobehaviorally to sleep curtailment. At least one interventional study in Japan did find that restricting television time to only 30 minutes per day advanced bedtime and increased total sleep time significantly in university students, whereas no effects were observed in elderly people (Asaoka, Fukuda, Tsutsu, & Yamazaki, 2007). This suggests that children, adolescents, and young adults should be the focus of prospective studies designed to increase sleep time, given the terrific risks to emotional, behavioral, and physical safety posed by inadequate sleep in these age groups (Carskadon, Acebo, & Jenni, 2004; Pack et al., 1995; Wolfson & Carskadon, 2003).

It is ironic that sleep loss is often quite high in educational settings, which are the very locations we should be teaching the next generation that adequate sleep is essential for learning, making good decisions, performing well, driving and operating machinery safely, and enjoying life, as well as for staying healthy. Yet there are major deterrents to obtaining adequate sleep in childhood, adolescence, and young adulthood. These include television, cellular phones, the Internet, too many extracurricular activities, and school start times that are too early. The latter are especially problematic for adolescents, who must be at school very early to satisfy logistical (e.g., too few school buses) and economic (e.g., labor contracts) priorities. They are also subject to performance demands without regard to sleep need; for example, it is not uncommon for high school students in the United States to be brought in for the Scholastic Aptitude Test, which is a key factor in access to colleges and universities, early on a Saturday morning, after a week of classes with an accompanying sleep debt.

Increasing physiological sleep time in adolescents could be quite beneficial. For example, a recent study demonstrated that a 1-hour delay in high school start times increased sleep duration and decreased extended sleep on weekends (Danner & Phillips, 2008). Average crash rates for teenage drivers in the study county in the 2 years after the change in school start time dropped by 16.5% compared with the 2 years prior to the change, whereas teenage crash rates for the rest of the state increased by 7.8% over the same time period.

Although many agree that it is important to avoid sleep deprivation in children, adolescents, and young adults, there is not always agreement on whether these cohorts should be allowed to sleep in (i.e., extend their sleep) on weekends. It is often worrisome to the parents of a teenager to find that their child is sleeping through the normal external (alarm clock) and internal (biological clock) wake-up signals on a Saturday and/or Sunday morning and extending their sleep through the morning and into the afternoon. However, our research has shown repeatedly that this is the normal homeostatic response of a young sleep-deprived brain.

Of course, it would be better if we prevented chronic partial sleep deprivation altogether in adolescents and young adults. If we cannot prevent it, we certainly should not prevent the ad libitum recovery sleep opportunities that adolescents and young adults get after chronic partial sleep deprivation. Surprisingly, there has not always been universal agreement on this point among sleep specialists. Approximately 15 years ago, I was asked to debate a colleague during a meeting on whether adolescents should be allowed to sleep in on weekends. I argued in favor of the value of the recovery sleep, and my opponent argued that it did emotional harm. Remarkably, at that time, neither of us could show data on the benefits of prolonged sleep periods for recovery (even though they commonly occur in adults) because sleep science had completely ignored the question of how much sleep is needed to effectively recover from chronic partial sleep deprivation. Only recently have studies begun to appear observing inadequate recovery. Thanks to the NINR support of our research, we have just completed the first large-scale experimental study on the effects of varying amounts of recovery sleep duration following chronic sleep restriction (Banks et al., 2009). These data will be published soon. Without divulging details that protect the copyright of the article to be published, suffice it to say that the findings thoroughly support the position I took 15 years ago.

A final comment on preventing sleep deprivation in children, adolescents, and young adults concerns the recognition that sleep curtailment in modern society often collides with inadequate policies, planning and practices, and public (mis)understanding of risks. Much more work needs to be done in educational settings to teach children, adolescents, and young adults that adequate sleep is vital for learning and performing at one's best. We also need better public communication to administrators, parents, teachers, coaches, and others, to encourage them to help ensure that children and young people have adequate time for sleep. Finally, we need prospective studies to support the prioritization of sleep time for improving the educational experience and its effectiveness at all grade levels.

Policies Should Focus on Sleep in Addition to Work Hours

Economic and logistical imperatives and policies dominate the human use of time in modern industrialized countries. The biology of sleep need and its optimal circadian timing is often forced to contort to these policies (Roenneberg, Kumar, & Merrow, 2007; Wittmann, Dinich, Merrow, & Roenneberg, 2006). The policy concept and legal language most widely used in government and industry as a very loose surrogate for the concept of "sleep" is "rest." The policy concept and legal language most widely used for inadequate "rest" is "fatigue." Hence, federal statutes and regulations talk about preventing and mitigating fatigue and about work-rest hours, or duty hours, or hours of service—all of which emphasize that government or nongovernment policies are written from the perspective of work hours in relation to fatigue, not sleep loss in relation to sleepiness.

Although the concept of fatigue overlaps substantially with that of sleepiness in terms of some performance manifestations (i.e., both can result in time on task decrements, performance variability, and subjective sense of being tired—see Dinges, 1995), it is obvious that rest need not include physiological sleep. It is still nearly impossible to find a single federal statute or regulation, state law, or private policy that uses the words "sleep" or "sleepiness." The ideas that how long one works is the only thing that makes one tired (or sleepy) and that rest (even without sleep) provides the same biological recovery as does healthy physiological sleep date back more than 90 years and are based on antiquated and scientifically unsound theories and no data.

These deeply entrenched ideas in statutes and regulations form a major barrier to effective policies for preventing catastrophic human error due to neurobehavioral performance deficits from inadequate sleep. In the last 50 years, there have been hundreds of published scientific studies in peer review journals (e.g., *Science, Nature, Sleep,* and *Journal of Sleep Research*) demonstrating that rest must involve physiological sleep for the brain to recover within each 24 hours (i.e., circadian cycle) and that the sleep must be adequate in duration and quality (continuity, depth, etc.) to ensure alert wakefulness (see the following comprehensive texts: Kryger, Roth, & Dement, 2005; Lee-Chiong, 2006). Although rest without sleep is important in providing some recovery to work again, and doing other work during rest periods may be essential or fiscally rewarding, neither can satisfy the genetically programmed need for sleep and its physiological benefits for restoring subsequent waking alertness and a range of cognitive functions essential for safe and effective performance on the job and in other aspects of life (Goel et al., 2009). In short, rest (without sleep) and rewarding work are not substitutes for satisfying the daily need for sleep. Sleep deprivation is a major unaccounted-for cause of fatigue not explicitly considered in most federal policies regarding fatigue risks to health and safety.

Scientific studies have proven the essential need for adequate sleep in humans to prevent waking neurobehavioral decrements that lead to mistakes and accidents, and no amount of rest (without sleep) or rewarding work can prevent the effects of inadequate sleep. In fact, the neurobiology of sleep cannot be prevented from destabilizing wakefulness when sleep is inadequate in physiological quality and/or duration or when wakefulness has been prolonged resulting in sleep deprivation. In these circumstances, sleep neurobiology will intrude uncontrollably into wakefulness, affecting a range of neurobehavioral and cognitive functions, as well as alertness (Goel et al., 2009; Harrison & Horne, 2000; Lim & Dinges, 2008). There is ample evidence that for the majority of people, sleep reduction directly causes increased sleep propensity and deficits in mood and neurocognitive functions including alertness and executive attention, cognitive speed and working memory, and executive functions (Harrison & Horne, 2000; Philibert, 2005). Sleep restriction also increases the risk of motor vehicle crashes (Barger et al., 2005; Horne & Reyner, 1999; Stutts, Wilkins, Osberg, & Vaughn, 2003) and workplace errors and accidents (Ayas et al., 2006; Dinges, 1995; Komada et al., 2008; Landrigan et al., 2004; Mitler et al., 1988), which are estimated to cost between $43 billion and $56 billion annually (Leger, 1994).

I have spent my professional career interacting with, and/or lecturing to, and/or testifying for, and/or performing research for, and/or advising a wide range of federal agencies and private organizations on the evidence that *daily adequate healthy sleep* is a critical factor for ensuring safe operators in 24/7 industries and that policies governing work hours must also prioritize sleep need.[4] Given the scientific evidence, one would expect that polices explicitly focused on ensuring that people obtain adequate sleep to be fit for work would be widespread, especially in safety-sensitive occupations involving security, energy plant operations, hazardous materials, all transportation modes, healthcare, leadership positions requiring critical decision making, and others. However, this is not the case. Virtually no regulation, statute, or policy intended to protect the public from unsafe fatigued workers focuses on sleep. Instead, the focus is nearly always on limiting work hours and providing time for rest (without regard to whether sleep is obtained). These policies are often ineffective at increasing sleep time because work hours are only moderately (inversely) correlated with sleep time.

An excellent example of the need to improve safety by both limiting excessive work hours and increasing sleep time is contained in the recommendations of a recent report from the IOM on how to improve patient and resident physician safety relative to resident (trainee) duty hours (Ulmer, Wolman, & Johns, 2009). I was a member of the IOM Committee on Optimizing Graduate Medical Trainee (Resident) Hours and Work Schedules that generated the report, and our NINR-funded research on chronic sleep deprivation was among the many findings discussed in the report. The IOM report acknowledged that the scientific literature makes clear that the risks of fatigue-related errors and accidents derive from multiple interacting variables of work and sleep. Chapter 7 in the report reviews the literature on sleep and human performance and recommends specific adjustments to the current Accreditation Council for Graduate Medical Education

---

[4] This includes the following federal entities: Federal Aviation Administration, Federal Motor Carrier Safety Administration, Federal Railroad Administration, NASA, National Highway Traffic Safety Administration, National Transportation Safety Board (and NTSB Academy), U.S. Air Force, U.S. Anti-Doping Agency, U.S. Coast Guard, U.S. Congress Office of Technology Assessment, U.S. Department of Justice, and U.S. Navy. It includes the following private entities: Accreditation Council for General Medical Education, Air Transport Association, American Trucking Association Foundation, Flight Safety Foundation, and International Life Sciences Institute North America. It includes the following international entities: Commonwealth of Australia House of Representatives, European Union, Transport Canada, and Transportation Workers Union.

resident duty hours to enhance the prevention and mitigation of resident fatigue as an unsafe condition. The report used the following scientifically based rationales for its specific recommendations:

(1) Work duration should be limited because human performance degrades after 16 hours of wakefulness whether one is working or not; (2) sufficient time for sleep needs to be incorporated into daily and weekly work schedules to prevent acute and chronic sleep deprivation, respectively, and to allow recovery from accumulated sleep debt; and (3) when extended duty periods are considered an essential aspect of resident training and continuity of care, a protected sleep period should be provided during that period to reduce the effects of acute sleep loss and to enhance performance. . . . The committee leaves some flexibility for programs, but urges that adequate protected sleep periods be maintained, and that fatigue prevention and mitigation be a matter of professionalism that requires attention by residents, attending physicians and all those charged with maintaining patient safety (Ulmer et al., 2009, p. 217).

This IOM report offers an important case for considering sleep need in human error in healthcare training of young physicians. It also reminds us that the prevalence of sleep curtailment in our 24/7 society often collides with inadequate policies even in the healthcare sector. Much more work needs to be done through public communication, interventional research, lifestyle changes, and public policies to reduce the burden that sleep curtailment places on public health and public safety.

REFERENCES

Asaoka, S., Fukuda, K., Tsutsu, Y., & Yamazaki, K. (2007). Does television viewing cause delayed and/or irregular sleep-wake patterns? *Sleep and Biological Rhythms, 5,* 23–27.

Ayas, N. T., Barger, L. K., Cade, B. E., Hashimoto, D. M., Rosner, B., Cronin, J. W., et al. (2006). Extended work duration and the risk of self-reported percutaneous injuries in interns. *JAMA: Journal of the American Medical Association, 296*(9), 1055–1062.

Banks, S., & Dinges, D. F. (2007). Behavioral and physiological consequences of sleep restriction in humans. *Journal of Clinical Sleep Medicine, 3*(5), 519–528.

Banks, S., Van Dongen, H. P. A., & Dinges, D. F. (2009). One night recovery from sustained sleep restriction: A dose-response study of neurobehavioral functions. *SLEEP, 32.*

Barger, L. K., Cade, B. E., Ayas, N. T., Cronin, J. W., Rosner, B., Speizer, E. F., et al. (2005). Extended work shifts and the risk of motor vehicle crashes among interns. *New England Journal of Medicine, 352*(2), 125–134.

Basner, M., & Dinges, D. F. (2009). Dubious bargain: Trading sleep for Leno and Letterman. *SLEEP, 32*(6), 747–752.

Basner, M., Fomberstein, K., Razavi, F. M., William, J., Simpson, N., Rosa, R., et al. (2007). American Time Use Survey: Sleep time and its relationship to waking activities. *SLEEP, 30*(9), 1081–1091.

Basner, M., Samel, A., & Isermann, U. (2006). Aircraft noise effects on sleep: Application of the results of a large polysomnographic field study. *Journal of the Acoustical Society of America, 119*(5), 2772–2784.

Belenky, G., Wesensten, N. J., Thorne, D. R., Thomas, M. L., Sing, H. C., Redmond, D. P., et al. (2003). Patterns of performance degradation and restoration during sleep restriction and subsequent recovery: A sleep dose-response study. *Journal of Sleep Research, 12,* 1–12.

Cappuccio, F. P., Taggart, F. M., Kandala, N-B., Currie, A., Peile, E., Stranges, S., et al. (2008). Meta-analysis of short sleep duration and obesity in children and adults. *Sleep, 31*(5), 619–626.

Carskadon, M., & Dement, W. (1981). Cumulative effects of sleep restriction on daytime sleepiness. *Psychophysiology, 18*(2), 107–113.

Carskadon, M. A., Acebo, C., & Jenni, O. G. (2004). Regulation of adolescent sleep: Implications for behavior. *Annals of the New York Academy Sciences, 1021,* 276–291.

Centers for Disease Control and Prevention. (2008). Perceived insufficient rest or sleep—Four states. 2006. *MMWR Morbidity, Mortality, Weekly Report, 57*(8), 200–203.

Chaput, J. P., Despres, J. P., Bouchard, C., & Tremblay, A. (2007). Short sleep duration is associated with reduced leptin levels and increased adiposity: Results from the Quebec family study. *Obesity, 15,* 253–261.

Cirelli, C., & Tononi, G. (2008). Is sleep essential? *PLoS Biology, 6*(8), 216.

Colten, H. R., & Altevogt, B. M. (Eds.), Committee on Sleep Medicine and Research. (2006). *Sleep disorders and sleep deprivation: An unmet public health problem.* Institute of Medicine, National Academy of Sciences Press.

Danner, F., & Phillips, B. (2008). Adolescent sleep, school start times, and teen motor vehicle crashes. *Journal of Clinical Sleep Medicine, 4,* 533–535.

Dinges, D. F. (1995). An overview of sleepiness and accidents. *Journal of Sleep Research, 4*(Suppl. 2), 4–14.

Dinges, D. F., Pack, F., Williams, K., Gillen, K. A., Powell, J. W., Ott, G. E., et al. (1997). Cumulative sleepiness, mood disturbance, and psychomotor vigilance performance decrements during a week of sleep restricted to 4–5 hours per night. *Sleep, 20*(4), 267–277.

Dinges, D. F., & Rogers, N. L. (2008). The future of human intelligence: Enhancing cognitive capability in a 24/7 world. In P. C. Kyllonen, R. D. Roberts, & L. Stankov (Eds.), *Extending intelligence: Enhancement and new constructs* (pp. 407–430). New York: Lawrence Erlbaum Associates.

Eguchi, K., Pickering, T. G., Schwartz, J. E., Hoshide, S., Ishikawa, J., Ishikawa, S., et al. (2008). Short sleep duration as an independent predictor of cardiovascular events in Japanese patients with hypertension. *Archives of Internal Medicine, 169*(20), 2225–2231.

Ferrie, J. E., Shipley, M. J., Cappuccio, F. P., Brunner, E., Miller, M. A., Kumari, M., et al. (2007). A prospective study of change in sleep duration: Associations with mortality in the Whitehall II cohort. *SLEEP, 30*(12), 1659–1666.

Goel, N., Rao, H., Durmer, J. S., & Dinges, D. F. (2009). Neurocognitive consequences of sleep deprivation. *Seminars in Neurology, 29*(4), 320–339.

Harrison, Y., & Horne, J. A. (2000). The impact of sleep deprivation on decision making: A review. *Journal of Experimental Psychology: Applied, 6*(3), 236–249.

Horne, J. A. (1988). *Why we sleep.* Oxford: Oxford University Press.

Horne, J., & Reyner, L. (1999). Vehicle accidents related to sleep: A review. *Occupational and Environmental Medicine, 56,* 289–294.

Hublin, C., Kaprio, J., Partinen, M., & Koskenvuo, M. (2001). Insufficient sleep: A population-based study in adults. *Sleep, 24*(4), 392–400.

Ikehara, S., Iso, H., Date, C., Kikuchi, S., Watanabe, Y., Wada, Y., et al. (2009). Association of sleep duration with mortality from cardiovascular disease and other causes for Japanese men and women: The JACC study. *Sleep, 32*(3), 259–301.

King, C. R., Knutson, K. L., Rathouz, P. J., Sidney, S., Liu, K., & Lauderdale, D. S. (2008). Short sleep duration and incident coronary artery calcification. *JAMA: Journal of the American Medical Association, 300*(24), 2859–2866.

Komada, Y., Inoue, Y., Hayashida, K., Nakajima, T., Honda, M., & Takahashi, K. (2008). Clinical significance of correlates of behaviorally induced insufficient sleep syndrome. *Sleep Medicine, 9*(8), 851–856.

Knutson, K. L., Spiegel, K., Penev, P., & Van Cauter, E. (2007). The metabolic consequences of sleep deprivation. *Sleep Medicine Reviews, 11*(3), 163–178.

Kripke, D. F., Garfinkel, L., Wingard, D. L., Klauber, M. R., & Marler, M. R. (2002). Mortality associated with sleep duration and insomnia. *Archives of General Psychiatry, 59,* 131–136.

Krueger, P. M., & Friedman, E. M. (2009). Sleep duration in the United States: A cross-sectional population-based study. *American Journal of Epidemiology, 169*(9), 1052–1063.

Kryger, M. H., Roth, T., & Dement, W. C. (2005). *Principles and practice of sleep medicine* (4th ed). Philadelphia: W. B. Saunders.

Landrigan, C. P., Rothschild, J. M., Cronin, J. W., Kaushal, R., Burdick, E., Katz, J. T., et al. (2004). Effect of reducing interns' work hours on serious medical errors in intensive care units. *New England Journal of Medicine, 351*(18), 1838–1848.

Lauderdale, D. S., Knutson, K. L., Yan, L. L., Liu, K., & Rathouz, P. J. (2008). Self-reported and measured sleep duration: How similar are they? *Epidemiology, 19,* 838–845.

Lee-Chiong, T. L. (2006). *Sleep: A Comprehensive Handbook*. Hoboken: John Wiley & Sons.

Leger, D. (1994). The cost of sleep-related accidents—A report for the National Commission on Sleep Disorders Research. *Sleep, 17*(1), 84–93.

Lim, J., & Dinges, D. F. (2008). Sleep deprivation and vigilant attention. In molecular and biophysical mechanisms of arousal, alertness, and attention. *Annals of the New York Academy of Sciences, 1129,* 1–18.

Meerlo, P., Mistiberger, R. E., Jacobs, B. L., Heller, H. C., & McGinty, D. (2009). New neurons in the adult brain: The role of sleep and consequences of sleep loss. *Sleep Medicine Reviews, 13*(3), 187–194.

Mitler, M. M., Carskadon, M. A., Czeisler, C. A., Dement, W. C., Dinges, D. F., & Graeber, R. C. (1988). Catastrophes, sleep, and public policy: Consensus report. *Sleep, 11*(1), 100–109.

National Sleep Foundation. (2006). *Sleep in America poll*. Washington: National Sleep Foundation.

Mollicone, D. J., Van Dongen, H. P. A., Rogers, N. L., & Dinges, D. F. (2008). Response surface mapping of neurobehavioral performance: Testing the feasibility of split sleep schedules for space operations. *Acta Astronautica, 63*(7–10), 833–840.

Pack, A. I., Pack, A. M., Rodgman, E., Cucchiara, A., Dinges, D. F., & Schwab, C. W. (1995). Characteristics of crashes attributed to the driver having fallen asleep. *Accident Analysis and Prevention, 27*(6), 769–775.

Philibert, I. (2005). Sleep loss and performance in residents and nonphysicians: A meta-analytic examination. *SLEEP, 28*(11), 1392–1402.

Roenneberg, T., Kumar, C. J., & Merrow, M. (2007). The human circadian clock entrains to sun time. *Current Biology, 17,* R44–R45.

Shankar, A., Koh, W-P., Yuan, J-M., Lee, J-M., & Yu, M. C. (2008). Sleep duration and coronary heart disease mortality among Chinese adults in Singapore: A population-based study. *American Journal of Epidemiology, 168*(12), 1367–1373.

Siegel, J. (2008). Do all animals sleep? *Trends in Neuroscience, 31*(4), 208–213.

Siegel, J. (2009). Sleep viewed as a state of adaptive inactivity. *Nature Reviews Neuroscience, 10*(10), 747–753.

Stutts, J. C., Wilkins, J. W., Osberg, J. S., & Vaughn, B. V. (2003). Driver risk factors for sleep-related crashes. *Accident Analysis and Prevention, 35*(3), 321–331.

Ulmer, C., Wolman, D. M., & Johns, M. M. E. (2009). *Resident duty hours: Enhancing sleep, supervision, and safety*. Washington, DC: Committee on Optimizing Graduate Medical Trainee (Resident) Hours and Work Schedules to improve Patient Safety. Institute of Medicine, National Academies Press.

Van Dongen, H. P. A., Rogers, N. L., & Dinges, D. F. (2003a). Understanding sleep debt: Theoretical and empirical issues. *Sleep and Biological Rhythms, 1,* 5–13.

Van Dongen, H. P., Maislin, G., Mullington, J. M., & Dinges, D. F. (2003b). The cumulative cost of additional wakefulness: Dose-response effects on neurobehavioral functions and sleep physiology from chronic sleep restriction and total sleep deprivation. *Sleep, 26*(2), 117–126.

Vgontzas, A. N., Liao, D., Bixler, E. O., Chrousos, G. P., & Vela-Bueno, A. (2009). Insomnia with objective short sleep duration is associated with a high risk of hypertension. *Sleep, 32*(4), 491–497.

Walsh, J. W., Dement, W. C., & Dinges, D. F. (2005). Sleep medicine, public policy and public health. In M. H. Kryger, T. Roth, & W. C. Dement (Eds.), *Principles and practice of sleep medicine* (4th ed., pp. 648–656). Philadelphia: W. B. Saunders.

Wittmann, M., Dinich, J., Merrow, M., & Roenneberg, T. (2006). Social jetlag: Misalignment of biological and social time. *Chronobiology International, 23,* 497–509.

Wolfson, A. R., & Carskadon, M. A. (2003). Understanding adolescents' sleep patterns and school performance: A critical appraisal. *Sleep Medicine Reviews, 7*(6), 491–506.

Young, T. (2008). Increasing sleep duration for a healthier (and less obese?) population tomorrow. *SLEEP, 31*(5), 593–594.

14

Transitional Care: Improving Health Outcomes and Decreasing Costs for At-Risk Chronically Ill Older Adults

Mary D. Naylor and Ellen T. Kurtzman

INTRODUCTION

Uneven, inequitable healthcare quality (Institute of Medicine [IOM], 2001); frequent, preventable adverse events (IOM, 2000); rapidly escalating healthcare costs (Anderson, Hussey, Frogner, & Waters, 2005); and growing rates of uninsurance (Center on Budget and Policy Priorities, 2006; Kaiser Family Foundation, 2008) characterize the current U.S. healthcare system. The consensus among major healthcare leaders is that transformation of the care delivery system is essential to improve health outcomes, reduce spending, and expand coverage (the Patient Protection and Affordable Care Act, 2010). Among the solutions to achieve these goals is transitional care, an innovative care delivery approach proven to more effectively and efficiently address the healthcare goals and needs of the growing population of chronically ill older adults in this country. This chapter describes the major shifts in demographic and illness patterns of older adults, the inadequacy of the current healthcare system in responding to the changing healthcare needs of older adults, the rationale and evidence base supporting the need for transitional care, and the implications of adopting the more rigorously tested transitional care models for healthcare policy, clinical practice, and future research.

SOCIETAL CONTEXT FOR TRANSITIONAL CARE

Today's population is both older and more chronically ill than that at any other point in our nation's history. According to a recent U.S. Census Bureau report (He, Sengupta, Velkoff, & DeBarros, 2005), the older adult population, which grew from 3 million to 35 million during the last century, will increase substantially during the next few decades when the first Baby Boomers turn 65 years old. From 2010 to 2030, the populations 65 years of age or older (the "older" population) and 85 years of age or older (the "older-old") are both expected to double—from 36 million to 72 million and from 4.7 million to

9.6 million, respectively. A larger segment of these elders will be healthier than earlier generations. However, as the older population expands, the incidence and prevalence of chronic illness and disability also will increase.

Chronic illness is defined as the co-occurrence of two or more diseases that are of long duration and slow progression (van den Akker, Buntinx, Metsemakers, Roos, & Knottnerus, 1998). Nearly 80% of the elderly have at least one chronic disease (Anderson, 2003), and these conditions are often the leading causes of disability and death (Kramarow, Lubitz, Lentzner, & Gorina, 2007). More than 20% of older adults suffer from more than five chronic diseases (AARP, 2009).

The demographic shifts alone are likely to result in an expanded burden to Medicaid, the state controlled healthcare program for people with low incomes and receiving long-term care. The physical, cognitive, and functional impairments resulting from multiple chronic conditions will be associated with increased utilization of acute care services among the burgeoning population of at-risk older adults, further taxing Medicare, the federally funded healthcare program for older adults. Older adults with multiple chronic illnesses already account for a disproportionate number of inpatient hospitalizations, home health care visits, prescription medications, and physician visits (Anderson & Knickman, 2001; Partnerships for Solutions for the Robert Wood Johnson Foundation, 2004).

Because of rapid and frequent changes in health status among these older adults, transitions among healthcare professionals and within and between healthcare settings are common and recurrent. Persons 65 years of age or older account for 229.8 million physician office visits, 16.5 million hospital outpatient visits, 17.2 million hospital emergency department visits, and 13.1 million hospital discharges (Cherry, Hing, Woodwell, & Rechtsteiner, 2008). A recent study of Medicare beneficiaries aged 65 years or older discharged from an acute care hospital found that nearly 13% of the episodes involved three or more transfers over a 30-day period (Coleman, Min, Chomiak, & Kramer, 2004).

These transition points are particularly vulnerable times for this cohort and have been linked to increased adverse clinical events (Forster, Murff, Peterson, Gandhi, & Bates, 2003; Moore, Wisnevesky, Williams, & McGinn, 2003; Wenger et al., 2003), serious unmet needs (Bowles, Foust, & Naylor, 2003; Naylor, 2003), and poor satisfaction with care (AARP, 2009; National Priorities Partnership, 2008). A recent study published by the AARP (2009), for example, found that patients and their families report stress and anxiety, poor communication, and problems with quality of care at these points of transition.

Reports reveal that chronically ill older adults also experience higher rates of avoidable hospitalization, often attributable to poor handoffs between these acute care settings and elders' homes or long-term care settings and inadequate attention to the root causes of patterns of poor outcomes. Jencks, Williams, and Coleman (2009) found that nearly 20% of Medicare beneficiaries discharged from hospitals are rehospitalized within 30 days; and 34%, within 90 days.

Beyond the tremendous human impact associated with avoidable rehospitalizations, there also is a huge economic toll. Healthcare spending is 15 times greater among elders with five or more chronic diseases compared with those without any chronic illness (AARP, 2009). This group of older adults consumes 75% of Medicare's total healthcare spending (Center for Disease Control and Prevention). The vast majority of these costs are due to high rates of hospital admission and readmission—a "churning" of patients that accounts for an estimated $15 billion annually in Medicare spending (Medicare Payment Advisory Commission [MedPAC], 2008). In addition to the impact of caring for older adults with multiple chronic conditions on healthcare spending, American businesses lose an estimated $34 billion each year due to employees' need to care for loved ones (Metlife Mature Market Institute and National Alliance for Caregiving, 2006).

WHAT IS TRANSITIONAL CARE?

Transitional care refers to a broad range of time-limited services and environments designed to ensure healthcare continuity, avoid preventable poor outcomes among at-risk populations, and promote the safe and timely transfer of patients from one level of care to another or from one type of setting to another (Coleman & Boult, 2003; Naylor, 2000). At-risk, chronically ill older adults are ideal candidates for transitional care because of their high healthcare utilization rates, frequent "handoffs," increased vulnerability, and disproportionately high healthcare costs.

Key Elements

Recent position and consensus statements (e.g., American Geriatrics Society, National Quality Forum, Agency for Healthcare Research and Quality) describe the core elements of transitional care, which include the following minimum, standard components:

- a comprehensive assessment of physical and mental condition, cognitive and functional capacities, medications, and social and environmental considerations;
- implementation of an evidence-based plan of transitional care;
- care that begins at hospital admission and extends beyond discharge;
- mechanisms to gather and appropriately share and distribute information across sites of care;
- involvement in and input from informal and family caregivers in planning and executing the care plan; and
- coordination of services during and after the hospitalization by a professional who has special preparation—typically a master's-prepared nurse.

Healthcare Context for Transitional Care

Transitional care is designed to complement high-quality primary care and/or care coordination. In contrast to discharge planning, which involves the development of a follow-up plan of care for older adults prior to leaving the hospital (Shepperd, Parkes, McClaren, & Phillips, 2004), transitional care services are designed to position the older adult to be in the best possible health condition at the hospital discharge. Additionally, these services extend well beyond discharge. Whereas disease management is "a system of coordinated healthcare interventions and communications for populations with conditions in which patient self-care efforts are significant" (DMAA: The Care Continuum Alliance), transitional care is not narrowly focused on specific diseases, nor does this approach focus solely on self-management. Unlike case management, which "is a collaborative process of assessment, planning, facilitation and advocacy for options and services to meet an individual's health needs through communication and available re-sources" (Case Management Society), transitional care involves the direct delivery of ser-vices in hospitals and older adults' homes. Finally, whereas care coordination is a term that is typically used to broadly define an interdisciplinary approach to care integra-tion for extended time periods covering multiple phases of the chronic illness trajectory (Brown, 2009), transitional care refers to time-limited services with a unique focus on the acute care episode (Figure 14.1).

Transitional care services begin at the onset of an acute event, continue through the postacute period, and end when the older adult is no longer at risk for poor outcomes such as adverse clinical events or acute hospitalizations. Unlike all of the aforementioned approaches, transitional care's foci are addressing the root causes of repeated poor out-comes and preventing the common breakdowns in care, including poor communication and inadequate preparation of older adults and their family caregivers.

Evolution of Evidence-Based Transitional Care

In 1980, a multidisciplinary team based at the University of Pennsylvania developed the Quality Cost Model of Advanced Practice Nurse (APN) Transitional Care. Concerned about the health of vulnerable patient groups and in response to changes in healthcare delivery resulting from managed care penetration, the model was initially designed to achieve early discharge of high-risk, high-cost, and high-volume patients by substituting a portion of hospitalization with a comprehensive program of home follow-up by nurse specialists.

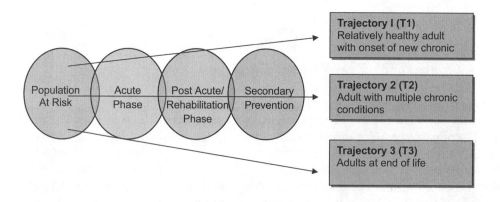

FIGURE 14.1   Context for transitional care: acute care episode.

Adapted with permission from the National Quality Forum's Measurement Framework: Evaluating Efficiency Across Episodes of Care (NQF, 2009).

Early tests of the model focused on low-birth-weight infants and women with high-risk pregnancies, unplanned cesarean births, and hysterectomy surgery. Results of four randomized clinical trials (RCTs) consistently demonstrated improved satisfaction, reduced rehospitalizations, and reduced healthcare costs among intervention group patients when compared with controls (Brooten et al., 1986; Brooten et al., 1994; Brooten et al., 2001; Hollingsworth & Cohen, 2000; York et al., 1997).

The introduction of Medicare's prospective payment system in 1983 provided hospitals with a substantial financial incentive to discharge older adults more quickly. By the late 1980s, the average length of hospital stay for Medicare beneficiaries was reduced by almost 2 days (Prospective Payment Assessment Commission, 1992). Unfortunately, this major change in hospital financing was not accompanied by any significant adjustment in the delivery of healthcare. Not surprisingly, shorter lengths of hospital stays were soon associated with growth in postdischarge services use (VanGelder & Bernstein, 1986; Wolock, Schlesinger, Dinerman, & Seaton, 1987). An unanticipated consequence of this policy change, however, included increased incidence of unmet needs for elders and their family caregivers (Naylor, 1986; Rogers et al., 1990) and higher rehospitalization rates among older adults (Anderson & Steinberg, 1984). To address these significant healthcare concerns, clinical scholars turned to the promise of transitional care.

MODELS OF TRANSITIONAL CARE

Since the introduction of the prospective payment system, researchers have pursued two major paths to advance knowledge related to the care and outcomes of vulnerable elders during challenging transitions from hospitals to the next care sites. Most teams have targeted interventions such as reengineering the discharge planning process, improving information transfer across sites, or reconciling medications (Jack et al., 2009; Konetzka, Spector, & Limcangco, 2008). In general, these one-dimensional strategies have yielded short-term positive impact. In a recent review of the empiric, peer-review literature, only two multidimensional models of transitional care tested in the U.S. were identified: The Care Transitions Program and the Transitional Care Model (TCM). The former emphasizes addressing gaps in care common during transitions, whereas the latter incorporates strategies to avoid such breakdowns but emphasizes interrupting the cycle of repeated hospitalizations with the goal of promoting long-term positive outcomes.

The Care Transitions Program

The Care Transitions Program is a patient-centered interdisciplinary team intervention designed to improve transitions across sites of care by educating and empowering older adults and their family caregivers to assure that their needs are met. This is accomplished by providing patients with tools that facilitate transitions as elders move from hospital to home, and promote elders' knowledge and ability to manage their conditions (Parry, Coleman, Smith, Frank, & Kramer, 2003).

During a 4-week program, patients with complex care needs receive specific tools, have Transition Coach support, and learn self-management skills to ensure that their needs are met during the transition from hospital to home. The tested model, which includes one hospital, one home visit, and telephone follow-up, is composed of the following components:

1. A patient-centered record that consists of the essential care elements for facilitating productive interdisciplinary communication during the care transition (referred to as the personal health record);
2. A structured checklist of critical activities designed to empower patients before discharge from the hospital or nursing facility; and
3. A patient self-activation and management session with a Transition Coach (a role assured by a variety of licensed and unlicensed health professionals) in the hospital, designed to help patients and their caregivers understand and apply the first two elements and assert their role in managing transitions

The intervention focuses on four conceptual areas, referred to as its pillars: medication self-management; use of a dynamic patient-centered record; primary care and specialist follow-up; and knowledge of "red flags," indications that the patient's condition is worsening, and how to respond (Parry, Kramer, & Coleman, 2006). Evidence supporting the Care Transitions Program is based on two studies, one quasi-experimental (Coleman et al., 2004) and one a foundation-supported RCT (Coleman & Chalmers, 2006). In the latter study, when the impact of the Care Transitions Program was compared with that of standard care received by a control group, the intervention resulted in lower all-cause rehospitalization rates through 90 days ($p = .04$). Without accounting for the cost of the intervention, mean hospital costs were approximately $500 lower for intervention patients compared with controls at 6 months postdischarge.

The Transitional Care Model

Based on the effectiveness of the Quality Cost Model of Advanced Practice Nurse Transitional Care (hereafter referred to as the TCM) among neonates and high-risk women, the model has been adapted and tested for at-risk older adults hospitalized for common medical and surgical conditions. The TCM provides comprehensive in-hospital planning and home follow-up to develop streamlined, rational care plans; interrupt patterns of frequent acute hospital and emergency department use; prevent health status decline; and promote long-term positive outcomes. The following are the core components of the model:

1. Continuity across the entire episode of acute care with a consistent master's-prepared nurse (APN) as the primary deliverer of the TCM protocol;
2. In-hospital assessment and collaboration with the healthcare team in the development of an evidence-based care plan;
3. Regular home visits with ongoing telephone support for an average of 2 months;
4. Comprehensive, holistic focus on each older adult's needs, including primary and coexisting chronic conditions and health risks, with particular emphasis on the root causes of poor outcomes;
5. Active engagement of older adults and family caregivers via identification of their health goals and desires, and active participation in care plan design;

6. Preparation of older adults and family caregivers to identify early and respond to healthcare risks and symptoms and avoid adverse events;
7. Multidisciplinary team approach to support the APN in addressing the complex care needs of older adults and family caregivers;
8. Physician–nurse collaboration with the APN accompanying the older adult to at least the first follow-up visit to primary care providers; and
9. Communication between and among older adults, family caregivers, and healthcare team.

Across three completed RCTs funded by the National Institute of Nursing Research, older adults in the intervention groups consistently demonstrated significant improvements in clinical and economic outcomes when compared with controls (Naylor et al., 1999; Naylor et al., 2004; Naylor et al., 1994). In the most recent multisite RCT (Naylor et al., 2004), for example, older adults who received the TCM demonstrated significant improvements in physical function and quality of life in the short-term, enhanced satisfaction with care, increased time to first readmission or death, and fewer total rehospitalizations through 1 year postdischarge. After accounting for the cost of the intervention, the mean savings in total healthcare costs of was $5,000 per older adult.

An ongoing clinical trial funded by the National Institute on Aging (NIA) is comparing the effects of the TCM to lower intensity interventions among cognitively impaired, hospitalized older adults and their family caregivers (NIA R01-AG023116; Marian S. Ware Alzheimer's Program, 2005–2010). Additionally, a longitudinal study (NIA and National Institute of Nursing Research, R01-AG025524; Marian S. Ware Alzheimer's Program, 2006–2011) is documenting changes in the trajectory of health and quality of life among frail elders who are newly transitioning to long-term care. The frequency, nature, and impact of transitions to and from hospitals for episodes of acute illness on the elders' trajectories also are being examined.

While the evidence base linking the TCM to improved health and cost outcome indicators continues to grow, translational research is providing important insights into the facilitators and barriers to implementing evidence-based care models in the "real world" of clinical practice (Naylor et al., 2009). With support of a number of foundations (The Commonwealth Fund, Jacob & Valeria Langeloth Foundation, The John A. Hartford Foundation, Inc., Gordon & Betty Moore Foundation, and California HealthCare Foundation) and guided by a national advisory committee of healthcare leaders, the University of Pennsylvania team formed a partnership initially with Aetna Corporation and subsequently with Kaiser Permanente Health Plan to translate and integrate TCM into a major insurance organization and a large integrated health plan and to determine if clinical and economic outcomes achieved in the RCTs could be replicated. To position the model for diffusion into these organizations, translation tools including a set of Web-based training modules to prepare nurses to implement the TCM, a clinical information system that houses the assessment tools, an intervention protocol and a documentation system, and a strategy for quality monitoring and improvement, were developed. Findings from a quasi-experimental study of the impact of the TCM among a high-risk Medicare managed care population in Aetna Corporation's mid-Atlantic region confirmed earlier results regarding the TCM's effectiveness, demonstrating that a rigorously tested transitional care model can be successfully translated into real-world organizations. The project with Kaiser Permanente Health Plan is ongoing.

IMPLICATIONS

Findings from the transitional care body of evidence, coupled with the lessons from integration of the TCM into real-world healthcare systems, have several implications for healthcare policy, research, and education and offer a roadmap for future efforts to translate research into practice.

Policy

Despite the growing body of evidence demonstrating transitional care's effectiveness, significant regulatory barriers exist to widespread implementation. Inconsistent and inflexible eligibility rules, financing models, and quality monitoring systems not only promote discontinuities in delivering care across settings, but also prevent the adoption of models proven to address the resulting fragmentation in care. The traditional Medicare and Medicaid programs are oriented to care delivered by individual providers in separate and distinct silos, contributing to duplication of services and gaps in care. Different funding streams, for example, pay for hospital, home health, and skilled nursing home care, and these systems are not aligned, consistent, or integrated. Under current models, financial incentives promote hospitalizations rather than positioning chronically ill older adults and their family caregivers with the knowledge, skills, and resources they need to prevent them. Furthermore, many of the longitudinal, team-based services that comprise evidence-based transitional care (e.g., care delivered by the same nurse in hospitals, skilled nursing facilities and elder's homes, nurse-accompanied physician visits, and 7-day-per-week availability) are not reimbursable under current public and private payment systems. Together, these policies pose significant barriers to the adoption of evidence-based transitional care.

Despite the significant and ongoing challenges, recent developments signal a shifting political climate that is "friendly" to transitional care:

- In 2007, MedPAC released a set of recommendations on healthcare delivery reform. Among the proposed strategies are those encouraging public reporting of hospital readmission rates, payment reform to stimulate reductions in rehospitalizations, and health system delivery reform to encourage the replication of proven strategies to reduce admissions (e.g., adoption of evidence-based best practice guidelines, improved patient communication, and medication reconciliation; MedPAC, 2007).
- Under its contract with quality improvement organizations, the Centers for Medicare & Medicaid Services recently emphasized reducing readmission rates through its Patient Pathways (Care Transitions) Theme. Fourteen quality improvement organizations have assumed active roles in reducing rehospitalizations at a community-wide level. Furthermore, as part of its broader commitment to transparency, the Centers for Medicare & Medicaid Services publicly reports 30-day risk standardized readmission rates for acute myocardial infarction, heart failure, and community-acquired pneumonia. Finally, through its value-based purchasing initiatives, home health providers are financially incentivized to reduce avoidable readmissions. Together, these policy directions have led to greater receptivity to transitional care.
- Under President Obama's administration and the 111th Congress' interest in healthcare reform, a number of bills and legislative initiatives have focused on improving

care to the chronically ill elderly and reducing costs to Medicare. Most notably, the Patient Protection and Affordable Care Act signed on March 23, 2010, establishes a 5-year, $500MM Community-Based Care Transitions Program. The Program targets high-risk Medicare beneficiaries, including those with multiple chronic conditions or who experience repeated hospital readmissions, and provides transitional care interventions, including in-hospital planning, self-management support, and medication review.

At a time when the Medicare Trust Fund is projected to be insolvent by 2017 (Boards of Trustees of the Federal Hospital Insurance and Federal Supplementary Medical Insurance Trust Funds, 2009) effective implementation of innovations that improve healthcare quality and reduce costs, such as the Community-Based Care Transitions Program, is vital.

Research

Despite the expanding scientific base reinforcing the promise of transitional care, many gaps in knowledge exist. For example, studies that distinguish the impact of these models on racially, ethnically, and socioeconomically diverse subgroups are essential. Additionally, although models have been studied in various geographic locations, additional evidence of their effectiveness in rural settings is needed to inform policy and practice. Finally, studies of these models among chronically ill patient groups of all ages transitioning to and from all care settings (e.g., skilled nursing facility to hospital and hospital to hospice) will inform their application and foster widespread adoption.

Most important, comparative effectiveness research that enables an apples-to-apples comparison of these evidence-based models is critical. Without studies that identify the most effective elements of these interventions and cost/benefit comparisons, policy makers, public and private payers, and consumers are unlikely to distinguish among them.

Education

Findings from these studies provide insights into the nature and preparation of the workforce that are required to implement transitional care. As recognized by the IOM's Committee on the Future Health Care Workforce for Older Americans, an adequate supply of healthcare practitioners is only part of the solution. Healthcare workforce competence needs dramatic improvement. This is especially true as it relates to care delivered within and, especially, across settings and practitioners:

> For the health care workforce, the challenges presented by the aging of America are multifaceted. . . . The vast majority of older adults have chronic illnesses that take them to multiple providers each year, and the management of chronic illness depends on better coordination and team-based care (IOM, 2008, p. ix).

Evidence from the translational work that has been conducted echoes the IOM's recommendations. Health professionals at all levels need didactic and clinical preparation in geriatrics and the skills, techniques, and competencies to deliver evidence-based care within and across care settings.

Because of the challenges anticipated and the inadequacies in health professions education, the next generation of healthcare professionals will need an enhanced understanding of this population's complexity, as well as clinical and system skills to address these needs. Evidence from these transitional care studies reveals the importance of preparation in comprehensive geriatric assessment, the integration of health and social services to meet the complex needs of elders with chronic disease management, and the appropriate and timely use of palliative and end-of-life care.

In addition to clinical skills, health professionals need mature and dynamic communication skills that foster collaboration with other health care team members in responding to older adults' and family caregivers' health goals and needs. In addition to interpersonal skills, communication skills must extend to the use of electronic exchanges that are meaningful, comprehensive, and supportive. Information technology, which will be relied on in these contacts, needs to facilitate the exchange of patient information that is accurate and comprehensive while appropriately maintaining privacy and confidentiality. Specific information to enable smooth and effective transitions of medications, diagnostic tests, and advance directives will be necessary. Although electronic medium will play a dominant role in future communications, interdisciplinary team training will be necessary to improve the person-to-person exchanges on which transitional care is dependent. Models such as those developed under the Hartford Foundation geriatric interdisciplinary team training programs are instructive.

Finally, although the chronically ill elderly experience a disproportionately high hospitalization rate, the majority of care is provided by family and an extended, informal caregiver network (e.g., relatives, friends, and neighbors). While preparation of the health professional workforce will need retooling, family caregivers provide the majority of care for this population and are largely untrained. Consistent with the IOM's recommendations, these authors recommend that systematic approaches to educating, counseling, and supporting family caregivers be developed and promoted.

CONCLUSION

The population in the United States is older and more chronically ill than ever before. Shifts in demographics and illness patterns, coupled with mounting healthcare expenditures, necessitate the adoption of care models that improve health outcomes at reduced costs. Two decades of research supports the effectiveness and efficiency of evidence-based models of transitional care for at-risk chronically ill elderly. Although signs point to this science already informing practice, additional investments in research and education accompanied by policy reform are necessary to accelerate translation and create a climate that is fully receptive to and supportive of transitional care.

REFERENCES

AARP. (2009). *Chronic care: A call to action for health reform.* Washington, DC: Author. AARP.

Anderson, G. (2003). Chronic care. *Public Health & Policy, 3*(2), 110–111.

Anderson, G. F., Hussey, P. S., Frogner, B. K., & Waters, H. R. (2005). Health spending in the United States and the rest of the industrialized world. *Health Affairs, 24*(4), 903–914.

Anderson, G., & Knickman, J. R. (2001). Changing the chronic care system to meet people's needs. *Health Affairs, 20*(6), 146–60.

Anderson, G., & Steinberg, E. (1984). Hospital readmissions in the Medicare population. *The New England Journal of Medicine, 311*, 1349–1353.

Boards of Trustees of the Federal Hospital Insurance and Federal Supplementary Medical Insurance Trust Funds. (2009). *The 2009 annual report of the Boards of Trustees of the Federal Supplementary Medical Insurance Trust Funds.* Washington, DC: Author. Retrieved on June 6, 2009, from http://www.cms.hhs.gov/ReportsTrustFunds/downloads/tr2009.pdf

Bowles, K. H., Foust, J. B., & Naylor, M. D. (2003). Hospital discharge referral decision making: A multidisciplinary perspective. *Applied Nursing Research, 16*(3), 134–143.

Brooten, D., Kumar, S., Brown, L., Butts, P., Finkler, S., Bakewell-Sachs, S., . . . Delivoria-Papadapoulos, M. (1986). A randomized clinical trial of early discharge and home follow-up of very low birth-weight infants. *The New England Journal of Medicine, 315*, 934–939.

Brooten, D., Roncoli, M., Finkler, S., Arnold, L., Cohen, A., & Mennuti, M. (1994). A randomized trial of early hospital discharge and nurse specialist home follow-up of women having cesarean birth. *Obstetrics and Gynecology, 84*, 832–838.

Brooten, D., Youngblut, J. M., Brown, L., Finkler, S., Neff, D. F., & Madigan, E. (2001). A randomized trial of nurse specialist home care for women with high risk pregnancies: Outcomes and cost. *American Journal of Managed Care, 7*, 793–803.

Brown, R. (2009). *The promise of care coordination: Models that decrease hospitalizations and improve outcomes for Medicare beneficiaries with chronic illnesses.* National Coalition on Care Coordination (NC3). Retrieved on June 6, 2009, from http://socialworkleadership.org/nsw/Brown_Full_Report.pdf

Case Management Society. Retrieved on June 13, 2009, from http://www.cmsa.org/Home/CMSA/WhatisaCaseManager/tabid/224/Default.aspx

Center on Budget and Policy Priorities. (2006). *The number of uninsured Americans is at an all-time high.* Washington, DC: Author.

Cherry, D. K., Hing, E., Woodwell, D. A., & Rechtsteiner, E. A. (2008). *National ambulatory medical care survey: 2006 summary.* National Health Statistics Reports, 3. Atlanta, GA: Center for Disease Control and Prevention. Retrieved on June 15, 2009, from http://www.cdc.gov/nchs/data/nhsr/nhsr003.pdf

Coleman, E. A., & Boult, C. (2003). Improving the quality of transitional care for persons with complex care needs. *Journal of the American Geriatric Society, 51*, 556–557.

Coleman, E. A., & Chalmers, S. (2006). The care transitions intervention: Results of a randomized controlled trial. *Archives of Internal Medicine, 166*, 1822–1828.

Coleman, E. A., Min, S., Chomiak, A., & Kramer, A. M. (2004). Posthospital care transitions: Patterns, complications, and risk identification. *Health Services Research, 39*(5), 1449–1465.

Coleman, E. A., Smith, J. D., Frank, J. C., Min, S., Parry, C., & Kramer, A. M. (2004). Preparing patients and caregivers to participate in care delivered across settings: The Care Transitions Intervention. *Journal of the American Geriatric Society, 52*, 1817–1825.

DMAA: The Care Continuum Alliance. Retrieved on May 31, 2009, from http://www.dmaa.org/dm_definition.asp

Forster, A. J., Murff, H. J., Peterson, J. F., Gandhi, T. K., & Bates, D. W. (2003). The incidence and severity of adverse events affecting patients after discharge from the hospital. *Annals of Internal Medicine, 138*(3), 161–167.

He, W., Sengupta, M., Velkoff, V. A., & DeBarros, K. A. (2005). U.S. Census Bureau, Current Population Reports, P23-209, *65+ in the United States: 2005.* Washington, DC: U.S. Government Printing Office.

Hollingsworth, A. O., & Cohen, S. M. (2000). Outcomes of early hospital discharge of women undergoing abdominal hysterectomy. In M. T. Nolan & V. Mock (Eds.). *Measuring patient outcomes* (pp. 155–167). Thousand Oaks, CA: Sage.

Institute of Medicine (IOM). (2000). *To err is human: Building a safer health system.* Washington, DC: National Academies Press.

Institute of Medicine (IOM). (2001). *Crossing the quality chasm: A new health system for the 21st Century.* Washington, DC: National Academies Press.

Institute of Medicine (IOM). (2008). *Retooling for an aging America: Building the health care workforce.* Washington, DC: National Academies Press.

Jack, B. W., Chetty, V. K., Anthony, D., Greenwald, J. L., Sanchez, G. M., Johnson, A. E., . . . Culpepper, L. (2009). A reengineered hospital discharge program to decrease rehospitalization: A randomized trial. *Annals of Internal Medicine, 150*, 178–187.

Jencks, S. F., Williams, M. V., & Coleman, E. A. (2009). Rehospitalizations among patients in the Medicare Fee-for-Service Program. *New England Journal of Medicine, 360*, 1418–1428.

Kaiser Commission on Medicaid and the Uninsured. (2008). *The uninsured and the difference health insurance markets.* Washington, DC: Kaiser Family Foundation. Publication #1420-10.

Konetzka, R. T., Spector, W., & Limcangco, M. R. (2008). Reducing hospitalizations from long-term care settings. *Medical Care Research and Review, 65,* 40–66.

Kramarow, E., Lubitz, J., Lentzner, H., & Gorina, Y. (2007). Trends in the health of older Americans, 1970–2005. *Health Affairs, 26*(5), 1417–1425.

Medicare Payment Advisory Commission (MedPAC). (2007). *Report to Congress: Promoting greater efficiency in medicare.* Washington, DC: MedPAC.

Medicare Payment Advisory Commission (MedPAC). (2008). *MedPAC Data Book, June 2008.* Washington, DC: MedPAC.

MetLife Mature Market Institute and National Alliance for Caregiving. (2006). *MetLife caregiving cost study: Productivity losses to U.S. business.*

Moore, C., Wisnevesky, J., Williams, S., & McGinn, T. (2003). Medical errors related to discontinuity of care from an inpatient to an outpatient setting. *Journal of General Internal Medicine, 18*(8), 646–651.

National Priorities Partnership. (2008). *National priorities and goals: Aligning our efforts to transform America's healthcare.* Washington, DC: National Quality Forum.

National Quality Forum (NQF). (2009). *Measurement framework: Evaluating efficiency across patient-focused episodes of care.* Washington, DC: NQF.

Naylor, M. (1986). *The health status and health care needs of older Americans.* Washington, DC: US Senate Special Committee on Aging. Serial 99-L.

Naylor, M. D. (2000). A decade of transitional care research with vulnerable elders. *Journal of Cardiovascular Nursing, 14*(3), 1–14.

Naylor, M. D. (2003). Transitional care of older adults. In J. J. Fitzpatrick, P. G. Archbold, & B. J. Stewart (Eds.), *Annual review of nursing research* (Vol. 20). New York: Springer.

Naylor, M. D., Brooten, D., Campbell, R., Jacobsen, B. S., Mezey, M. D., Pauley, M. V., Schwartz, J. S. (1999). Comprehensive discharge planning and home follow-up of hospitalized elders: A randomized clinical trial. *JAMA. Journal of the American Medical Association, 281,* 613–620.

Naylor, M. D., Brooten, D. A., Campell, R. L., Maislin, G., McCauley, K. M., & Schwartz, J. S. (2004). Transitional care of older adults hospitalized with heart failure: A randomized, controlled trial. *Journal of the American Geriatric Society, 52,* 675–684.

Naylor, M., Brooten, D., Jones, R., Lavizzo-Mourey, R., Mezey, M., & Pauley, M. (1994). Comprehensive discharge planning for the hospitalized elderly. *Annals of Internal Medicine, 120,* 999–1006.

Naylor, M. D., Feldman, P. H., Keating, S., Koren, M. J., Kurtzman, E. T., MacCoy, M. C., & Krakauer, R. (2009). Translating research into practice: Transitional care for older adults. *Journal of Evaluation in Clinical Practice, 15,* 1164–1170.

Parry, C., Coleman, E. A., Smith, J. D., Frank, J. C., & Kramer, A. M. (2003). The care transitions intervention: A patient-centered approach to facilitating effective transfers between sites of geriatric care. *Home Health Services Quarterly, 22*(3), 1–18.

Parry, C., Kramer, H. M., & Coleman, E. A. (2006). A qualitative exploration of a patient-centered coaching intervention to improve care transitions in chronically ill older adults. *Home Health Care Services Quarterly, 25,* 39–53.

Partnership for Chronic Disease. Retrieved on April 13, 2009, from http://www.fightchronicdisease.org/issues/about.cfm

Partnerships for Solutions for the Robert Wood Johnson Foundation. (2004). *Chronic conditions: Making the case for ongoing care.* Baltimore, MD: Johns Hopkins University. September 2004 Update.

The Patient Protection and Affordable Care Act, Pub. L. No. 111–118, § Sec. 3026.

Prospective Payment Assessment Commission. (1992). *Medicare prospective payment and the American health care system: Report to Congress.* Washington, DC: Prospective Payment Assessment Commission.

Rogers, W. H., Draper, D., Kahn, K. L., Keeler, E. B., Rubenstein, L. V., Kosecoff, J., & Brook, R. H. (1990). Quality of care before and after implementation of the DRG-based prospective payment system. A summary of effects. *JAMA. Journal of the American Medical Association, 264,* 1989–1994.

Shepperd, S., Parkes, J., McClaren, J., & Phillips, C. (2004). Discharge planning from hospital to home. *Cochrane Database of Systematic Reviews, 2004*(1).

The Patient Protection and Affordable Care Act. (2010), Pub. L. No. 111–148, Sec. 3026.

VanGelder, S., & Bernstein, J. (1986). Home health care in the era of hospital prospective payment: Some early evidence and thoughts about the future. *Pride Institute Journal of Long-Term Home Health Care, 5,* 3–11.

van den Akker, M., Buntinx, F., Metsemakers, J. F., Roos, S., & Knottnerus, J. A. (1998). Multimorbidity in general practice: Prevalence, incidence, and determinants of co-occurring chronic and recurrent diseases. *Journal of Clinical Epidemiology, 51*(5), 367–375.

Wenger, N. S., Solomon, D. H., Roth, C. P., MacLean, C. H., Saliba, D., Kamberg, C. J., et al. (2003). The quality of medical care provided to vulnerable community- dwelling older patients. *Annals of Internal Medicine, 139*(9), 740–747.

Wolock, I., Schlesinger, E., Dinerman, M., & Seaton, R. (1987). The posthospital needs and care of patients: Implications for discharge planning. *Social Work Health Care, 12*, 61–76.

York, R., Brown, L. P., Samuels, P., Finkler, S., Jacobsen, B., Armstrong, C., . . . Robbins, D. (1997). A randomized trial of early discharge and nurse specialist transitional follow-up care of high risk childbearing women. *Nursing Research, 46*, 254–261.

15

Nursing: Saving Lives, Improving Patient Care Outcomes

Linda H. Aiken

INTRODUCTION

The term *reality shock* aptly captured my experiences as a new nurse graduate specializing in bedside care at a major teaching hospital (Kramer, 1974). I had excellent professional and clinical education and I was practicing in a hospital with a record of innovation in nursing. However, in my first position as a registered nurse (RN) I found that the nurse practice environment worked against my very best efforts to provide excellent care to patients. That perception has been repeated in every hospital in which I have practiced and has motivated me to study how the organizational context of nursing care affects patient and nurse outcomes. My studies of hospital bedside care nurses in the United States and internationally, reflect my own clinical experiences and suggest that the environment in most hospitals is not as supportive of professional nursing care as it could be, leading to uneven quality of care, patient safety hazards, and high rates of nurse burnout (Aiken et al., 2001).

In 1990, with the establishment of the Center for Health Outcomes and Policy Research at the University of Pennsylvania School of Nursing, I set out to contribute to the development of a scientific basis for motivating and informing changes in clinical, managerial, and public policies regarding the organizational context in which nursing care is delivered. My research has focused on many different settings in which nurses provide care, but hospitals have been of particular concern because that is where the largest share of nurses practice and where the risk of life-threatening adverse outcomes for patients is greatest This chapter is a summary of my program of research and highlights some of our findings, discusses how we made our research policy-relevant, and provides examples of policy responses.

RESEARCH AND THE POLICY PROCESS

There are at least two types of strategies for influencing policy changes. Although they overlap to some degree, they generally require two different career paths. One type of strategy is advocacy, often achieved through knowledge about the legislative process, understanding of politics, and organizing stakeholder coalitions. Understanding and interpreting research are effective political advocacy skills. The second, the path I chose, is influencing decisions through policy-relevant research. This is a path that requires rigorous research training, usually at the doctoral and postdoctoral levels. An understanding of current events and public debates is also required, which necessitates broad reading outside of one's own specialty area and opportunities for interdisciplinary discourse.

Over my career, research and evidence have begun to take on greater importance in legislative debates, serving to balance to some extent the use of personal stories and anecdotes that have traditionally motivated political action. The increased prominence of research is both an opportunity and a challenge. Researchers who have answers to questions *relevant* to political debate (and managerial debate in the private sector) at the *time* decision making is taking place have the opportunity to impact those decisions. However, having answers that are relevant and timely to legislative debate require researchers to *anticipate* the information that will be needed to motivate action and to undertake studies well in advance of public consensus that a topic is important. Another challenge that has accompanied the growing role of research in policy and managerial debates is increased scrutiny of research findings, particularly by stakeholders who seek to discredit findings that are not favorable to their perceived interests. Thus, it is extremely important to select in advance a defensible research design that is understandable and credible and that also has scientific validity and merit as evidenced by publication in a respected, peer-reviewed scientific journal. The findings must be clear and believable to informed generalists, including the media, in order to move from statistical significance to action.

Influencing change in policy and practice is much more likely if the research question selected for study is already of interest to the public, policy makers, managers, or practitioners. This seems self-evident. However, much of nursing research focuses on topics that do not have clear implications outside of nursing and/or are not framed in a larger context that would help others appreciate their significance.

We tend to follow one of three strategies in selecting topics for study and for framing our results once the studies have been completed to increase the policy relevance of our research findings: (1) selecting topics of health policy interest that have not been examined through the lens of nursing; (2) myth busting, which involves objectively investigating the validity of commonly held beliefs; and (3) translating research findings into a current policy context.

HEALTH SERVICES RESEARCH THROUGH A NURSING LENS

Nurse Staffing

There is a robust literature on the correlates of hospital mortality dating back to at least the early 1960s, when the National Halothane Study was undertaken to examine the impact of anesthetic agents on surgical mortality (Moses & Mosteller, 1968). One of the most surprising findings was that surgical mortality varied significantly across hospitals irrespective of the type of anesthesia. This observation resulted in many subsequent studies exploring explanations for the variation in hospital mortality. A careful reading of this literature shows that nursing was usually included in multivariate predictive models, often measured by nurse-to-bed ratios, and commonly found to be associated with variation in surgical mortality but not emphasized in the published findings (see, e.g., Hartz et al., 1989). Published policy papers on variation in hospital mortality tended to emphasize findings associated with national policy debates, such as whether hospital outcomes varied by ownership status in for-profit versus nonprofit hospitals (Shortell & Hughes, 1988) because at that time, nurse staffing in hospitals was not a topic attracting policy interest.

A similar example is a publication that examined hospital mortality rates by whether anesthesia providers were nurse anesthetists, physician anesthesiologists, or interdisciplinary teams, a topic of contentious debate over Medicare reimbursement policy (Silber et al., 2000). Most of the emphasis in that paper was in the main findings about the anesthesia providers, whereas little attention was given to the finding that nurse staffing ratios in hospitals had a larger effect on surgical mortality than did the qualifications of the anesthesia provider.

Hospital nurse staffing was found to be a significant correlate of hospital mortality in the early health services research literature on variation in hospital mortality outcomes, but nursing was treated as a statistical control rather than a variable of interest and was rarely included in the discussion and policy sections of published papers. Despite a number of papers published in leading interdisciplinary scientific journals that demonstrated the effect of hospital nurse staffing on variation in hospital mortality, the lack of development of the nurse staffing findings resulted in little recognition of the potential importance of nurse staffing in reducing variation in hospital mortality.

My program of research set out to look directly at the effect of nurse staffing on hospital mortality. My interest was in the net effect of nurse staffing after taking into consideration other possible explanations of hospital mortality, whereas previous research was interested in the net effects of variables, such as ownership, controlling for nurse staffing. It was my contention that nurse staffing was a modifiable feature of hospital organization and therefore merited attention. Nurse staffing levels could be changed if research findings underscored their importance in patient outcomes in contrast to relatively immutable characteristics like ownership and teaching status that had been the focus of earlier published papers. In order to make my point, I replicated earlier research with the same rigor as previously published papers, including using state-of-the-science methods of controlling for differences in illness severity of patients across hospitals (Iezzoni, 2003). In essence, I looked at a researchable question through the lens of nursing and, in doing so, produced a body of research findings that had been obscured by the policy context selected for emphasis by other investigators (Aiken, Clarke, Sloane, Sochalski, & Silber, 2002; Aiken, Smith, & Lake, 1994).

Higher Volume and Better Outcomes

Another example of reexamining a large body of research through a nursing lens is our ongoing research on the impact of nursing on the "volumes/outcomes relationship." There are hundreds of published research papers documenting that hospitals with larger annual volumes of patients undergoing specific surgical procedures, such as aortic aneurysm repair, or with particular medical diagnoses, such as AIDS, have lower mortality than do hospitals with lower patient volumes (Luft, Garnick, Mark, & McPhee, 1990). There is also evidence that the better outcomes associated with higher volumes produce care at lower overall costs. This literature has been very influential in motivating quality standards that require hospitals to meet volume thresholds to conduct some surgical procedures and payer policies that encourage providers to refer patients to high-volume hospitals. Two primary hypotheses have been offered to explain the volumes–outcomes association. One is that practice makes perfect; that is, personnel who participate in the same procedures over and over again gain knowledge and skill that contribute to better patient outcomes. The second hypothesis is one of selective referral; that is, hospitals develop reputations for good outcomes and/or high volume of a certain procedure and attract patients because of the reputation. The patients attracted by hospitals' reputations include a high proportion of low-risk patients, resulting in better overall outcomes because of the lower risk status of the patients. Regardless of the explanation for the volumes–outcomes relationship, the findings have been used to promote the regionalization of care for certain types of patients. Regionalization is not without its human costs, often requiring patients to obtain care far from home and their social support network.

Of the more than 300 published papers on the volumes–outcomes relationship, we found only two that mention nursing. We find that surprising because of the assumption that the experience of the "team" is important to achieving good patient outcomes, and nurses are the most numerous members of the team. Additionally, the results of one of our early studies of AIDS care gave us reason to evaluate the volumes–outcomes literature through a nursing lens.

We published the results of our national evaluation of AIDS hospital care in the interdisciplinary journal *Medical Care* (Aiken et al., 1999) in the same month and year that another paper was published on the outcomes of AIDS care (Cunningham, Tisnado, Lui, Nakazono, & Carlisle, 1999). The two papers reached the opposite conclusions on what should be done to improve inpatient AIDS outcomes.

Our study included 20 hospitals with large numbers of AIDS patients in cities with high AIDS incidence. Our study was designed to compare hospital mortality for AIDS patients in terms of three comparison groups: (1) within-hospital comparisons of AIDS patients receiving care on dedicated versus general medical units; (2) between-hospital comparisons of AIDS mortality in hospitals with and without dedicated AIDS units; and (3) comparison of outcomes for AIDS patients in Magnet hospitals (see McClure, Poulin, Sovie, & Wandelt, 1983, for a description of Magnet hospitals) compared with hospitals with and without dedicated AIDS units (Aiken, Lake, Sochalski, Sloane, 1997). We found that (1) AIDS mortality was significantly lower in dedicated AIDS units than in general medical units in the same hospitals; (2) AIDS mortality was significantly lower in hospitals with dedicated AIDS units than in matched hospitals without such units; and (3) Magnet hospitals had the lowest AIDS mortality without having dedicated AIDS units, specialty HIV/AIDS services, or high volume of AIDS patients (Aiken et al., 1999). We were able to show that the mortality advantage and higher patient satisfaction levels associated with both Magnet hospitals and dedicated AIDS units could be attributed to more generous RN staffing and an organizational context of care that supported professional nursing practice. We concluded that the outcomes of inpatient AIDS care could be improved by better nurse staffing and improved nurse practice environments in all hospitals providing AIDS care regardless of volume of HIV patients.

The contrast in conclusions between the two papers could not have been greater. The paper by Cunningham et al. (1999) examined the relationship between volume of AIDS care in all California hospitals and mortality. Higher volume AIDS hospitals were found to have significantly lower mortality. There was no mention of nursing and the authors recommended regionalization of AIDS care. Our paper recommended investments in nursing in all hospitals.

Our work "unpacking" the link between nursing and the volumes–outcomes relationship is continuing. Most of the research on the volumes–outcomes relationship is limited to specific surgical procedures. We are replicating those studies, but in addition, we are examining the contribution of nursing factors to outcomes. Our preliminary findings so far suggest that (1) the volumes–outcomes mortality advantage does not seem to persist over time, suggesting that volume is less important as new knowledge and technologies disseminate more broadly; (2) in procedures where a volumes–outcomes relationship can still be demonstrated, nursing factors such as staffing and the nurse work environment are associated with mortality independent of volume; and (3) hospitals with better nurse work environments, including better staffing, have superior outcomes for a wide range of patients admitted with common medical and surgical treatments, not just in narrow subspecialties where volumes explain better outcomes.

Our findings over multiple studies led us to conclude that policies to promote volume thresholds and regionalization have been promulgated without regard to other strategies, particularly strengthening nursing in hospitals. Volume thresholds, as implemented, affect relatively small proportions of patients in few hospitals, whereas improving nursing could potentially affect large proportions of patients in most hospitals, thus having a greater impact on improving hospital outcomes than do volume thresholds. Interest by the policy world in the volumes–outcomes relationship is not only in the potential of volume thresholds to produce better outcome, but also because there may be cost savings also. In contrast, there are insufficient data as yet to establish whether nursing investments can produce better outcomes *and* lower costs. Our program of research is now focusing on determining whether investments in nursing offset other types of hospital costs, including fewer intensive care unit days, fewer laboratory tests and drug expenditures, and shorter lengths of stay resulting from complications prevented. Better cost data may be the key to translating into practice those nursing interventions shown to be effective. My point in this discussion is that researchers serve the public interest by persistently pursuing promising approaches to improving care even in the face of widespread support for other options.

Nurse Work Environment

My presidential address to the American Academy of Nursing in 1980 was a call to action to improve nursing practice in hospitals and nursing homes (Aiken, 1981). Members of the academy responded with what became one of the most important ideas in nursing: Magnet hospitals (McClure & Hinshaw, 2002; McClure, Poulin, Sovie, & Wandelt, 1983). Magnet hospitals were able to attract and retain nurses even when other hospitals in their local labor markets were experiencing nurse shortages because of the organizational culture they had developed to support the professional practice of nursing. Our program of research was the first to show that Magnet hospitals also had lower mortality rates than other similar hospitals (Aiken et al., 1994). Thanks to innovative research by Marlene Kramer, mentioned at the outset of this chapter for her influential book, *Reality Shock*, we developed a research plan for measuring in all hospitals the organizational attributes found in Magnet hospitals. We modified a survey instrument originally developed by Kramer to measure nurse satisfaction and quality to document the presence of organizational attributes found in Magnet hospitals, such as decentralized decision making, a visible chief nursing officer, and good relationships between nurses and doctors.

The instrument, called the Modified Nurse Work Environment (NWI-R) (Aiken & Patrician, 2000) and the Practice Environment Scale (PES) of the NWI-R (Lake, 2002), enabled us to empirically measure the quality of a work environment supportive of professional nursing practice using survey research.

Once we had a good survey-based measure of the nurse work environment, we were able to conduct large-scale studies of hospitals that were never before possible. We typically draw a large random sample of RNs from state licensing boards and survey the nurses at their home addresses, asking them to complete the NWI-R and other information relating to their current hospital employer. We ask each nurse to provide the name of her or his employer and we aggregate responses of all nurses who work in the same hospital to create a hospital-level empirical measure of the quality of the nurse work environment. In our latest study, we surveyed 80,000 nurses in four states (Pennsylvania, New Jersey, California, and Florida) who filled out the NWI-R on more than 850 hospitals. We asked the nurses in the survey about how many patients they cared for on their last shift, creating a common patient-to-nurse ratio across the 850 hospitals. Additionally, the nurses provided us with their highest educational attainment, which then allowed us to create a new variable also missing from existing databases; that is, the proportion of nurses in each of the 850 hospitals who had obtained at least a baccalaureate degree. We combined these primary survey data from nurses with standardized patient discharge information from the same hospitals and then were able to study the impact of the work environment on patient outcomes including mortality across the 850 hospitals. A major advantage of this design is that all hospitals can be studied without having to seek the permission of hospital administrators, thus eliminating bias in the hospital sample that could be associated with nursing factors. That is, hospitals with poor nurse staffing or work environments could not opt out of the study.

The findings from our research on the nurse work environment have been the most innovative and path breaking in our program of research because we have been able to empirically study in hundreds of hospitals an organizational/cultural phenomenon previously thought of as "soft" or subjective. We have used the PES-NWI in a number of papers where we have been able to demonstrate that the quality of the nurse work environment is a significant factor in patient outcomes, even after controlling for differences among hospitals in nurse staffing (Aiken, Clarke, Sloane, Lake, & Cheney, 2008; Friese, Lake, Aiken, Silber, & Sochalski 2008). For example, surgical patients in hospitals with better nurse work environments have 13% lower odds of dying than do patients in hospitals with poor nurse work environments. Similarly, patients in hospitals with better staffing have 11% lower odds of dying. Better nurse work environments and better staffing are independent and additive, meaning that patients in hospitals with the best work environments and the best staffing have 24% lower odds of dying (Aiken et al., 2008).

Our research has helped propel the importance of organizational culture into the mainstream of the thought about how to improve patient safety. For example, the prestigious Institute of Medicine (IOM, 2004) of the National Academy of Sciences released a major report in its quality series entitled *Keeping Patients Safe: Transforming the Nurse Work Environment*. Prior to our research, there was no empirical measure of the nurse work environment, and hence, most health services research on nursing focused only on nurse staffing. We are still one of the few research programs to include a measure of the quality of the nurse work environment in nursing outcomes research. Thus, we are trying to make information on the nursing work environment more readily available to researchers and practicing nurses. The American Nurses Association's (ANA's) National

Database of Nursing Quality Indicators now includes the PES-NWI in its hospital data benchmarking program (www.nursingquality.org). The PES-NWI has also been adopted as one of 15 National Quality Forum nurse-sensitive quality indicators recommended for routine collection by hospitals (National Quality Forum, 2007).

MYTH BUSTING

Despite considerable emphasis on moving toward more evidence-based decision making in health services, two common scenarios persist. First, science-based practices are not consistently followed in day-to-day healthcare, resulting in preventable adverse outcomes for patients. My focus here is on the second phenomenon, which involves acting on closely held beliefs that are not evidence based and possibly not true. Myths abound in healthcare, and myth busting can be a very effective way of bringing attention to newly emerging research. Two examples from our research illustrate the point.

Nurses' Education

The first example of myth busting involves the widely held belief that in nursing, experience is the most important factor in producing good patient outcomes. Some would go even further in their belief that experience is a substitute for higher education. At a time when other health professions (social work, pharmacy, clinical psychology, and physical and occupational therapy) have moved entry into practice to the master's or doctoral levels, a growing share of nurses—two-thirds now—get their basic education from associate degree programs, and most get no further education. Whether this pattern of educational attainment for nurses is in the public interest depends upon whether care outcomes are associated with nurses' educational qualifications.

In keeping with our practice stated earlier—to frame nursing research questions in a broader context to attract greater interest—we reviewed the research literature on professional qualifications and hospital patient outcomes. We found a number of studies suggesting that hospitals with a greater proportion of physicians with board certification had lower risk-adjusted mortality, controlling for other factors (Brennan et al., 2003). There were no comparable large-scale studies examining the composition of hospitals' nurse workforces by educational attainment. Thus, we replicated the physician board certification research and added two new variables. One measured the percentage of nurses by hospital who had a baccalaureate or higher degree, and the other measured mean years of experience of nurses by hospital. We were able to create these new variables from large-scale surveys of nurses that we had conducted in the state of Pennsylvania with National Institute of Nursing Research funding with the aim of understanding the association between nurse factors and patient outcomes.

Our nurse survey requested information from respondents on their highest educational degree plus the name of each nurse's employing hospital. We aggregated individual nurse's responses to his or her employing hospital, thus creating a hospital-level variable for all hospitals in Pennsylvania of percentage of staff nurses with a bachelor of science in nursing (BSN) or higher educational attainment, a measure similar conceptually to percentage of board-certified physicians in each hospital. The health services research literature on physician board certification gave us the idea of studying nurses' qualifications as a property of the hospital versus most other studies of nurses' education and experience that conceptualized nursing education and experience as properties of individual nurses.

Our first finding was that hospitals varied dramatically in the proportion of bedside care nurses with BSN or higher educational preparation; the range was from under 10% to over 90%. Usually in health services, when there is that much variation across hospitals in an input variable, outcomes also differ. In contrast, nurses' average years of experience by hospital did not vary significantly. We applied predictive models using robust regression techniques that account for the nesting of nurses and patients within hospitals to determine the independent effects of percentage BSN nurses and mean years of RN experience on variation in hospital mortality. We controlled statistically for patient illness severity, percentage of board-certified physicians, and other possible explanations for differences in hospital mortality, including teaching hospital status and high technology availability.

Our findings, reported in the *Journal of the American Medical Association*, suggested that each 10% increase in the proportion of staff nurses with BSNs was associated with a 5% decline in mortality (Aiken, Clarke, Cheung, Sloane & Silber, 2003). Mean years of nurse experience was not significantly associated with hospital mortality. The proportion of board-certified physicians was also significantly associated with mortality. Thus, nurses' qualifications and physician qualifications were equally important determinants of patient mortality. We are presently extending this research to examine the effects of nurse specialty certification over and above the effects of BSN education. Our education result has been replicated by our international collaborators in Canada (Estabrooks, Midodzi, Cummings, Ricker, & Giovannetti, 2005; Tourangeau et al., 2007) and in Belgium (Van den Heede et al., 2009). These research findings have changed the tenor of the longstanding debate over minimum educational requirements for nurses because they provide compelling evidence that experience is not a substitute for education, a widely held belief but apparently not a valid one.

Supplemental Nurse Staffing

Another widely held belief is that the use by hospitals of temporary or supplemental nurses employed by agencies negatively affects the quality of care and patient outcomes. This belief is so strongly held that the use of supplemental nurses has become a commonly used proxy indicator for poor care quality; that is, some investigators now use employment of supplemental nurses as *the* negative outcome (Burnes Bolton et al., 2007). Unfortunately, in retrospect, we contributed to the perception of supplemental nurse staffing as a negative factor by reporting in a study of the exposure of nurses to blood-borne pathogens through needlestick injuries that the odds of needlestick injuries were higher in hospitals that employed more temporary nurses (Aiken, Sloane, & Klocinski, 1997).

However, as our program of research advanced, and we demonstrated that hospitals with more favorable patient-to-nurse ratios had lower mortality (Aiken et al., 2002), we began to examine more critically the hypothesis that temporary nurses "cause" poor patient and nurse outcomes. If having more nurses is a good thing for patients, as demonstrated by our research, how could obtaining higher favorable patient-to-nurse ratios by employing RNs from private agencies result in poorer outcomes? We reasoned that the agency nurses would have to be less qualified to have a negative impact. When we empirically examined the qualifications of temporary nurses using the National Sample Survey of Registered Nurses conducted every 4 years, we found that they were as qualified as nurses employed directly by hospitals. Moreover, over half of nurses who sometimes worked for agencies also were employed by hospitals, so there were no significant differences in qualifications of nurses who were "temporary" versus permanent employees of hospitals (Aiken, Xue, Clarke, & Sloane, 2007).

Another possible explanation for poor outcomes associated with the employment of supplemental nurses is the lack of continuity in nursing care that might result from temporary nurse assignments. Upon further reflection, that explanation seems to lack validity given the reality that a majority of nurses in hospitals now work approximately three 12-hour shifts per week, and thus, there may be little continuity of patient care assignments whether nurses are employed by the hospital or by an agency.

Most health outcomes research is cross-sectional, including most studies that we have conducted; that is, the studies are undertaken at a single point in time. No matter how big the studies are, single-point-in-time studies can establish whether associations exist between factors but cannot determine causation. In our cross-sectional study of needlestick injuries to hospital staff nurses and employment of temporary nurses, we demonstrated a statistically significant relationship between the odds of a needlestick injury and the proportion of nurses who were temporary employees. But we could not establish that temporary nurses "caused" more injuries. Likewise, other studies that have demonstrated an association between poor outcomes and the employment of more temporary nurses cannot establish causation, but a misreading of their results has led nurses and others to believe that there is evidence that temporary nurses cause poor outcomes.

We thought that a possible explanation for the association between poor patient outcomes and the employment of a large proportion of temporary nurses could be a third unmeasured factor in most studies of the outcomes of supplemental nurse staffing. To us, the most obvious unmeasured factor in most research on the topic was the quality of the nurse work environment across hospitals. We reasoned that hospitals with poor work environments would have difficulty recruiting and retaining permanently employed nurses and thus would turn to supplemental staffing agencies to fill their vacant positions. If this were the case, the poor outcomes associated with supplemental nurses could be "caused" by poor work environments and not by the supplemental nurses. We tested that hypothesis and found it to be true (Aiken et al., 2007). We found that almost all hospitals, even those with the best reputations, employ some supplemental nurses. In most hospitals, temporary nurses constitute fewer than 10% of all bedside care nurses, but in some hospitals, more than 20% of nurses were temporary nurses. We looked to see whether the quality of the nurse work environment was poor in hospitals in which a significant portion of their nurse workforce was temporary, and the answer was yes. Then, we tested empirical models that examined the extent to which the poor outcomes associated with temporary nurses could be explained by poor work environments. The answer was that when the quality of the work environment was taken into account, there was no longer an association between temporary nurses and poor outcomes, suggesting that poor work environments, not temporary nurses, are responsible for poor patient outcomes, although longitudinal studies will be required to further test causation.

In summary, things are not always as they appear. Often, beliefs without a strong empirical basis turn out to be false or at least questionable. A "research imagination" can help sort out beliefs that are evidence based from those that are not, and thereby often improve practice and efficient use of resources.

TRANSLATING RESEARCH FINDINGS

Nursing research is conducted to advance knowledge development and to inform the decisions of the public, clinicians, health services administrators, and/or health policy makers. The greatest challenge for researchers, besides conducting excellent research on important topics, is to effectively communicate their findings to the broad research community as well as to those in positions to act on the findings. Publishing scientific findings that others are likely to see and read is important but often not sufficient. Scientific papers are not easy for most of us to interpret even if we are motivated to read them. And most of those in positions to act on scientific findings do not have the time or academic background to read scientific papers. With these challenges in mind, we have several strategies that have helped us get our messages to the target audiences. (1) We end every scientific paper with a discussion section that interprets the findings for a general audience. (2) We try to interest the media in writing about our findings because, often, the target audience is more likely to read their summary than our paper, and journalists are often excellent at targeting the most significant aspects of the research from the public's perspective. In order to get media coverage, we have to write the discussion section in the scientific paper to capture their attention. (3) We invest heavily in communicating our results directly to target audiences like nurse clinicians and administrators, educators, non nurse stakeholders, and public policy makers. We try to do this strategically by getting our message to those who will pass it on. But again, we generally need to identify a reason why the target audience should be interested in our findings.

The next examples show how we try to locate our research within a contemporary professional or policy debate in the introductions and discussion sections of scientific papers and in media communications. We have found this to be a very useful strategy in helping to translate our research findings into actionable information.

Nurse Staffing Legislation

For almost three decades, nurses have been reporting that patient-to-nurse staffing ratios in hospitals are dangerously high (Aiken & Mullinix, 1987; Aiken, Sochalski, & Anderson, 1996). Nurses lobbied the Congress in the early 1990s to request a study by the IOM, National Academy of Sciences, on whether nurse staffing levels in hospitals and nursing homes were adequate. The IOM report (Wunderlich, Sloan, & Davis, 1996) recommended minimum nurse staffing standards for nursing homes but cited insufficient evidence to reach a similar conclusion about hospitals; instead, the IOM recommended additional research on hospital staffing. Over the next decade, a number of studies were undertaken on nurse staffing, resulting in a recently published meta-analysis of close to 30 published studies concluding that there is strong evidence that less favorable (to patients) nurse staffing in hospitals is associated with higher mortality (Kane, Shamliyan, Mueller, Duval, & Wilt, 2007). Even as more studies were being undertaken, nurses turned to policy strategies, including lobbying their elected state representatives for legislative regulations, to compel hospitals to improve nurse staffing and to eliminate employer requirements of mandatory nurse overtime. As of March 2009, 13 states and the District of Columbia had enacted nurse staffing legislation and/or adopted regulations addressing nurse staffing, and another 18 states had introduced legislation (ANA, 2009). In 1999, California passed legislation to become the first state to establish minimum nurse-to-patient staffing requirements in acute care hospitals, with implementation in 2004 (Coffman, Seago, & Spetz, 2002; Spetz, 2004).

Our study of the impact of variation in nurse workloads and surgical mortality was undertaken with 1999 data and included all the hospitals in Pennsylvania. As noted earlier, we found a significant association between how many patients nurses cared for, on average, in a hospital and the hospital's risk-adjusted mortality (Aiken et al., 2002). Although we made every attempt to write the paper clearly, the analytic techniques used—logistic regression models—were too complex for the average reader who might be interested in the topic. To make the paper more understandable and relevant to contemporary issues, we included in the discussion section examples illustrating the magnitude of the effect sizes of nurse staffing on mortality. The illustration was based upon the nurse staffing ratios being hotly debated at that time in California. The minimum ratio legislation had already passed, but the actual ratios were still being determined by the California Department of Health. Nurse stakeholder groups were asking for the ratios to be set between four and six patients per nurse on medical and surgical units, whereas interest groups representing hospitals wanted the ratio set closer to 10 patients per nurse.

Using a technique called direct standardization, we estimated the differences in the number of deaths under different staffing scenarios, applying our findings to the ratios under debate in California. Remember that our study was of hospitals in Pennsylvania, where there was no legislation; but by using the staffing scenarios under debate in California, our study became highly relevant. As indicated in Figure 15.1, we estimated that for every 100 patients who died after common surgeries in hospitals in which nurses, on average, cared for four patients each, 107 would die where nurses cared for five patients; 114 patients would die where nurses cared for six patients; 123 would die where nurses cared for seven patients; and 131 would die where nurses cared for eight patients each. This illustration made the paper come alive to the general reader and resulted in great media attention, and probably influenced the decision about mandated ratios in California,

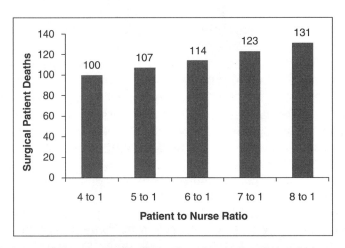

FIGURE 15.1 For every 100 surgical patients who die in hospitals with 4 to 1 patient to nurse ratios, the number that would die in hospitals with higher nurse to patient ratios increases linearly.
Source: Based upon findings in Aiken, L.H., Clarke, S.P., Sloane, D.M., Sochalski, J., & Silber, J.H. (2002). hospital nurse staffing and patient mortality, nurse burnout and job dissatisfaction. *Journal of the American Medical Association, 288*(16):1987–1993.

which were ultimately set at no more than five patients per nurse on medical and surgical units when the ratios were fully implemented in 2005.

Nursing Education Policy

Within nursing, and higher education more broadly, there has been a longstanding debate about the educational requirements for nurses. When I graduated from a baccalaureate nursing program in 1964, I was among the minority of nurses. Over 85% of new nurses in 1964 graduated from hospital diploma programs. In 1965, the ANA set 1985 as the target date by which entry into professional nursing should be standardized at the baccalaureate level. For reasons having little to do with the ANA and more to do with social trends, including women enrolling in higher education in large numbers as well as the increasing cost of nursing education to hospitals, enrollments in diploma schools declined precipitously over the subsequent decades, until now when less than 5% of new nurses graduate from diploma schools. At the same time, community colleges began to flourish, helped by public subsidies, student preferences for pursuing education in an institution of higher learning rather than in a trade school, and the accessibility and lower costs of community college education. Nursing became an increasingly popular student choice and source of revenue for the colleges. A very different scenario developed than the one envisioned by the ANA in 1965: Associate degree nursing education became dominant rather than baccalaureate education.

As noted earlier, our outcomes research has shown that patients benefit from a more educated hospital workforce in terms of lower risk of death (Aiken et al., 2003). Our paper reporting these results was widely covered by the press. The *Newark Star Ledger*, for example, published a ranking of major New Jersey hospitals by the proportion of their nurses who were qualified at the baccalaureate level. As a result of the published ranking, we know of several New Jersey hospitals that began recruitment policies to increase employment of nurses with baccalaureate degrees. Also, the American Organization of Nurse Executives passed a resolution stating that baccalaureate education was the desired standard of education for nurses in the future, a significant event because the American Organization of Nurse Executives represents the major employers of nurses. Additionally, our results have been cited by the New York State Nurses Association in their proposed state legislation to give all nurses at the time of their initial licensure a limit of 10 years to obtain a baccalaureate degree in order to retain their licenses.

In keeping with our goal of framing our research in a context relevant to contemporary issues, we are also examining whether the trend toward a higher proportion of nurses receiving their initial education in associate degree programs is likely to influence the future supply of nurses. In particular, we are examining whether there is a link between type of initial education and the nurse faculty shortage that is currently serving as a major barrier to the expansion of nursing school enrollments.

Nursing has become a popular career choice in the United States, so popular that tens of thousands of qualified applicants to nursing schools are being turned away because of capacity limitations associated with a faculty shortage and financial constraints. In the past, national nursing shortages have resulted from too few Americans wanting to be nurses. Now that there are sufficient numbers of qualified applicants, nursing schools have not been able to expand their enrollments to accommodate them. Solving the nurse faculty shortage is imperative to expanding nursing school enrollments. Projections suggest a large nursing shortage in the future.

We conducted a study of how educational attainment over a nursing career is affected by type of initial education (Aiken, Cheung, & Olds, 2009). Using National Sample Surveys of Registered Nurses conducted by the federal government, as of 2004 we determined the highest educational attainment of nurses who received their initial nursing education between 1970 and 1994. We found that about 20% of nurses got an additional academic degree beyond their initial education. For nurses with an associate degree, 80% of those getting additional education stopped at the baccalaureate degree, whereas almost all nurses pursuing a second degree starting with a baccalaureate degree ended up with a graduate degree. Almost all nurse faculty positions require a graduate degree, at least a master's and, often, a doctoral degree. Thus, three times as many nurses who started with a baccalaureate degree ultimately got the credential qualifying them to be faculty members compared with nurses who started with an associate degree. Or another way to look at the results: More than three times as many associate degree nurses would have to be educated to produce the same number of nurses with a graduate degree as nurses with an initial baccalaureate degree.

Taking the example one step further for ease of translating the findings for the general reader, we created a scenario in which the proportions of nurses with associate degrees and baccalaureate initial education were reversed from what exists at present. That is, we assumed in the scenario that two-thirds of nurses graduated initially from a baccalaureate program and one-third graduated from associate degree programs. Note that this was the recommendation of the National Advisory Council on Nurse Education and Practice in 1996 that was obviously not followed. If the proportions had been reversed between 1970 and 1994, there would be over 50,000 more nurses today with graduate degrees qualifying them to be faculty members, which would have likely made a big difference in preventing the current faculty shortage.

We concluded from these analyses that it was a "mathematical improbability" that the shortage of nursing faculty could be solved unless the distribution of nurses by type of initial education was changed (Aiken et al., 2009). Thus, we have shown with our two studies that it is in the public's interest to have more baccalaureate nurses at the hospital bedside, but that is unlikely to happen unless educational policies are enacted that promote a shift in initial nurse education from associate to baccalaureate degree programs. Can public policies encourage such a shift? Yes, the composition of the nursing workforce can be shaped by targeting public (federal and state) subsidies to students graduating from initial programs with a baccalaureate degree. If public funding followed the students, it is likely that community colleges and universities would collaborate to find more efficient and affordable options for students entering nursing to graduate from initial programs with a baccalaureate degree.

CONCLUSIONS

This is an exciting time for nursing. Research on many aspects of nursing care is accumulating to document the positive impact of nurses on improving the quality and safety of care, access to appropriate services, and getting more value for monetary investments—all goals of national health reform. Numbers count in public debates and in decisions of healthcare organizations on how to best provide health care and which strategies will yield the best health outcomes. Traditionally, the numbers have come from financial ledgers. Nursing's contributions to health care have been constrained by financial assumptions that nursing care is a cost but not a revenue source. However, the accumulated evidence base is now producing counterbalancing numbers that are beginning to make a compelling case that nursing is key to achieving better health outcomes at affordable costs. Nurse researchers can continue to advance the health of the public by conducting studies of the highest quality, anticipating the answers that will be needed in the future to create more effective healthcare services, and translating their findings so that those in clinical practice and decision-making positions can act on the basis of the new knowledge they create.

REFERENCES

Aiken, L. H. (1981). Nursing priorities for the 1980s: Hospitals and nursing homes. *American Journal of Nursing, 81*(2), 324–330.

Aiken, L. H., Cheung, R., & Olds, D. (2009). Education policy initiatives to address the nurse shortage. *Health Affairs, 28*(4), w646–w656.

Aiken, L. H., Clarke, S. P., Cheung, R. B., Sloane, D. M., & Silber, J. H. (2003). Educational levels of hospital nurses and surgical patient mortality. *Journal of the American Medical Association, 290*(12), 1617–1623.

Aiken, L. H., Clarke, S. P., Sloane, D. M., Lake, E. T., & Cheney, T. (2008). Effects of hospital care environments on patient mortality and nurse outcomes. *Journal of Nursing Administration, 38*(5), 220–226.

Aiken, L. H., Clarke, S. P., Sloane, D. M., Lake, E. T., Sochalski, J., & Weber, A. L. (1999). Organization and outcomes of inpatient AIDS care. *Medical Care, 37*(8), 760–772.

Aiken, L. H., Clarke, S. P., Sloane, D. M., Sochalski, J. A., Busse, R., & Clarke, H. (2001). Nurses' reports of hospital quality of care and working conditions in five countries. *Health Affairs, 20*(3), 43–53.

Aiken, L. H., Clarke, S. P., Sloane, D. M., Sochalski, J. A., & Silber, J. H. (2002). Hospital nurse staffing and patient mortality, nurse burnout, and job dissatisfaction. *Journal of the American Medical Association, 288*(16), 1987–1993.

Aiken, L. H., Lake, E. T., Sochalski, D., & Sloane, D. M. (1997). Design of an outcomes study of the organization of hospital AIDS care. *Research in the Sociology of Health Care, 14*, 3–26.

Aiken, L. H., & Mullinix, C. F. (1987). The nurse shortage: Myth or reality? *New England Journal of Medicine, 317*(10), 641–646.

Aiken, L. H., & Patrician, P. A. (2000). Measuring organizational traits of hospitals: The revised nursing work index. *Nursing Research, 49*(3), 146–153.

Aiken L. H., Sloane D. M., & Klocinski J. L. (1997). Hospital nurses' occupational exposure to blood: Prospective, retrospective, and institutional reports. *American Journal of Public Health, 87*, 103–107.

Aiken, L. H., Smith, H. L., & Lake, E. T. (1994). Lower Medicare mortality among a set of hospitals known for good nursing care. *Medical Care, 32*(8), 771–787.

Aiken, L. H., Sochalski, J., & Anderson, G. F. (1996). Downsizing the hospital workforce. *Health Affairs, 15*(4), 88–92.

Aiken, L. H., Xue, Y., Clarke, S., & Sloane, D. (2007). Supplemental nurse staffing in hospitals and quality of care. *Journal of Nursing Administration, 37*(7), 335–342.

American Nurses Association. (2009). Safe nurse staffing laws in state legislature. Retrieved March 19, 2009, from http://www.safestaffingsaaveslives.org/WhatisANADoing/StateLegislation.com

Brennan T. A., Horwitz, R. I., Duffy, F. D., Cassel, C. K., Goode, L. D., & Lipner, R. S. (2003). The role of physician specialty board certification status in the quality movement. *Journal of the American Medical Association, 290*, 1183–1189.

Burnes Bolton, L., Aydin, C. E., Donaldson, N., Storer Brown, D., Sandhu, M., Fridman, M., et al. (2007). Mandated nurse staffing ratios in California: A comparison of staffing and nursing-sensitive outcomes pre- and postregulation. *Policy, Politics, & Nursing Practice, 8*(4), 238–250.

Coffman, J. M., Seago, J. A., & Spetz, J. (2002). Minimum nurse-to-patient ratios in acute care hospitals in California. *Health Affairs, 21*(5), 53–64.

Cunningham, W. E., Tisnado, D. M., Lui, H. H., Nakazono, T. T., & Carlisle, D. M. (1999). The effect of hospital experience on mortality among patients hospitalized with acquired immunodeficiency syndrome in California. *American Journal of Medicine, 107*(2), 137–143.

Estabrooks, C. A., Midodzi, W. K., Cummings, G. G., Ricker, K. L., & Giovannetti, P. (2005). The impact of hospital nursing characteristics on 30-day mortality. *Nursing Research, 54*(2), 74–84.

Friese, C. R., Lake, E. T., Aiken, L. H., Silber, J. H., & Sochalski, J. (2008). Hospital nurse practice environments and outcomes for surgical oncology patients. *Health Services Research, 43*(4), 1145–1163.

Hartz, A. J., Krakauer, H., Kuhn, E. M., Young, M., Jacobsen, S., Gay, G., . . . Rimm, A. (1989). Hospital characteristics and mortality rates. *New England Journal of Medicine, 321,* 1720–1725.

Iezzoni, L. I. (2003). *Risk adjustment for measuring health care outcomes* (3rd ed.). Chicago: Health Administration Press.

Institute of Medicine. (2004). *Keeping patients safe: Transforming the work environment of nurses* (Report of the Committee on the Work Environment for Nurses and Patient Safety). Washington, DC: National Academies Press.

Kane, R. L., Shamliyan, T. A., Mueller, C., Duval, S., & Wilt, T. J. (2007). The association of registered nurse staffing levels and patient outcomes: Systematic review and meta-analysis. *Medical Care, 45*(12), 1195–1204.

Kramer, M. (1974). *Reality shock: Why nurses leave nursing.* St. Louis: C.V. Mosby Company.

Lake, E. (2002). Development of the practice environment scale of the Nursing Work Index. *Research in Nursing and Health, 25,* 176–188.

Luft, H. S., Garnick, D. W., Mark, D. H., & McPhee, S. J. (1990). *Hospital volume, physician volume, and patient outcome.* Ann Arbor: Health Administration Press Perspectives.

McClure, M. L., & Hinshaw, A. S. (2002). *Magnet hospitals revisited: Attraction and retention of professional nurses.* (pp. 83–103). Washington, D.C.: American Nurses Publishing.

McClure, M. L., Poulin, M. A., Sovie, M. D., & Wandelt, M. A. (1983). *Magnet hospitals: Attraction and retention of professional nurses.* Washington, DC: American Nurses Association.

Moses, L. E., & Mosteller, F. (1968). Institutional differences in post-operative death rates. *JAMA: Journal of the American Medical Association, 203,* 492–494.

National Advisory Council on Nurse Education and Practice. (1996). *Report to the secretary of the Department of Health and Human Services on the basic registered nurse workforce.* Rockville, MD: DHHS.

National Quality Forum. (2007). Nursing performance measurement and reporting: A status report. *NQF Issue* Brief. Number 5, June 2007.

Shortell, S. M., & Hughes, E. F. (1988). Effects of regulation, competition and ownership on mortality rates among hospital inpatients. *New England Journal of Medicine, 318*(17), 1100–1107.

Silber, J. H., Kennedy, S. K., Even-Shoshan, O., Chen, W., Koziol, L. F., Showan, A. M., & Longnecker, D. E. (2000). Anesthesiologist direction and patient outcomes. *Anesthesiology, 93,* 152–163.

Spetz, J. (2004). California's minimum nurse-to-patient ratios: The first few months. *Journal of Nursing Administration, 34,* 571–578.

Tourangeau, A. E., Doran, D. M., McGillis Hall, L., O'Brien Pallas, L., Pringle, D., & Tu, J. V., & Cranley, L. A. (2007). Impact of hospital nursing care on 30-day mortality for acute medical patients. *Journal of Advanced Nursing, 57*(1), 32–41.

Van den Heede, K., Lasaffre, E., Diya, L., Vleugels, A., Clarke, S. P., Aiken, L. H., & Sermeus, W. (2009). The relationship between inpatient cardiac surgery mortality and nurse numbers and educational level: Analysis of administrative data. *International Journal of Nursing Studies, 46*(6), 796–803.

Wunderlich, G., Sloan, F., & Davis, C. K. (Eds.) (1996). *Nursing staff in hospitals and nursing homes: Is it adequate?* Washington, DC: National Academy Press.

16

Nursing Workforce and Health Policy

Linda O'Brien-Pallas and Laureen Hayes

INTRODUCTION

One of the most challenging tasks for healthcare administrators and policy makers is to ensure that there are enough skilled nurses to provide needed care. Canada, like many other countries, is facing a nursing shortage due to an aging nursing workforce and early retirements, limited number of new recruits, and unsatisfactory work environments (Blakeley & Ribeiro, 2008; O'Brien-Pallas et al., 2003). An inadequate nursing workforce will jeopardize the functioning of the healthcare system as increasing evidence shows a relationship between registered nurse (RN) care and patient outcomes. The negative impact of insufficient nurse staffing has driven health researchers and decision makers to examine nurses' work environments to determine factors amenable to policy change and to produce increased stability in the workforce.

This chapter illustrates how research is shaping health human resources (HHR) strategies for nursing in Ontario, Canada, and describes policy responses to alleviate widespread fears about a looming nursing workforce shortage. An account is given of the state of nursing in the 1990s and government initiatives to begin resolving the situation. The HHR theoretical framework and its application in research and policy are discussed. Researchers should understand the nature of the policy cycle in order to promote effective collaboration with policy makers; therefore, the policy cycle is explained. This chapter also conveys how research evidence, using a continuous quality improvement process, is contributing to current strategies aimed at strengthening the nursing workforce in Ontario and highlights some considerations for the future of nursing that are proposed in current literature.

THE CONTEXT: INITIATIVES TO ADDRESS THE SHORTAGE

In the 1990s, healthcare organizations in North America had undergone dramatic changes as a result of extensive downsizing, restructuring, and merging (Burke & Greenglass, 2000). The recession and the need for cost constraints resulted in shorter lengths of stay in hospitals, reductions in the number of hospital beds, and increased patient acuity. As a consequence of workforce cuts, RNs were replaced by less educated practical nurses and nursing assistants (Burke, 2001; Robertson & Dowd, 1996). Nurses less than 30 years old were increasingly employed in part-time and casual positions, therefore lacking opportunities to be socialized into the profession. Many Canadian RNs migrated to the United States as healthcare restructuring in many provinces eliminated full-time nursing positions, effectively forcing nurses to find stable employment elsewhere. Declining enrollments in nursing programs and reduced supply of new nursing graduates, nurse layoffs, and an aging baby boomer generation were contributing to a looming shortage. As a result of all these changes, the 1990s produced the largest displacement of nurses in Canadian history and a marked decrease in continuity of nursing care (Grinspun, 2002). For the nurses who remained, the work environment became increasingly "unhealthy" as morale declined and a significant number chose to leave the profession (Commission on the Future of Health Care in Canada, 2002). Our research and that of others suggested that the work environment and the nature of nursing work were leading to the poorer physical health in our mature nurses and limited emotional hardiness in the younger nursing population in our country (O'Brien-Pallas, Duffield, & Alksnis, 2004; O'Brien-Pallas et al., 2005).

From a country-level policy perspective, a nurse shortage is usually defined in relation to that country's own historical staffing levels, resources, and estimates of demand for health services (Buchan, 2006). It involves a lack of nurses willing to work as nurses in the present conditions; therefore, retention of senior experienced nurses has been suggested as a key factor in solving the shortage (Baumann et al., 2001; Buchan & Aiken, 2008). Given the major concern around the aging of the workforce, O'Brien-Pallas et al. (2003) generated estimates of the number of RNs in Canada aged 50 years or older who could be expected to leave the RN workforce due to death or retirement by 2006. Retirement at age 65 years would result in an estimated loss of almost 30,000 RNs, equivalent to 13% of the 2001 workforce. Retirement at age 55 years would result in a loss of 64,248 RNs to retirement or death by 2006, equivalent to 28% of the RN workforce in 2001. As senior nurses leave the workforce, immense intellectual capital is lost; therefore, incentives were recommended to encourage them to stay longer in employment. For example, Blakeley and Ribeiro (2008) explored factors that influence nurses to retire early and found that many could be addressed by employers (e.g., flexible hours, recognition, lighter work, and in-service support).

Within the broad HHR planning (HHRP) agenda, two approaches used in many countries to address the nursing shortage are to recruit nurses from overseas and to increase the enrollment of nursing students in schools of nursing (Aiken, Buchan, Sochalski, Nichols, & Powell, 2004; Baumann, Blythe, Kolotylo, & Underwood, 2004). Duffield and O'Brien-Pallas (2002) noted that recruiting from overseas creates ethical problems when recruits are from countries that are also lacking nurses. Canada's approach should follow sound national HHRP frameworks based on principles agreed to by the various policy makers at all levels (Little, 2007). Increasing enrollment in nursing schools raises other concerns with the delay in its actual impact on nurse supply, the limited clinical placement options for students, and dwindling numbers of experienced faculty (O'Brien-Pallas, Tomblin-Murphy et al., 2004). Moreover, there is no guarantee that graduating nurses will stay in nursing or work in the country where they obtained their education (Blakeley & Ribeiro, 2008).

Recent years have seen some improvement in nurse supply, attributed to government policy initiatives around HHRs. In Ontario, the Minister of Health and Long-Term Care (MOHLTC) established the Nursing Task Force (NTF) in 1998 in response to growing concerns about the instability of the nursing workforce and nurses' concerns about their ability to provide safe care. In its report *Good Nursing, Good Health: An Investment for the 21st Century* (NTF, 1999), recommendations were to create new nursing positions, reform basic education, increase clinical education, support research to guide human resources planning for nurses, develop an aggressive recruitment and retention strategy, and promote professional development and practice for nurses. The MOHLTC accepted the recommendations, and the NTF charged the Joint Provincial Nursing Committee (JPNC) with responsibility for implementation.

Two years later, the progress report *Good Nursing, Good Health: A Good Investment* (JPNC, 2001) highlighted the positive trends in addressing nursing issues: improved employment opportunities for nursing, improvements in research in nursing human resources, and reforms in basic education for nurses. However, remaining unresolved issues were high rates of casualization and part-time employment, underutilization of nurses to their full scope of practice, overtime and absenteeism, wage disparity, and problems with inconsistent nursing human resource data. In 2003, progress was again highlighted in *Good Nursing, Good Health: The Return on Our Investment* (JPNC, 2003). By 2002, all RN education programs were at the baccalaureate level through the development of collaborative programs between universities and colleges. The Best Practice Guidelines project was underway for nurses, and the role of the nurse practitioner was supported. Retention initiatives focused on improving the working environment, minimizing casualization, reducing part-time and agency work, creating more full-time jobs for nurses, and ensuring strong nursing leadership. Ontario's recruitment initiatives focused on creating new opportunities for nurses, attracting nurses who left the system to return, and encouraging recruitment into the profession.

The nursing research unit, funded by the MOHLTC since 1991 and codirected by Drs. Linda O'Brien-Pallas and Andrea Baumann, contributed to the work of the NTF. Also, as a newly minted Canadian Health Services Research/Canadian Institute of Health Services Research chair in 1990, Dr. O'Brien-Pallas had a 10-year salary support to research and build capacity on HHRs and to work with decision and policy makers in a special way; these experiences will be shared as part of this chapter. At inception of the research unit, the research focused on quality of nursing work life. Subsequently, the emphasis switched to human resource issues to study the impact of restructuring on the nursing workforce and workforce planning and projection, particularly issues of recruitment, retention, effective use of nurses, and the result of the current nursing shortage (Nursing Effectiveness, Utilization, and Outcomes Research Unit, 2004). The research unit contributes to the knowledge of policy decision makers and makes recommendations about future data collection. Thus, a central component is a joint mechanism for knowledge transfer between the MOHLTC and the research unit to ensure that evidence is used to guide policy and management decision making. Evidence-based decisions require linkages between policy makers and researchers to ensure that findings are communicated in a policy-relevant manner.

LINKING RESEARCH AND POLICY

Researchers and policy makers need to work together on shared issues and understand the nature of each other's roles to promote use of findings in practice. Researchers can become familiar with frameworks that have been developed to describe the policy cycle.

For example, Tarlov (1999) described a framework that separates policy development into two phases. The initial phase leads to the development of a public consensus and the later political phase is when specific policy actions are taken. According to the framework, there needs to be public understanding that the problem can be addressed to everyone's advantage. The problem must be evident and be a priority among a sufficient proportion of the population to create a national agenda and momentum for action, which is then followed by political process to pursue policy.

A similar policy cycle consisting of two phases is the framework adopted by the Office of Nursing Policy at Health Canada (Shamian & Griffin, 2003). Phase 1, Getting to the Policy Agenda, is concerned with beliefs and values and has four conditions: It must embrace an issue consistent with the values and beliefs of the society; the issue must be problematic, visible, and important to more than those directly involved and have some urgency; there must be high-quality evidence to support giving attention to the issue; and the public must be made aware of the issue and the strategy to address it. Phase 2, Moving Into Action, consists of political engagement, involvement of interest groups, issue debate and policy formulation, and development of actual policy, law, or regulation. Implementation of action and evaluation can begin after the eight steps.

Linkage between research and policy is vital because a lack of research in key areas and gaps in data can hinder optimum use of research findings in policy initiatives. However, as Lomas (2000) states, collaboration between research environments and decision making is not without obstacles. Lack of time due to heavy workloads and full schedules, decision makers needing results faster than the research process can produce them, the resources required to tailor a project to the agendas of multiple decision-maker partners, and changes in policy personnel may discourage establishment of linkages. Decision makers do not always understand what is involved in the research process and may not have the opportunity to learn. Lomas refers to the different cultures surrounding those doing research and those who might be able to use it. Decision makers might claim that researchers produce irrelevant, poorly communicated "products," and, in turn, researchers might accuse decision makers of political expediency that results in inappropriate outcomes.

If decision makers are to use the "evidence to make decisions," they need firsthand knowledge of the issues, the research process, and its limitations and also need to be aware of existing research and participate in planning future research with the researcher (Lomas, 2000). Following the NTF, the HHR chair and researchers from the research unit were added to the membership of the JPNC. This was to ensure that in the process of deliberation and advisement to the government and the key players, the latest research was made available to the decision makers.

THE RESEARCH: HHRs IN NURSING

Continuous cycles of oversupply and undersupply of health manpower in North America reflect the inadequate projection methods used to estimate future requirements. There is no unambiguous "right" number and mix of health professionals (O'Brien-Pallas, Birch, Baumann, & Tomblin Murphy, 2001). Health provider requirements are determined by broad societal decisions concerning the commitment of resources, funding and delivery of programs, and level and mix of services. Health human resource planners have traditionally considered only supply variables, or the actual number, type, and geographic distribution of care providers available to deliver health services at any given point. The supply of HHRs makes up only one important piece of an HHRP framework. The adequacy of any particular level of supply depends on the health needs of the population, the financial resources devoted to healthcare, and the prevailing values of the population.

Three distinctive approaches to HHRP and their related assumptions, questions, and methods have been described (Lavis & Birch 1997; O'Brien-Pallas, Baumann, Birch, & Tomblin Murphy, 2000). In the utilization-based approach, the current quantity, mix, and distribution of healthcare resources in the population are adopted as a baseline for estimates of future requirements, regardless of this baseline's adequacy and effectiveness. In the needs-based approach, future requirements are based on the estimated health needs of the population as well as the potential for addressing these needs using healthcare services. In the effective demand-based approach, economic considerations are introduced to complement the needs-based approach. Health human resource planning has assumed that population structure alone determines the service needs of the population and that the age of the providers determines the quantity of care provided (Birch, O'Brien-Pallas, Alksnis, Tomblin Murphy, & Thomson, 2003). The main limitation of such approaches is the failure to reflect the complex nature of the processes underlying the needs for services (population health) and the delivery of services (healthcare provision), as well as the effects of HHRP on population, provider, and system outcomes (Birch et al., 2003).

HHR Framework

The HHR conceptual framework (Figure 16.1) considers the key elements of the HHRP process and is helpful to policy makers and health services researchers and planners in planning a healthcare workforce to meet the health needs of the population (O'Brien-Pallas, Tomblin Murphy, Birch, & Baumann, 2001). The dynamic system-based framework incorporates each of the three methodological approaches for planning and forecasting HHR described by Birch et al. (2003) but places these approaches in the context of assessment of needs and outcomes of service provision. Human resource planning needs to be placed within the broader system in which healthcare services are provided and take to into account the impact of social, political, geographical, technological, and economic factors. Health human resource planning must reflect the complex nature of the processes underlying the needs for services (population health) and the delivery of services (healthcare provision), as well as the effects of HHRP on population, provider, and system outcomes (Birch et al., 2003).

At the core of the framework is the recognition that HHR must be matched as closely as possible to the health needs of the population (O'Brien-Pallas, 2002). Building on the work of Andersen's (1995) service utilization model, Donabedian's (1966) quality-of-care framework, Leatt's conceptualization of technology in human services organizations (Leatt & Schneck, 1981), and the human resources decision support model reported by Kazanjian, Pulcins, and Kerluke (1992), the HHR framework considers the following key elements (O'Brien-Pallas, 2002):

• *Population characteristics related to health levels and risks* (needs-based factors) reflect the multivariate characteristics of individuals in the population that create the demand for curative and preventive health services.

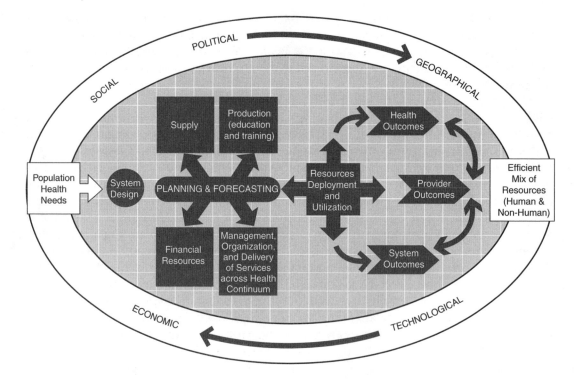

FIGURE 16.1 Health Human Resources Conceptual Framework (O'Brien-Pallas, Tomblin Murphy, Birch, 2005; adapted from O'Brien-Pallas, Tomblin Murphy, G., Baumann, A., & Birch, S., 2001; and O'Brien-Pallas, Baumann, 1997).

- *Planning and forecasting* reflect the array of methodologies used to predict service requirements and the numbers of providers needed to deliver these services. The choice of the modelling approach is often influenced by data availability.
- *Supply* reflects the actual number, type, and geographic distribution of regulated and unregulated providers available to deliver health services at a given point.
- *Financial resources* reflect the overall portion of the gross domestic product that is dedicated to health and education.
- *Production* involves the education and training of future health providers.
- *Management, organization, and delivery of health services* influence the amount and quality of care provided, provider health and satisfaction, and associated costs. Organizational characteristics such as structural arrangements, degree of formalization and centralization, environmental complexity, and culture influence the way work gets done and impacts on outcomes.
- *Resource deployment and utilization* reflect the amount and nature of the resources deployed to provide health services to the population at large.
- *Health outcomes* refer to the health status of the population.
- *Provider outcomes* include the health status of providers, retention rates, turnover rates, sick time, job satisfaction, and levels of burnout and other responses to the work environment.

• *System outcomes* include the costs associated with resources dedicated to health services. These include hospitalization and readmission rates, home visits, expenditures on the various health sectors, the number of people treated in each health sector, the neediness of the population being treated, case intensity, cost efficiency, discharge efficiency, proportion of acute versus nonacute care, outpatient/inpatient surgery rates, and occupancy rates.

• *Context* includes political, social, geographical, technological, and economic factors and "shocks to the system." At the population level, there are many determinants of health besides medical care. Physical environment, social environment, individual behavior, genetic endowment, and medical care are all factors in the health of a population.

• *Efficient mix of human and nonhuman resources* reflects the number and type of resources that must be deployed in order to achieve the best population, provider, and system outcomes.

• In 2006, after a review by the federal/provincial/territorial committee on human resources, the term *system design* was added to the model to reflect the unique characteristics of the system for which human resources were being planned.

Although this conceptual framework may seem easy to understand, the underpinning data requirements for the mathematical model are complex and must be defined carefully. In this framework, simulations of the health system are used to provide needs-based estimates that are aimed at optimizing outcomes. The model builds on research conducted at the macro- and micro-levels in order to reflect the complexity of relationships in the HHR process.

Needs-Based Studies in HHRs

Planning for HHRs should be based on the health needs of the population and consider factors that affect use of healthcare services. Using secondary data sources and employing both longitudinal and cross-sectional designs, O'Brien-Pallas and colleagues tested elements of the HHR conceptual framework in Health Human Resources Planning: An Examination of Relationships Among Nursing Service Utilization, an Estimate of Population Health and Overall Health Status Outcomes in the Province of Ontario (Tomblin Murphy et al., 2003). The study explored the relationship between the health needs of Ontarians, their use of community and hospital nursing services, and variations in outcomes. The findings suggest that greater intensity of nursing resources is associated with shorter lengths of stay (other things being equal). Use of nursing services can be predicted by using factors that indicate need for healthcare, such as health status, disability, chronic conditions, and socioeconomic factors.

Understanding the complex relationships between health, age, and birth year as well as social indicators is vital to ensure accurate and efficient planning for future HHR requirements. The research program "Health Human Resources Modeling: Challenging the Past, Creating the Future" (O'Brien-Pallas, Tomblin Murphy, et al., 2007) demonstrated that the effect of age on health has changed over time; therefore, direct independent measures of health and health risks at the population level are needed to adequately inform HHRP. It is also important to consider the role of productivity, referring to service rendered per unit of time worked by the healthcare provider. The study demonstrated that the employment levels of other staff are associated with the average productivity of nurses. As such, the required number of nurses to deliver a planned level of service (or manage a particular patient mix) will depend on the configuration of other hospital inputs (i.e., it is context specific) and on the methods of production. Thus, plans to change other inputs (e.g., number of beds) must consider implications for nurse human resource requirements to achieve desired levels of *services*.

Nurse Staffing and Workload: Patient Care Delivery Model

Nurse staffing and work overload are key sources of dissatisfaction and concern for nurses working in hospitals. Hospital administrators rely on measures of workload, cost, and nurse productivity to guide organizational planning decisions, which should be informed by evidence of the relationships between nurse staffing standards and outcomes. Within the HHR conceptual framework, staffing and workload data inform the component "Management, Organization, and Delivery of Services Across the Health Continuum." As illustrated by the Patient Care Delivery Model (Figure 16.2), provision of nursing services results from a complex array of health system inputs (characteristics of patients, nurses, and organizations), throughputs (e.g., work environment and nursing utilization), and outputs (patient, nurse, and organizational outcomes).

The influence of environmental complexity factors refers to the extent to which unanticipated disruptions in nurses' daily assignments impact outcomes (O'Brien-Pallas et al., 2002). The complexity of the caring environment is hypothesized to include three dimensions: (a) unanticipated and delayed events and the subsequent resequencing and coordination in which the nurse is involved; (b) multiple and long procedures that are a function of increased patient acuity; and (c) the characteristics and composition of the caregiving team, such as being short staffed or having students, relief staff, and absence of administrative support (O'Brien-Pallas, Irvine, Peereboom & Murray, 1997).

At the organizational level, deployment and utilization of nursing human resources cannot be considered in isolation from the system in which nursing care is delivered. Calculated at the unit level as patient workload divided by nurse worked hours, nursing unit utilization measures how well an organization is staffed to meet patient care standards and needs (O'Brien-Pallas, Thomson et al., 2004). The more a unit is understaffed (reflected by high utilization levels), the lower the amount of actual nursing time available for each patient. Decision makers in healthcare organizations need evidence to support nursing staffing decisions, which includes both the volume and mix of nurses required to provide efficient and effective care.

The Evidence Based Standards for Measuring Nurse Staffing and Performance study (O'Brien-Pallas, Thomson et al., 2004), which tested the Patient Care Delivery Model, broke new ground in providing empirical evidence of the link between nurse staffing levels and provider outcomes and system effectiveness. The principal objective of this study was to examine the interrelationships among variables thought to influence patient, nurse, and system outcomes. In Canada, 93% is the maximum work capacity of any nursing unit because 7% of the shift consists of paid mandatory breaks during which time no work is contractually expected. At a 93% level of utilization, nurses have no flexibility to meet unanticipated demands or rapidly changing patient acuity. The Evidence Based Standards for Measuring Nurse Staffing and Performance study found that nursing utilization should be kept at 85%, plus or minus 5%. When rates rise above 80%, costs increase and quality of care decreases. Patient health is more likely to be improved at

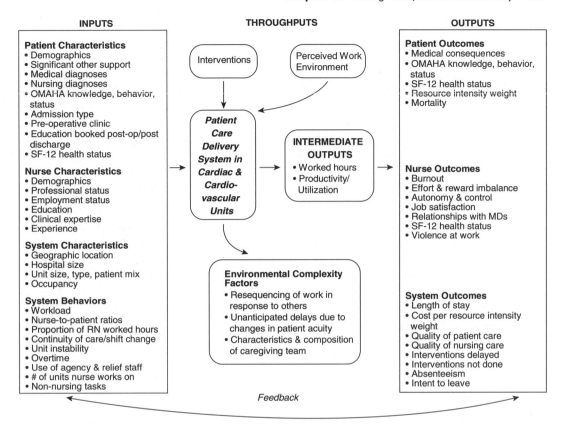

FIGURE 16.2 Patient Care Delivery Model (O'Brien-Pallas, L., Thomson, D., McGillis Hall, L. Pink, G., Kerr, M., Wang, S., et al., 2004).

discharge if levels are below 80% and if patients are cared for by nurses who work less overtime. When utilization levels are kept below 80%, nurses are more likely to be satisfied with their jobs and absenteeism is reduced, and nurses are less likely to want to leave their jobs when utilization is less than 83%. Costs are lower when hospitals maintain levels below 90% and implement strategies to improve nurse health and incentives to retain experienced nurses. The findings of this study suggest that to actually reduce the cost and improve the quality of patient care, organizations will benefit from hiring experienced, full-time, baccalaureate-prepared nurses; staffing enough nurses to meet workload demands; and creating work environments that foster nurses' mental and physical health, safety, security, and satisfaction.

Nurses' Work Environment

It is important for decision makers to understand how nurses perceive their work environment as they consider strategies to promote nurse retention and staffing stability. As part of the Nursing Labour Market in Canada: An Occupational/Sector Study, a Canadian survey of RNs, practical nurses, and registered psychiatric nurses was conducted. The purpose of the survey was to determine and describe the perspectives of nurses regarding factors in their work environments that influence the nature and effectiveness of their nursing care. O'Brien-Pallas et al. (2005) highlight a number of findings that underscore the importance of HHR initiatives. For example, nurses were less likely to leave their current position if they were mentally healthy and satisfied with their current positions. Satisfaction with current position was more likely with more autonomy, work empowerment, resources, and leadership. Nurses were less likely to be physically or mentally healthy when they worked involuntary overtime or preferred to reduce their work hours and when there was violence at the workplace. Nurses working with frequent shift changes (more than twice within 2 weeks) reported poorer mental health.

Preferred policy initiatives for nurse retention are explored in "Health Human Resources Modeling: Challenging the Past, Creating the Future" (O'Brien-Pallas, Tomblin Murphy et al., 2007). A cross-sectional survey design sampled three groups of nurses from six Canadian provinces: former RNs who have left nursing and do not maintain registration; RNs who maintain registration but do not work in nursing or are unemployed; and RNs who remain in practice, with special attention to oversampling in the under 35 years age cohort. Highly ranked retention policies by all three groups of nurses related to appropriate workload, benefits package, better salary, support for continuing education, and improved work environment. Highly ranked policies to attract former nurses back to nursing included appropriate workload, better salary, and improved work environment. Those under age 35 years valued full-time employment, whereas those in midcareer prioritized workplace safety. Having preferred shifts was highly ranked by those under age 50 years, and position availability was very important to those aged 35 years or older. The study results suggest that policies to increase retention of the workforce need to consider ways to tailor the options based on the age distribution of the providers.

The recently completed Nursing Turnover Study provided evidence about the incidence of nurse turnover and its predictors and its impact on patient and nurse outcomes and associated system costs. Participating healthcare organizations consisted of 18 sites representing over 41 hospitals and 181 nursing units across 10 provinces in Canada. Data were collected from nurses, patients, medical records, personnel, and financial departments over two waves. The study findings indicate that nurse turnover is a major problem in Canadian hospitals, with a mean turnover rate of 19.9% and an average cost of $25,000 (O'Brien-Pallas et al., 2008). The temporary replacement and decrease in initial productivity of new hires contribute to the highest cost components. The overall study findings will inform strategies to promote leadership, orientation and mentorship, reasonable work hours, role clarity, autonomy, and adequate staffing resources within healthcare organizations.

THE ACTION: USE OF RESEARCH IN POLICY

Health human resource planning has become an area of intense interest in Canada and there have been investments made by governments and employers since the early part of this decade. HealthForceOntario is the province's strategy to ensure that Ontarians have access to the right number and mix of qualified healthcare providers. The nursing secretariat at the MOHLTC provides strategic advice on health, the healthcare system, and public policy issues from a nursing perspective. Created in December 1999, the secretariat supports and monitors the implementation of the Nursing Strategy for Ontario (MOHLTC, Nursing Secretariat). It informs the government and external stakeholders of the status of the implementation of the NTF recommendations and provides policy and administrative support to the JPNC in its responsibilities.

The Ontario Nursing Strategy

The Nursing Strategy, a component of HealthForceOntario, is described as a comprehensive, multifaceted, cross-sectoral strategy that is intended to address the core reasons for instability in the nursing workforce and to improve access to care, reduce wait times, and improve patient, client, and resident outcomes by increasing recruitment and retention of healthcare professionals (Ministry of Health and Long-term Care, n.d.). Retirement projections aimed to assist nursing resource planners and decision makers by understanding the severity and impact that retirement would have on the RN workforce and provide a foundation upon which to plan for the future nursing supply. The findings contributed to recommendations to recruit new nurses into the workforce, retain current nurses aged 55 years and over in the workforce, create full-time jobs for new graduates, improve the work environment for nurses, and expand current administrative databases to enable needs-based analysis for all sectors in the healthcare system.

New Graduate Initiative

The Nursing Enhancement Fund, as part of the Ontario Nursing Strategy to create new permanent nursing positions, was in response to the recommendation of the NTF to enhance healthcare delivery by stabilizing the nursing workforce and improving retention of existing nurses. The New Graduate Initiative in Ontario was created to assist graduates in gaining full-time experience, helping to ease the transition into the workforce and ensure that nursing graduates remain working in Ontario (Ontario Ministry of Health and Long-term Care, n.d.). An online employment portal links new nursing graduates with employers interested in hiring them through an online application and matching process. This policy represents a first step toward addressing the fundamental issues around nurse recruitment and retention and how to solve a long-term nursing shortage (McGillis Hall et al., 2009).

As highlighted in *Employment of Nursing Graduates: Evaluation of a Provincial Policy Strategy,* since 2005 the Nursing Graduate Guarantee has influenced an upward trend of full-time employment in Ontario (Baumann, Hunsberger, Idriss, Alameddine, & Grinspun, 2008). The preference of graduates for acute care hospitals has remained stable over time for both RNs and registered practical nurses (RPNs). However, as indicated in its evaluation report, opportunities for RPNs are still primarily in the long-term care sector, where fewer full-time positions are available and employers are disadvantaged in terms of their ability to participate in the initiative. Overall, employers and new graduates rated the initiative as satisfactory and made suggestions upon which to build in maintaining the initiative. Based on stakeholder feedback, Baumann et al. (2008) formulated recommendations that included focusing on specific employment initiatives for RPNs, retaining orientation and mentorship for all new graduates, focus on rural areas, alternative initiatives to assist long-term care, and follow-up research of new graduates.

Late-Career Initiative

The experience and knowledge gained by nurses through their years of participation in the healthcare system are invaluable. Even if staffing numbers meet reasonable thresholds, quality of care will suffer if the skill levels of nursing personnel are inadequate. Beyond the basic numbers of personnel present on units and their qualifications, the critical elements of experience and expertise of nurses in caring for particular populations and of team stability are also important (Clarke, 2007). Unfortunately, many older experienced nurses are considering early retirement because of the physical demands of nursing work.

As part of the 2005–2006 Ontario Nursing Strategy, the MOHLTC provided hospitals and long-term care facilities with funding for projects to support the work of late-career nurses (LCNs). The Late Career Initiative (LCNI) allows nurses over the age of 55 years to spend 20% of their time in less physically demanding nursing roles such as patient teaching or staff mentoring. An impact evaluation was conducted to identify what aspects of their work life changed for the LCN and the impact of the LCNI on organizations (O'Brien-Pallas, Mildon, et al., 2007). Nurse participants documented ways in which the initiative had a made a difference for them. Some of their perceptions were as follows: increased respect and recognition, decreased physical workload, improved job satisfaction, opportunities for professional development, empowerment through new knowledge, recognition for their expertise, and having time to spend with patients. Some nurses indicated that continuation of the initiative might influence them to delay plans for retirement. Challenges with implementing the LCNI occurred when fewer staff nurses were available to replace LCNs for their "late-career" days. Overall, the initiative was considered successful, with the recommendation to continue implementing such programs aimed at enhancing the late-career nursing workforce.

Other MOHLTC Initiatives to Enhance the Nursing Workforce

Other initiatives have also been implemented as part of the Ontario Nursing Strategy to promote healthy work environments and a stable nursing workforce. As outlined on the government Web site (Ministry of Health and Long-term Care, n.d.), these include the Clinical Simulation Initiative to help prepare nurses for practice, and the Mentorship/Preceptorship Initiative, Patient Lift Initiative, and Safety Engineered Sharps to help create positive work environments. The Clinical Simulation Equipment initiative provides funding to schools of nursing for the purchase of equipment that will give students more opportunity to enhance their skills and increase their confidence as they enter the workforce. The Mentorship/Preceptorship Initiative is aimed at promoting appropriate supports for nurses who have just graduated or are changing roles in nursing practice. The patient/resident lift strategy focuses on the prevention of musculoskeletal injuries and improved safety in the workplace through the purchase of mechanical lifting and transferring equipment. Government funding for the Safety Engineered Sharps is to help hospitals move to safer medical equipment such as needleless systems, blunt suture needles to replace sharp ones, and plastic blood collection tubes to replace breakable glass tubes.

A possible setback of the Ontario Nursing Strategy is a concern with the current economic situation. The Ontario Nurses Association is relaying reports of provincial employers laying off nurses and reducing their hours in attempts to balance their budgets. This trend, combined with a nursing shortage and the province's recent announcement that the promised 9,000 additional nurses will be delayed from 4 to 5 years due to the economic downturn, is claimed to be putting patients' health at risk (from *Nurses' Voice*, Canadian Federation of Nurses Unions, February 2009). Therefore, researchers and decision makers across the country need to collaborate in their efforts to determine ways to maintain the momentum created by recent policy implementations.

DIRECTIONS FOR NURSING IN CANADA

Numerous studies over the past decade substantiated the benefits of healthy workplaces on nurse retention, health and well-being, patient outcomes, and organizational performance. National initiatives to address the nursing shortage in Canada involved the creation of the Canadian Nursing Advisory. Its report, *Our Health, Our Future: Creating Quality Workplaces for Canadian Nurses* (Canadian Nursing Advisory Committee, 2002), contained 51 recommendations designed to resolve workforce management issues and create professional practice environments that would attract people into the profession and retain nurses. Shamian and El-Jardali (2007) highlight policy changes in many of the provinces: increased number of seats in nursing education programs, creation of new full-time nursing positions, workload measurement systems, phased-in retirement programs, and the Registered Nurses' Association of Ontario Healthy Work Environments Best Practice Guidelines project. Influential to this progress was the increased understanding that high-quality healthcare cannot occur without an adequately sized and well-prepared nursing workforce.

There is warning of some outcomes that can be expected within the context of the current recession: Vacant RN positions will be filled, and many healthcare organizations will report an end to the nurse shortage; new nursing graduates will experience difficulty finding jobs; nursing education programs could experience an increase in demand due to the perceived relative job security and earnings of nurses; and the capacity of some education programs could be affected negatively by budget reductions (Buerhaus, Auerbach, & Staiger, 2009). If employers and policy makers interpret such outcomes as an end to the nursing problem, attention could shift away from the nursing workforce at a time when continued efforts are needed more than ever. In view of the projected nurse shortage, researchers are urging that the priorities should be to strengthen the current nurse workforce and expand long-term supply and implement strategies to promote positive work environments and nurse retention.

The Nature of Nursing Work

In addition to the quality of the work environment, the nature of the role of the nurse can influence a decision whether to remain in a position. Needleman and Hassmiller (2009) suggest that nurses' knowledge and commitment to their patients and institutions be more effectively mobilized to enable them more decision-making responsibility for process improvement. In other words, nurses' perspectives should be represented at the highest levels of leadership and integrated into organizational decision making. Active involvement of nurses in making and sustaining change, and processes for engaging nurses and other frontline staff need to be expanded. For example, Buerhaus (2008) suggests that at a micro-level, efficiency gains are possible by reengineering nursing processes and improving documentation, medication administration systems, and care coordination. Reconfiguring the physical workspace to reduce time spent searching for supplies and equipment results in nurses spending more time providing direct patient care and increased likelihood of professional fulfillment.

Nurse administrators should explore factors that could motivate nurses to acquire relevant new knowledge and apply it to their care delivery. For example, Estabrooks, Midodzi, Cummings, and Wallin (2007) found that Internet use and emotional exhaustion influence research utilization and suggested that further investigation of these variables is warranted. Also, the increasing importance of nurse-sensitive performance measures support the case for more effective use and retention of nurses. In order to facilitate improvement of care for individual patients, nurses should have the opportunities to see the relationships between their nursing interventions and patient outcome achievements (Doran & Sidani, 2007). Providing nurses with readily accessible best practice guidelines, embedding the information in decision support tools, and delivering real-time feedback to nurses will stimulate nurses' interest in reflecting on their practice and adopting best practices (Doran & Sidani, 2007). Nurses who are actively engaged in planning the care of their patients and are supported in the care outcomes are more apt to continue in their nursing role.

Evidence-Based Staffing Patterns

Determining nurse staffing requirements is not straightforward, and the number of budgeted positions may vary widely for institutions with similar patient profiles, depending on the patient classification system used (Reinier et al., 2005). Increases in hospital occupancy and decreases in the average length of stay have resulted in increased average patient acuity and an increased number of patients to admit and discharge per shift. Allocation of staffing should consider the changing patient profile, experience and expertise of nurses, stability of the healthcare team, leadership, availability of clinical resources, care delivery systems, and management decisions such as use of overtime and type of equipment. As asserted in the Patient Care Delivery Model, recommendations for staffing decisions must be interpreted in light of broader professional and health system trends and decision makers' value systems and then considered within the context of local institutional realities (Clarke, 2007; O'Brien-Pallas, Thomson et al., 2004). In one study, patient-to-nurse ratio was found to be one of the most consistent unit characteristics to have a harmful affect on nurse outcomes, with high patient-to-nurse ratios negatively impacting nurses' perceptions of work and the work environment, unit-based nursing leadership, and nurses' job stress (McGillis Hall et al., 2008). Therefore, appropriate staffing measures are indicated, such as the use of part-time nurses as a resource at the unit level to reduce workload and improve nurse and patient outcomes.

Retention of Senior Nurses

The more experienced and older nurses are a key resource, and it is not yet know if older nurses will be willing to remain in the workforce when they reach the age of 60 years or so (Clarke, 2007). McGillis Hall et al. (2008) found that older nurses experience more job stress and concern with the quality of their work and work environment; therefore, workplace strategies should be directed at determining the sources of the stress. As a group, the senior nurses possess the most knowledge and clinical experience, which are needed in detecting patient complications and intervening to prevent the complication from worsening (Buerhaus et al., 2009). The knowledge and clinical skills of older nurses can help offset the increased risk of adverse patient outcomes as future shortages increase and persist for several years (Buerhaus, 2008). Thus, efforts to retain older nurses are needed to ensure that enough experienced nurses are available in the future to mentor younger nurses. Because the proportion of older RNs in the workforce is increasing and because they are more susceptible to injury and take longer to recover, now is the time to concentrate on improving their working conditions to promote their retention. Their continued presence would reinforce overall nurse supply and also make an important difference in the quality and safety of patient care.

Investment in Quality Data for HHRP

There are many nursing workforce issues that need to be explored further to help HHR planners understand how the nursing workforce affects patient access to care, utilization of health services, and healthcare outcomes. Some gaps in evidence are the longitudinal micro- and macro-level economic and organizational influences on RN workforce participation, demographic RN characteristics, and other factors that influence nursing workforce participation (Brewer, 2005). Data on supply, production, and financial resources can inform the planning and forecasting functions of the broader HHR conceptual framework. Predicting national or regional need for nurses is difficult because there is no consensus on the optimal number of health professionals necessary to meet the population's healthcare needs (O'Brien-Pallas, Birch, & Tomblin Murphy, 2001; Reinier et al., 2005). Analysis is based on a complex model including measures of current healthcare use (e.g., inpatient days, number of visits, and number of nursing facility residents) and factors that affect healthcare use (population age, gender, and urban/rural characteristics; the healthcare operating environment; economic conditions; and population health). To ensure appropriate allocation of nursing resources and advancement of HHRP beyond simple supply/demand forecasting, investment is needed in creating and maintaining readily accessible databases that allow comparison between and among jurisdictions. Policy options must be informed by evidence that is of good quality, comparable, and readily accessible.

Investment is also needed for infrastructure to collect data that will monitor and improve care delivery processes and measurement of performance outcomes. Because many policy initiatives began their implementation only within the past 5 years or so, researchers and decision makers should consider how to ensure that changes are sustainable and efficient (Shamian & El-Jardali, 2007). Healthcare organizations should track whether healthy workplace initiatives are achieving their desired effects through evaluation research of implementations (El-Jardali & Fooks, 2005). Research evidence should be portrayed in a way that links improved nurse work life to better patient outcomes and more efficient healthcare spending (Brewer, 2005). Public reporting of measurable results from healthy workplace initiatives would increase accountability and sharing of information on successes and barriers (Shamian & El-Jardali, 2007). Availability of administrative databases would facilitate better research, with improved data collection and analysis of relationships between the input factors and outcomes, such as how outcomes are influenced by nurse staffing decision.

CONCLUSIONS

This chapter portrayed how research is shaping HHR strategies for nursing in Ontario. The HHR framework has been applied in research, and the evidence is contributing to policy aimed at building a healthy nursing workforce. Strategies are being recommended to produce a sufficient supply of qualified RNs, to create work environments that support their practice, and to deploy their skills effectively. In addition to producing a supply of new nurses, attention should be paid to older nurses who are more likely to be retained in settings that offer flexible schedules and less strenuous jobs that use their knowledge and experience. Problems facing the nursing workforce should be higher on the health policy agenda so that effective actions can be implemented promptly. Given the projected nursing losses, it may take years before the workforce reaches a level stable enough indicate an end to the shortage. Thus, it is critical that healthcare organizations use the current workforce more efficiently, retain older RNs, and expand the size of the future RN workforce.

This chapter highlights the importance of the interaction of researchers and policy makers in planning for the number of human resources required in the future and how to retain nurses in the workforce once they have entered. What must be remembered is that this type of planning is not a one-time exercise and must be repeated over time. If we review researching and managing human resources as a continuous quality-improvement process, then the estimates and push-and-pull strategies must be revised regularly (at least every 3–5 years) as technology changes, generational differences emerge, or even the needs of the population change.

REFERENCES

Advisory Committee on Health Human Resources. (2002). *Our health, our future—Creating quality workplaces for Canadian nurses.* Final Report of the Canadian Nursing Advisory Committee. Author.

Aiken, L., Buchan, J., Sochalski, S., Nichols, B., & Powell, M. (2004). Trends in international nurse migration. *Health Affairs, 23*(3), 69–77.

Andersen, R. M. (1995). Revisiting the behavioral model and access to health care: Does it matter? *Journal of Health and Social Behavior, 36*(1), 1–10.

Baumann, A., Blythe, J., Kolotylo, C., & Underwood, J. (2004). *The international nursing labour market.* Building the future: An integrated strategy for nursing human resources in Canada. Nursing sector study corporation.

Baumann, A., Hunsberger, M., Idriss, D., Alameddine, M., & Grinspun, D. (2008). *Employment of nursing graduates: Evaluation of a provincial policy strategy.* Health Human Resources Series Number 10. Nursing Health Services Research Unit.

Baumann, A., O'Brien-Pallas, L., Armstrong-Stassen, M., Blythe, J., Bourbonnais, R., Cameron, S., et al. (2001). *Commitment and care: The benefits of a healthy workplace for nurses, their patients and the system.* Canadian Health Services Research Foundation and the Change Foundation.

Birch, S., O'Brien-Pallas, L., Alksnis, C., Tomblin Murphy, G., & Thomson, D. (2003). Beyond demographic change in health human resources planning: An extended framework and application to nursing. *Journal of Health Services Research and Policy, 8*(4), 225–229.

Blakeley, J. A., & Ribeiro, V. E. S. (2008). Early retirement among registered nurses: Contributing factors. *Journal of Nursing Management, 16*(1), 29–37.

Brewer, C. S. (2005). Health services research and the nursing workforce: Access and utilization issues. *Nursing Outlook, 53*(6), 281–290.

Buchan, J. (2006). Evidence of nursing shortages or a shortage of evidence? *Journal of Advanced Nursing, 56,* 457–458.

Buchan, J., & Aiken, L. (2008). Solving nursing shortages: a common priority. *Journal of Clinical Nursing, 17*(24), 3262–3268.

Buerhaus, P. I. (2008). Current and future state of the US nursing workforce. *JAMA: Journal of the American Medical Association, 300*(20), 2422–2424.

Buerhaus, P. I., Auerbach, I., & Staiger, D. O. (2009). The recent surge in nurse employment: Causes and implications. *Health Affairs, 28*(4), w657–w668. Retrieved June 23, 2009, from http://content.healthaffairs.org/cgi/reprint/hlthaff.28.4.w657v1

Burke, R. J. (2001). Nursing staff survivor responses to hospital restructuring and downsizing. *Stress and Health, 17,* 195–205.

Burke, R. J., & Greenglass, E. R. (2000). Organizational restructuring: Identifying effective hospital downsizing procedures. In R. J. Burke & C. L. Cooper (Eds.), *The Organization in Crisis* (pp. 284–303). London: Blackwell.

Canadian Federation of Nurses Unions. (2009, Feb). Cross country checkup. *Nurses' Voice,* 5–7. Retrieved June 4, 2009, from http://www.nursesunions.ca/media.php?mid=892

Canadian Nursing Advisory Committee. (2002). *Our health, our future: Creating high quality health care workplaces for Canadian nurses.* Author.

Clarke, S. P. (2007). Nurse staffing in acute care settings: Research perspectives and practice implications. *Joint Commission Journal on Quality and Patient Safety, 33*(Suppl. 11), 30–44

Commission on the Future of Health Care in Canada. (2002). *Building on values—The future of health care in Canada.* Final Report of the Commission on the Future of Health Care in Canada. Author.

Donabedian, A. (1966). Evaluating the quality of medical care (Part 2). *Milbank Memorial Fund Quarterly, 44*(3), 166–203.

Doran, D. M., & Sidani, S. (2007). Outcomes-focused knowledge translation: A framework for knowledge translation and patient outcomes improvement. *Worldviews on Evidence-Based Nursing, 4*(1), 3–13.

Duffield, C., & O'Brien-Pallas, L. (2002). The nursing workforce in Canada and Australia: Two sides of the same coin. *Australian Health Review, 25*(2), 136–144.

El-Jardali, F., & Fooks, C. (2005). *An environmental scan of current views on health human resources in Canada: Identified problems, proposed solutions and gap analysis.* Toronto: Health Council of Canada.

Estabrooks, C. A., Midodzi, W. K., Cummings, G. G., & Wallin, L. (2007). Predicting research use in nursing organizations: a multilevel analysis. *Nursing Research, 56*(4 Suppl), S7–S23.

Grinspun, D. (2002). A flexible nursing workforce: Realities and fallouts. *Hospital Quarterly, 6*(1), 79–84.

Joint Provincial Nursing Committee. (2001). *Good nursing, good health: A good investment.* Progress Report on the Nursing Task Force Strategy in Ontario.

Joint Provincial Nursing Committee. (2003). *Good nursing, good health: The return on our investment.* Progress Report of the Implementation Monitoring Subcommittee.

Kazanjian, A., Pulcins, I. R., & Kerluke, K. (1992). A human resources decision support model: Nurse deployment patterns in one Canadian system. *Hospital Health Services Administration, 37*(3), 303–319.

Lavis, J. N., & Birch, S. (1997). Applying alternative approaches to estimating nurse requirements. The answer is . . . Now what was the question? *Canadian Journal of Nursing Administration, 10*(1), 24–44.

Leatt, P., & Schneck, R. (1981). Nursing subunit technology: A replication. *Administrative Science Quarterly, 26*(2), 225–236.

Little, L. (2007). Nurse migration: A Canadian case study. *Health Services Research, 42*(3 Part 2), 1336–1353.

Lomas, J. (2000). Using 'linkage and exchange' to move research into policy at a Canadian foundation. *Health Affairs, 19*(3), 236–240.

McGillis Hall, L., Doran, D., & Pink, L. (2008). Outcomes of interventions to improve hospital nursing work environments. *Journal of Nursing Administration, 38*(1), 40–46.

McGillis Hall, L., Pink, G., Jones, C., Leatt, P., Gates, M., & Peterson, J. (2009). Is the grass any greener? Canada to United States of America nurse migration. *International Nursing Review, 56*(2), 198–205.

Ministry of Health and Long-term Care. (n.d.). Guidelines for application to the Ontario nursing strategy. Retrieved May 15, 2009, from www.health.gov.on.ca/english/providers/program/nursing_sec/strategy_app_mn.html

Ministry of Health and Long-term Care. (n.d.). Nursing secretariat. Retrieved May 15, 2009, from www. health.gov.on.ca/english/providers/program/nursing_sec/nursing_sec_mn.html

Needleman, J., & Hassmiller, S. (2009). The role of nurses in improving hospital quality and efficiency: Real-world results. *Health Affairs, 28*(4), w625–w633. Retrieved June 23, 2009, from http://content. healthaffairs.org/cgi/reprint/hlthaff.28.4.w625v1

Nursing Effectiveness, Utilization and Outcomes Research Unit. (2004). *Final report July 1, 1999–June 30, 2004*. Submitted to MOHLTC. Author.

Nursing Task Force. (1999). *Good nursing, good health: An investment for the 21st century*. Report of the Nursing Task Force. Author.

O'Brien-Pallas, L. (2002). Where to from here? (Editorial & Discourse). *Canadian Journal of Nursing Research, 33*(4), 3–14.

O'Brien-Pallas, L., Alksnis, C., Wang, S., Tomblin Murphy, G., & Birch, S. (2003). *Bringing the future into focus: Projecting RN retirement in Canada*. Toronto, Ontario: Canadian Institute for Health Information.

O'Brien-Pallas, L., Baumann, A., Birch, S., & Tomblin Murphy, G. (2000). Health human resource planning in home care: How to approach it—that is the question. *Healthcare Papers, 1*(4), 53–59.

O'Brien-Pallas, L., Birch, S., Baumann, A., & Tomblin Murphy, G. (2001). Integrating workforce planning, human resources, and service planning. *Human Resources Development Journal, 5*(1–3), 2–16.

O'Brien-Pallas, L., Birch, S., & Tomblin Murphy, G. (2001). Workforce planning and workplace management. *International Nursing Perspectives, 1*(2–3), 55–65.

O'Brien-Pallas, L., Duffield, C., & Alksnis, C. (2004). Who will be there to nurse? Retention of nurses nearing retirement. *Journal of Nursing Administration, 34*(6), 298–302.

O'Brien-Pallas, L., Irvine Doran, D., Murray, M., Cockerill, R., Sidani, S., Laurie-Shaw, B., et al. (2002). Evaluation of a client care delivery model part 2: Variability in client outcomes in community home nursing. *Nursing Economics, 20*(1), 13–21.

O'Brien-Pallas, L., Irvine, D., Peereboom, E., & Murray, M. (1997). Measuring nursing workload: Understanding the variability. *Nursing Economics, 15*(4), 171–182.

O'Brien-Pallas, L., Mildon, B., Tomblin Murphy, G., Bookey-Bassett, S., Hiroz, J., Hayes, L., et al. (2007). *The MOHLTC late career nurse funding initiative results of the phase 2 impact evaluation final report*. Toronto, Nursing Health Services Research Unit, University of Toronto.

O'Brien-Pallas, L., Thomson, D., McGillis Hall, L. Pink, G., Kerr, M., Wang, S., et al. (2004). *Evidence based standards for measuring nurse staffing and performance*. Report for the Canadian Health Services Research Foundation. Toronto, Ontario: Nursing Effectiveness, Utilization and Outcomes Research Unit.

O'Brien-Pallas, L., Tomblin Murphy, G., Birch, S., & Baumann, A. (2001). Framework for analyzing health human resources. In *Future development of information to support the management of nursing resources: Recommendations* (p. 6). Ottawa: Canadian Institute for Health Information.

O'Brien-Pallas, L., Tomblin Murphy, G., Birch, S., Kephart, G., Meyer, R., Eisler, K., et al. (2007). *Health human resources modelling: Challenging the past, creating the future*. Submitted to the Canadian Health Services Research Foundation.

O'Brien-Pallas, L., Tomblin Murphy, G., Laschinger, H., White, S., Wang, S., & McCulloch, C. (2005). *Canadian survey of nurses from three occupational groups*. The Nursing Labour Market in Canada: An Occupational Sector Study. Ottawa, Canada: Nursing Sector Study Corporation.

O'Brien-Pallas, L., Tomblin Murphy, G., Shamian, J., Li, X. M., Kephart, G., Laschinger, H., et al. (2008). *Understanding the costs and outcomes of nurses' turnover in Canadian hospitals (Nursing Turnover Study)*. Submitted to the Canadian Institutes of Health Research. Toronto, Ontario: Nursing Health Services Research Unit.

O'Brien-Pallas, L., Tomblin-Murphy, G., White, S., Hayes, L., Baumann, A. & Higgin, A., et al. (2004). *Research synthesis report*. Building the future: An integrated strategy for nursing human resources in Canada. Nursing Sector Study Corporation, Canada.

Reinier, K., Palumbo, M. V., McIntosh, B., Rambur, B., Kolodinsky, J., Hurowitz, L., et al. (2005). Measuring the nursing workforce: Clarifying the definitions. *Medical Care Research and Review, 62*, 741–755.

Robertson, R., & Dowd, S. (1996). The effects of hospital downsizing on staffing and quality of care. *Health Care Supervisor, 14*(3), 50–56.

Shamian, J., & El-Jardali, F. (2007). Healthy workplaces for health workers in Canada: Knowledge transfer and uptake in policy and practice. *HealthcarePapers, 7*(Sp), 6–25.

Shamian, J., & Griffin, P. (2003). Translating research into health policy. *Canadian Journal of Nursing Research, 35*(3), 45–52.

Tarlov, A. R. (1999). Public policy frameworks for improving population health. *Annals of the New York Academy of Sciences, 896*, 281–293.

Tomblin Murphy, G., O'Brien-Pallas, L., Alksnis, C., Birch, S. Kephart, G., Pennock, et al. (2003). *Health human resources planning: an examination of relationships among nursing service utilization, an estimate of population health and overall health status outcomes in the province of Ontario.* CHSRF.

17

Research Technology: Home Telehealth and Remote Monitoring

Stanley M. Finkelstein and Rhonda G. Cady

INTRODUCTION

Considerable interest in recent years on "fixing" the healthcare system in the United States has focused on how technology can be leveraged to increase safety, improve quality, increase productivity, and contain cost. The technology most often cited in these discussions has been the development, implementation, and use of electronic health records and personal health records by clinical centers and individual patients, respectively. New and improved imaging technologies also enter the discussion, but often are cited as examples of excessive costs accompanying newer technology rather than as examples of the potential of using new technology to improve both diagnostic and therapeutic functions. Telemedicine is a more recent player in these discussions, with promises of increasing access to care, improving satisfaction, improving quality, and containing cost. Home telehealth not only accomplishes these goals but, more importantly, also has the potential to change the way healthcare is delivered by making it accessible to individuals regardless of their physical location.

Home telehealth systems provide remote care delivery between healthcare providers or systems and clients or patients in their homes. These systems may include simple e-mail reminders or telephone communications between provider and client, remote monitoring of physiological variables which provide to assess acute interventions or to monitor chronic disease progression, and interactive video consisting of two-way audio and video transmissions, often called virtual visits, which provide ongoing assessment of patients with chronic diseases or as-needed assessment for acute problems that can benefit from face-to-face interactions without the patient being physically present in the clinic setting. In some cases, these are extensions of home monitoring programs that people have been using for many years, such as monitoring weight, blood pressure, and blood glucose. The major difference between these "traditional" programs and current home telehealth applications is the direct involvement of the healthcare provider in assessing the home measurements. Rather than relying on the subject to detect potential problems in their measurements and contacting their provider, the providers are now participating in the process by directly reviewing data transmitted from subjects' homes or by reviewing cases that have been identified as a potential problem by a prescreening triage system. Home telehealth can also be extended to the smart home concept, where environmental and motion monitoring can alert and trigger a response to unsafe conditions in a client's living area, such as a client being unable to get up after falling or a gas burner left unattended when a forgetful client leaves the kitchen for an extended period of time.

Home telehealth uses telecommunications and information technology to deliver support and services directly to individuals in their homes. The convergence of increasing broadband availability and less costly, user-friendly remote physiological monitoring devices has increased the potential impact of home telehealth programs on the healthcare delivery system and the lives of healthcare consumers. These systems typically use some or all of the following equipment to deliver home telehealth services: remote monitoring devices, Web camera, computer or equivalent video monitor, software for data collection, compression protocol, transmission/communication media (i.e., telephone or broadband Internet connection), and a Health Insurance Portability and Accountability Act (HIPAA) compliant transmission protocol. These applications have been implemented using both the plain old telephone system (POTS) and broadband connectivity via digital subscriber line (DSL) or cable service delivery. Applications may use POTS or cellular phones for basic telephone functions such as messaging or completing survey instruments, store and forward technologies using computer or equivalent personal digital assistants that can save information (e.g., e-mails, images, and monitoring data) for later transmission when immediate responses are not necessary, or interactive video between providers in a clinic/agency and patients at home.

Remote monitoring of physiological or behavioral conditions can be a part of the previous applications or can be stand-alone using either POTS or broadband connectivity. An advantage of POTS is its almost universal availability throughout the developed world, whereas broadband is still not as widely accessible, particularly in rural areas where infrastructure implementation costs may make it economically less desirable. However, the goal of most home telehealth applications is to be broadband-ready to take advantage of the high bandwidth, enabling faster communications for large amounts of information and better quality images for interactive video. In many developing regions of the world where traditional landline services have not been available, governments and private providers are moving directly to mobile or cellular phone technologies. Remote monitoring systems have typically been designed to transmit data over a landline using a telephone jack, but they will need to be designed for mobile data transmission if they wish to be part of the growing worldwide move to telemedicine and home telehealth.

When describing home telehealth systems, it is important to understand the differences among POTS, broadband, and wireless transmission media. In the United States, POTS or landline is the most widely available transmission medium. This medium was designed for voice transmission, and as a result, data transmission speeds are slow (56 Kbps or kilobits per second) and generally are unable to support high-quality video transmissions. Broadband was designed to support large data packet transmission common with Internet communication. The current broadband transmission media include DSL, cable, satellite, and wireless. Existing landlines are used by DSL to provide high-speed transmissions ranging from 128 Kbps to 7 Mbps (megabits per second), with rural DSL falling in the lower transmission ranges. Cable broadband offers transmission speeds in the 1.5 to 15.0 Mbps range, but requires a cable-ready home. Unlike landlines, which access nearly 96% of households in the United States (Federal Communications

Commission, 2009b), cable access has been slow to rural areas. Wireless or mobile transmission, which uses radio technology, was initially designed to support voice communication, with data transmission speeds similar to that of POTS. The current 3G technology supports high-speed, mobile data transmissions similar to cable broadband, but availability and transmission speed vary widely from urban to rural areas. Satellite wireless transmission speeds are faster than that of POTS (80 to 500 Kbps) but do not provide the high-speed data transmissions of other broadband media (Federal Communications Commission, 2009a).

Broadband Internet service utilizes two types of connection speeds, upload and download. The download speed is the rate at which data are received by a computer from another source. The upload speed is the rate at which data are sent from a computer to another source. Because the majority of Internet activity involves downloading data, this speed is often two to three times faster than upload speed. The differences in speeds are an important consideration for telehealth interactive video applications, as both upload and download speeds affect audio and video quality. The rate at which data (audio and video) are downloaded and displayed during a video conference is dependent on the upload speed of the sending computer. A minimum upload speed of 384 Kbps is needed for both quality audio and video clarity (Cady, Kelly, & Finkelstein, 2008).

The primary potential for home telehealth systems is to provide the needed support as the healthcare system shifts from institution-centric to patient-centric care and healthcare delivery changes from primarily acute care provision to encompass chronic care management. Such systems can "go home" with the patient and provide easier and more useful contextual information, as well as graphical and interactive instructions for following home care directives. A virtual visit would allow a care provider to observe and correct technique in filling and administering the correct insulin dose for a newly diagnosed diabetic patient, for example, or to correct the technique that an asthma or lung transplant recipient might employ in doing home spirometry. These approaches provide the continuity of care often lacking when a patient returns home after a hospitalization, often without a clear understanding of how to manage his or her newly acquired health needs (Frankl, Breeling, & Goldman, 1991; Naylor et al., 1999). The socialization made possible by virtual visits is another often overlooked, but critically important, benefit of these systems. The potential for regular visits with distant family members is an obvious benefit of interactive video, but virtual visits between elderly, home-bound patients and their home care nurses have emerged as important new avenues for socialization. Subjects in several of our research studies have been reluctant to give up their virtual visit equipment at the conclusion of the study because they did not want to lose the regular visits made possible by this technology.

Research on the impact of home telehealth systems on subject outcomes has shown positive results. A study of newly diagnosed cancer patients discharged with new ostomies showed that supplementing traditional home health nursing visits with twice weekly ostomy nurse virtual visits increased patient satisfaction and resulted in fewer pouch changes (Bohnenkamp, McDonald, Lopez, Krupinski, & Blackett, 2004). A randomized trial of usual care, usual care plus telephone, and usual care plus virtual visits for newly discharged congestive heart failure (CHF) patients showed a statistically significant drop in readmissions and emergency room visits for both intervention groups (Jerant, Azari, Martinez, & Nesbitt, 2003). The Internet Chronic Disease Self-Management Program utilized interactive Web-based English-language instruction and Web-based bulletin board discussion groups and successfully replicated the health status improvement results of a successful community-based, small-group Chronic Disease Self-Management Program (Lorig, Ritter, Laurent, & Plant, 2006). A systematic review of Interactive Health Communication Applications (Web-based tools that combine health information with social, decision, and/or behavior change support) showed a significant positive effect on social support and knowledge (Murray, Burns, See Tai, Lai, & Nazareth, 2005). The Veterans Health Administration developed a care coordination program that uses telehealth technology to facilitate self-management of chronic conditions (Bendixen, Levy, Olive, Kobb, & Mann, 2009; Joseph, 2006). The themes emerging from a content analysis of virtual visits for patients with chronic conditions were similar to the patterns of home care nurse and patient interactions described by Vivian and Wilcox (2000), and included small talk and psychosocial issues that facilitate socialization (Demiris, Speedie, Finkelstein, & Harris, 2003). A virtual visit pilot study for neurologically impaired children and their families showed decreased feelings of isolation (Guest, Rittey, & O'Brien, 2005). The depth and breadth of home telehealth research reveal a growing use and acceptance of the technology.

Is the time right for home telehealth? There are a growing number of healthcare and consumer electronic businesses that are entering the field, suggesting that there is the potential for successful business plans in the merging of healthcare, communications, and information technologies. Pushing the issue is a rapidly expanding aging population with multiple chronic conditions and a costly centralized healthcare system facing a shortage of trained providers, who are trying to empower patients by "outsourcing" their care to patients and families within their homes. Pulling the issue is the growing availability of fast, secure telecommunications and information technologies; the development of less expensive, easy-to-use remote monitoring devices; and the mounting evidence that home telehealth can increase access, improve quality, and contain cost in managing both acute and chronic healthcare problems from the home.

Our research group has been investigating the use of remote patient monitoring and home telehealth technologies in diverse populations for the past 25 years. Our home telehealth focus has been on the development and evaluation of systems combining information, instrumentation, and telecommunications technology to enable or support healthcare delivery services directly to the client at home. The goals for these studies were to improve access while providing quality care with cost-effective systems that are satisfactory to patients and providers. In most studies, a randomized controlled trial methodology has been used so that home telehealth results can be compared with standard care when policy decisions that impact the transition from the research laboratory to the community setting are considered. Four studies will be highlighted, as they cover a broad range of technology capabilities supporting home telehealth for a wide range of subject populations. They are (1) the lung transplant home monitoring program, using POTS-based remote monitoring for lung transplant recipients; (2) the TeleHomeCare Program, employing POTS-based remote monitoring and virtual nursing visits for elderly home-bound subjects; (3) the VALUE (Virtual Assisted Living Umbrella for the Elderly) program, utilizing broadband-based virtual visits and remote monitoring in support of independent living for elderly clients managing multiple chronic diseases; and (4) the U Special Kids program, using POTS-based care coordination and case management (CC/CM) for children with complex special healthcare needs. Subjects in all studies provided written informed consent, following the guidelines of the University of Minnesota Institutional Review Board.

HOME TELEHEALTH PROGRAMS

Lung Transplant Home Monitoring Program

The lung transplant program at the University of Minnesota has performed more than 600 lung transplants since its inception in 1986. Our lung transplant home monitoring research program, which began in 1992, provides a framework for conducting telehealth research that facilitates clinical translation. The underlying premise of remote home monitoring was, and still is, that timely information from clinically informative variables that are remotely acquired could lead to early detection and, thus, early intervention before problems become more intractable. Ideally, this early intervention would improve the patient's health status and increase survival while containing cost (Finkelstein et al., 1996).

For lung transplantation, home monitoring is designed to provide early indications of the onset of infection or rejection episodes. In the initial home monitoring study, subjects performed full spirometry and recorded vital signs and symptoms daily at home, using an electronic spirometer/diary instrument (Figure 17.1) designed by a local medical device manufacturer to the investigators' specifications. These data were stored in the device until downloaded by the subject once a week, over their regular landline telephone, to the study data center. Symptom data included frequency of coughing and wheezing, sputum production and color, shortness of breath at rest and after exercise, and amount (in minutes) and type of daily exercise. Vital signs included blood pressure, weight, pulse, and temperature. Transmitted data were reviewed weekly by home monitoring study nurse clinical coordinators to identify bronchopulmonary events that might need follow-up treatment. Home spirometry reliability and validity were evaluated throughout the study to ensure that subject training, nursing follow-up, and subject skills remained satisfactory. Validity analysis showed that clinic spirometry values could be reliably estimated from home monitoring spirometry (Finkelstein et al., 1993; Lindgren et al., 1997).

The next step in the home monitoring research program was the development of computer-based triage algorithms derived from the home monitoring data (spirometry, vital signs, and symptoms). Two rule-based decision support algorithms were evaluated for clinical implementation. One identified the development of chronic rejection and the other identified early signs of acute rejection or infection. The chronic rejection algorithm, using the progressive stages of bronchiolitis obliterans syndrome as the marker for rejection, identified initial movement into the various bronchiolitis obliterans syndrome stages earlier than could be obtained only from clinic visit spirometry (Finkelstein et al., 1999). A computerized decision support system (CDSS), using weekly home monitoring data and based on the heuristic rules established by the home monitoring nurse coordinators, triaged lung transplant recipients for potential acute bronchopulmonary events. The CDSS had excellent sensitivity and specificity using nurse triage decisions as the gold standard (Finkelstein, Scudiero, Lindgren, Snyder, & Hertz, 2005).

In the current home monitoring research study, we are conducting a randomized controlled trial comparing a Bayesian predictive model with nurse-based triage for early detection of validated acute bronchopulmonary disease events (Troiani & Carlin, 2004). The success of the Bayesian model would support the use of such a decision support tool in this triage function. Incorporating the CDSS into clinical use would have important

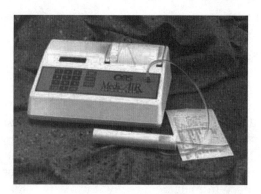

FIGURE 17.1 Home spirometer used in the lung transplant study.

implications for the economic and clinical factors related to chronic disease management, home monitoring, and the growing shortage of skilled nurses caring for the burgeoning "chronic disease" population. However, barriers to the diffusion of home spirometry monitoring exist. Reimbursement of home spirometry was added by the Centers for Medicare and Medicaid Services (CMS) in 1998, but the amount rarely covers the cost of providing the service (Health Care Financing Administration, 2 Nov. 1998). Patient adherence to home spirometry requires frequent monitoring and follow-up is needed to support long-term behavioral change, but the lack of sufficient reimbursement makes it unlikely that crucial follow-up to support home monitoring will be available.

The TeleHomeCare Program

The TeleHomeCare Program was a collaboration among the University of Minnesota, four rural and urban home health care (HHC) agencies, and several technical industry partners (Finkelstein et al., 2004). TeleHomeCare combined actual and virtual HHC visits with the goal of delivering quality care at an acceptable cost for patients receiving skilled nursing care at home. Virtual visits consisted of two-way audio and video interactions between a healthcare provider at a central site and the patient at home, transmitted over POTS (Figure 17.2). The overall objectives were to demonstrate that such a program can improve the quality and reduce or contain costs of skilled home healthcare while increasing patient access to care and satisfaction with the HHC intervention.

A randomized controlled trial to assess the effectiveness of virtual visits, Internet access, and remote physiological monitoring within an HHC setting was conducted from 1998 to 2001 (Finkelstein et al., 2004). Outcome measures included mortality and morbidity, need to transfer to a higher level of care (e.g., hospitalization or long-term care facility), patient and caregiver satisfaction, patient utilization of services, and cost. Sixty-eight patients with CHF, chronic obstructive pulmonary disease (COPD), or chronic wound care were randomized as subjects in the three arms of the study. The control group received standard HHC as determined by their underlying condition. Two intervention groups received varying levels of telehealth. One intervention group received standard HHC supplemented with virtual visits and Internet access. A second intervention group received standard HHC supplemented with virtual visits, Internet access, and remote physiological monitoring. Subjects in the second intervention group received pulse

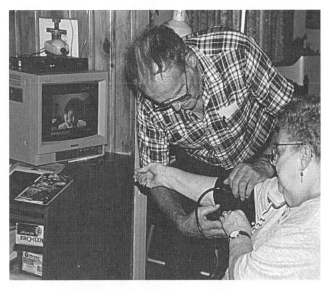

FIGURE 17.2 A subject in the TeleHomeCare study during a virtual visit with her homecare nurse.

oximeters (for oxygen saturation), electronic spirometers (for pulmonary function), and blood pressure cuffs depending on their underlying condition. After installation of equipment and a general review of telehomecare, the use of the interactive video equipment was taught during the next home visit, and the use of the monitoring equipment was taught in a third home visit. Training was done incrementally so as not to overwhelm the subjects, already often facing new home care procedures. All subjects used the interactive video, monitoring, and symptom reporting applications with little difficulty after receiving training from their HHC nurse. All subjects were followed for the length of the HHC episode and for 6 months after discharge from HHC to track their need for higher levels of care. They either returned to their home or to a relative, were admitted to a higher level of care facility (hospital or nursing home), or were deceased.

Study outcome measures indicated that home telehealth increased the satisfaction of both nurses and clients, was less costly than in-person HHC visits, and may reduce the need for increasing levels of care after discharge from the HHC program (Finkelstein, Speedie, & Potthoff, 2006). Subjects in all three groups were satisfied with their home care; those in the intervention groups showed equal or higher levels of satisfaction than did the control group. Subjects in the two intervention groups had an increased perception that the nurse can get a good understanding of the medical problem in a virtual visit, that virtual visits can save time for the nurse, that the telehomecare equipment is easy to use and is reliable, and that telehomecare does not violate one's privacy. Perception decreased in the area of saving the patient time and making it easier to contact the nurse. These results indicate that experience with telehomecare leads to a generally positive change in the patient's perception of this technology (Demiris, Speedie, & Finkelstein, 2000). The HHC nurses involved in this project rated the technical quality of virtual visits as acceptable to excellent in 94% of the cases. Nurses reported that in 92% of cases, the visit would not have been significantly better had it been performed with an actual home visit. In less than 5% of virtual visits, the nurses reported that there were questions not asked because of privacy or confidentiality concerns because they did not know who else was present in the subject's home at the time of the virtual visit (Demiris et al., 2003). The difference in discharge locations between the control and intervention subjects was on the border of statistical significance ($p = .053$); 8 of the 19 control subjects entered a higher level of care (42%), whereas 6 of the 34 intervention subjects entered a higher level of care (17.6%). Despite this difference in discharge destination between groups, there was no statistically significant difference in mortality (26.3% of control subjects; 20.6% of intervention subjects).

A cost analysis of actual HHC nurse visits versus virtual HHC nurse visits was conducted (Finkelstein et al., 2006). The average cost of actual visits was based upon the mileage traveled to each patient's home, the time spent during travel, and the time of the visit itself. Calculations conducted to determine the average virtual visit cost were more complex and based on nursing personnel time, amortized equipment costs, technical support costs, and administrative overhead. Virtual visits were divided into three categories depending upon whether they had only a videophone or a videophone plus monitoring equipment for either CHF or COPD. The virtual visit costs were higher for the COPD intervention subjects doing remote monitoring compared with the CHF intervention subjects also doing monitoring due to the large differential in the cost of the monitoring devices. The actual visit cost exceeded the cost of any of the types of virtual visits. The cost difference was attributed primarily to the amount of additional nursing time related to an actual visit, primarily transportation.

The TeleHomeCare Program demonstrated the technical feasibility of extending telehealth services to home-bound elderly; new avenues for socialization between elderly, home-bound patients and their home care nurses; and the potential for improved clinical outcomes at a lower cost. However, policy that reimburses HHC nurses for interactive audio and video communication within a beneficiary's home is currently ineligible for Medicare reimbursement. Lacking a sustainable payment mechanism, programs such as the TeleHomeCare Program must find new financial support after grant funding ends.

The VALUE Program

The VALUE program was a collaboration among the University of Minnesota, a rural healthcare agency, and an urban healthcare agency. The VALUE program provided virtual visits with a home care nurse, physiological remote monitoring, and a Web-based portal for ordering health related services, messaging between client and health provider, and Internet access, all via a broadband connection. The overall objective of the project was to evaluate the impact of a home telehealth program on maintaining frail elderly individuals in their home environment.

The VALUE program was a two-armed randomized controlled trial to evaluate the effectiveness of virtual visits, physiological monitoring, and a Web-based portal (Finkelstein et al., 2006). Outcome measures included usability and satisfaction with the telehealth platform components and utilization of health and related services. Eligible subjects were at least 60 years old, were managing one or more chronic conditions, were not receiving Medicare home health benefits at the time of enrollment but had functional limitations, could use a computer keyboard or manipulate a mouse, and had broadband connectivity available in their geographic area. A total of 99 eligible individuals participated in the study. Control group subjects continued with their regular living accommodations, obtaining supportive services as they do ordinarily, by telephone or visits to senior and community centers. Intervention group subjects received the VALUE workstation consisting of a PC platform with broadband (DSL or cable) connectivity, a HIPAA-compliant interactive video software, and a Web camera. Intervention group subjects also received physiological monitoring devices appropriate to their underlying health condition or continued using monitoring devices that they were already utilizing as part of their standard care.

The VALUE program organizers created a Web portal customized for each intervention group subject that facilitated access to Web-based health education resources, a telehealth nurse, and electronic ordering of various health and community services. The welcome page of the Web site is illustrated in Figure 17.3.

It was designed for improved accessibility for the elderly using the design principles proposed by Demiris, Finkelstein, and Speedie (2001). Fonts are large, colors are simple, and navigation can be accomplished either by a mouse pointer or by using the arrow keys. The screen identifies the user with both a name and a picture, and identifies the assigned project nurse. The portal provides messaging, educational content, and ordering/scheduling for services such as meals, transportation, house chores, medical/nurse appointments, drug refills (through the telehealth nurse), and ordering merchant coupons. The merchant coupons were included as a non-health-related activity to motivate subjects to practice using the portal for ordering services. The education link connects to a page that contains a variety of links to health-related educational sites suitable for this population. From this point, the user goes out onto the Internet to browse these educational sites.

The results of this study indicated that frail elderly persons can successfully utilize a telehealth platform that includes virtual visits, a Web-based information portal, and physiological monitoring. All subjects completed the Telemedicine Perception Questionnaire at baseline and after 60 days of participating in the study (Demiris et al., 2000). Both groups had similar baseline scores showing a similar level of attitudes to such technology. At 60-day follow-up, the intervention group scores were statistically significantly more positive toward technology compared with their baseline scores and the 60-day

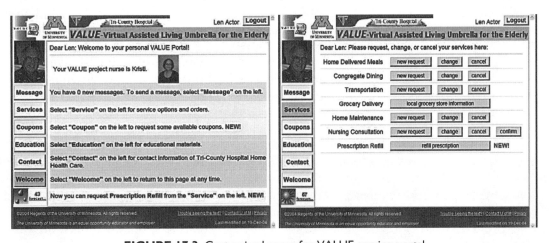

FIGURE 17.3 Customized pages for VALUE service portal.

scores for the controls (Finkelstein et al., 2007). The largest gains were for items relating to ease of use, improving general health, and cost. All subjects were able to use the portal after a brief instructional session with the VALUE nurse. They accessed all portal functions without difficulty. Prescription refills accounted for 65% of all service orders, and coupon book orders accounted for another 15% of all orders placed by intervention subjects. Remaining orders were for a wide range of needs. Virtual visits were conducted with all intervention subjects and consisted of two-way audio and video interactions between the project nurse at the agency site and the subject at home. There was an average of 26 virtual visits conducted with each of 40 intervention subjects who participated for at least 9 months. At the conclusion of the study, intervention subjects reported that they were very satisfied with the VALUE technology, virtual visits, and nurse interactions (Finkelstein et al., 2007). These subjects indicated that VALUE program met their expectations (9 of 10 points) and they would recommend the VALUE program to others (9.5 of 10 points).

Utilization measures included use of health and related services, such as visits with healthcare providers, use of emergency department and urgent care clinics, hospitalizations, pharmacy orders/delivery, transportation, dining services, and homemaker visits. Compared with control group subjects, the intervention group subjects had significantly fewer emergency department visits, higher use of pharmacy delivery services, and lower use of transportation services.

Although no new healthcare policy initiatives emerged from this study, it did provide further guidance into how society should think of the capabilities of an aging population. This study demonstrated that frail elderly individuals can use the home telehealth technology employed by the VALUE program when the proper modifications and user-focused training are addressed. Perception of the technology improved after hands-on experience and suggests acceptance of the VALUE technology by frail elderly persons. Earlier studies showed similar results using simpler and more familiar POTS connectivity (Finkelstein et al., 2004; Johnston, Weeler, Deuser, & Sousa, 2000; Mair et al., 2005).

The U Special Kids Program

The U Special Kids program at the University of Minnesota was a Medical Home Center (Kelly, Golnik, & Cady, 2008) that used a team of two advanced practice nurses (APNs) and a pediatrician to provide telephone-based CC/CM services to children with multiple, complex health conditions. Children enrolled in the program had four or more chronic health conditions, multiple specialists, numerous medications or rare pharmaceuticals, repeated hospitalizations and/or emergency room visits, and were dependent on technology (i.e., feeding tube, tracheotomy, central line, or oxygen). The CC/CM services provided by the U Special Kids program were delivered primarily by telephone, fax, and e-mail; these low-tech interventions fall under the broad definition of telehealth. The overall objectives of this research were to evaluate the impact of the telehealth intervention on hospitalization rate and assess the feasibility of incorporating CC/CM virtual visits.

A retrospective review measured the impact of low-tech, telephone-based CC/CM in reducing unplanned or emergency hospitalizations for children enrolled in the U Special Kids program (Cady, Finkelstein, & Kelly, 2009). An analysis of data from hospitalizations that occurred during the first 5 years of enrollment for 43 children showed a statistically significant reduction in unplanned hospitalizations (e.g., acute illness or injury and complications from underlying conditions) from Year 1 to Year 2, and a subsequent stabilization of unplanned hospitalization frequency. In contrast, planned hospitalizations (e.g., scheduled device insertion/replacement) remained relatively stable over the 5-year period (Cady, Finkelstein, & Kelly, 2009).

A pilot study evaluated the feasibility of conducting virtual visits between the U Special Kids APNs and families of children enrolled in the program (Cady et al., 2008). The quality of audio and video transmissions over different types of Internet connections in urban and rural areas was assessed, and a protocol for initiating and conducting CC/CM virtual visits was established. Over a 6-month period, two APNs conducted 23 scheduled video sessions with a convenience sample of three urban and two rural families. The study found that interactive video home telehealth was feasible with an Internet upload speed of 384 Kbps or greater. Although all families participating in this study had a broadband Internet connection, the families in rural locations had low-speed DSL or satellite connections that did not meet the 384 Kbps minimum for audio and video quality.

Three unscheduled sessions were initiated by the APNs and indicate that supplementing telephone-based CC/CM with virtual visits increases the amount of data communicated (Cady et al., 2008). In one session, a mother called to report a new rash on her child. The APN and pediatrician assessed the rash visually and determined that it was not serious enough to warrant a trip to the child's primary care provider. A second video session was initiated to observe a child for signs of a local reaction to a new oral supplement. The mother spoke limited English and the nurse was concerned that a verbal description of the child's reaction would be inadequate. The third unscheduled session occurred when a mother called to show her child walking for the first time with new assistive technology. These sessions provide explanatory validation that home-based, interactive video could increase the effectiveness of CC/CM for children with multiple, complex health conditions.

The U Special Kids program demonstrated that APN-delivered, telephone-based CC/CM reduces unplanned hospitalizations in children with multiple, complex health conditions. Currently, this is not a reimbursable service through Medicaid or third-party payers because the program does not provide in-person, primary-type care. Without a sustainable funding mechanism, the program was dependent on state appropriations and support from the affiliated tertiary medical center. The recent economic troubles faced by all segments of society resulted in program termination due to a lack of funding.

POLICY IMPLICATIONS

Lung Transplant Home Monitoring Program

As monitoring and communications technology improved over the years, it became clear that availability of patient-friendly devices was no longer the major problem initially thought to hinder the development and clinical use of remote monitoring systems. The two major barriers to technology diffusion are now adherence and reimbursement. Adherence to protocols requiring behavioral change such as diet, exercise, and following medication orders continues to be an issue, particularly when dealing with long-term adherence, as is the case with home lung function monitoring. We have investigated subject adherence to the home monitoring protocol and developed basic approaches to promote adherence among our subjects (Chlan et al., 1998; Sabati, Snyder, Edin-Stibbe, Lindgren, & Finkelstein, 2001). The basic elements of adherence promotion are frequent monitoring of protocol use with necessary telephone follow-up, assessing and resolving barriers to protocol use, correcting equipment problems, and contracting for a mutually agreed upon number of measurements each week. All are labor intensive and generally become the responsibility of the remote monitoring nurse. Investigation of Internet-based adherence promotion methods is ongoing (Karl, Finkelstein, & Robiner, 2006). Although adherence concerns fall within the study design, addressing the reimbursement question will require changes in healthcare policy.

A cost analysis of home monitoring in our lung transplantation population showed that outpatient costs increased modestly and inpatient costs decreased considerably with increasing adherence, suggesting an economic incentive to include remote monitoring as a regular part of postsurgery home care for transplant recipients. The shift from inpatient to outpatient episodes for adherent home monitoring subjects should be expected, because the home monitor identifies early signs of potential problems and recommends a clinic visit, often avoiding a more costly hospitalization (Adam, Finkelstein, Parente, & Hertz, 2007). As in our lung transplant research program, similar findings in other studies have shown that remote monitoring and virtual visits can reduce costly hospitalizations with more frequent but less expensive outpatient visits (Bendixen et al., 2009; Darkins et al., 2008).

Results from these and other spirometry home monitoring investigations were cited by the CMS in their 1998 decision (Health Care Financing Administration, 2 Nov. 1998) to provide reimbursement for home monitoring of pulmonary function for patients with asthma and for lung transplant recipients. Unfortunately, the reimbursement levels rarely covered the cost of the service, but it was the start of support for clinical remote monitoring. Our clinical center at the University of Minnesota, Fairview, initiated a clinical home spirometry program based on the success of the research program, patient satisfaction with home monitoring, and availability of reimbursement. Unfortunately, the clinical program was recently closed due to the worsening economic outlook in 2008–2009, since patient copayments and insurer reimbursement did not provide sufficient support to cover the cost of the program. This typifies the transitory nature of support for home telehealth and other programs in which potential healthcare benefits do not directly generate revenue for their institution. Policy changes that take a long-term view of the potential clinical and cost-savings benefits of such new, technology-supported programs are needed if these programs are to be transferable from the research setting to standard clinical practice.

The TeleHomeCare Program

Initial Medicare reimbursement for telehealth services focused on payments to a provider when telehealth consultation replaced in-person consultation. In 2009, reimbursement for telehealth services was expanded to include the location of an eligible Medicare beneficiary at the time of service provision. These locations, termed *originating sites*, are limited to rural health professional shortage areas and counties outside of a Metropolitan Statistical Area or telemedicine demonstration projects, and include practitioner offices, hospitals, rural health clinics, federally qualified health centers, hospital-based dialysis centers, skilled nursing facilities, and community mental health centers (CMS, 13 July 2009). Reimbursement is provided only for real-time, interactive audio and video communication between a practitioner and beneficiary at approved sites; store and forward telehealth is reimbursable only in Hawaii and Alaska demonstration projects. Although this policy change facilitates the expansion of Medicare telehealth services to a broader base of originating sites, it does not provide for practitioner reimbursement when the originating site is a beneficiary's home. The TeleHomeCare Program demonstrated the technical feasibility of extending telehealth services to home-bound elderly persons and illustrated new avenues for socialization between elderly people, home-bound patients, and their home care nurses, as well as the potential for improved clinical outcomes at a lower cost. A policy that reimburses practitioners for audio and video communications from a beneficiary's home is needed to support such programs. Lacking a sustainable payment mechanism, programs such as TeleHomeCare must develop new sources of financial support after research grant funding ends, and this is rarely successful.

The VALUE Program

There is a general belief that elderly individuals otherwise unfamiliar and inexperienced with computer-like technology will not use such systems, but this study has shown that this issue can be satisfactorily addressed with proper technology modifications and user-focused training. There was widespread concern among many eligible study candidates about using a "computer," but those who agreed to try the program generally became strong supporters and were reluctant to give up the system at the conclusion of the study.

The TeleMedicine Perception Questionnaire (TMPQ) results demonstrate that hands-on experience with the technology improves user perception and suggest the importance of such exposure to the acceptance and successful use of programs like VALUE in the future. The decrease in perception in the control group after 60 days suggests how short a time one may recall the details of new telehealth programs based solely on a short introduction without the opportunity for direct contact and use of the system. These are important lessons in user perception that should be addressed with the rollout of new telehealth technologies.

The service portal utilization results also point to an important aspect of systems use. Although all subjects were able to navigate the portal with little difficulty, few of them used the portal to order needed health-related services for which they had previously developed a satisfactory ordering process. Consumer candidates for such home telehealth programs must be able to identify the potential benefits of the programs beyond simply replacing a working application with new technology.

The U Special Kids Program

The retrospective review of hospitalization frequency provided preliminary validation of the cost impact of the U Special Kids model and highlighted two important policy implications. Hospitalizations, due to a lack of home care, comprised only 1% of the total admissions, yet their occurrence warrants further discussion. These hospitalizations result from unmet social service needs (e.g., child neglect, lack of housing, and lack of home care help), not health needs, and CC/CM that focuses only on healthcare interventions will not prevent this type of hospitalization. Incorporating a social services framework into the CC/CM model could eliminate these unnecessary hospitalizations (Cady et al., 2009). Inherent to this approach is new policy that mandates the coordination of county and state social service agencies with CC/CM providers to eliminate unnecessary duplication of services and adequate funding to support the care of children with complex health conditions in their home.

The second policy implication involves the financial misalignment of nurse-delivered, telephone-based CC/CM programs. For children with complex health conditions, a reduction in hospitalizations has a positive financial impact on the agency responsible for the child's health-related costs (e.g., Medicaid and third-party payers), but no financial support is received by the program providing the CC/CM. Equally as important, nurse-delivered, telephone-based CC/CM services are not reimbursable under current Medicaid or third-party payer guidelines. This misalignment of financial incentives where nonreimbursable, low-cost care delivered from an outpatient setting leads to a reduction in reimbursable, high-cost inpatient utilization, has to be revised. Otherwise, the shift from high-cost inpatient care to more frequent but less costly outpatient care as demonstrated by programs like TeleHomeCare and U Special Kids will not be sustainable.

Federal policy that expanded broadband service to both urban and rural areas made home-based, interactive video feasible. However, the start-up costs for interactive video CC/CM are higher than the start-up costs for telephone-based CC/CM, and the technology may not be needed for all children receiving CC/CM services. Identifying the subgroups of children that benefit from interactive video CC/CM must precede efforts to establish policy for the provision and reimbursement of the service.

Similar to the lung transplant home monitoring program, the U Special Kids program was recently closed. The worsening economic outlook of 2008–2009 in the absence of reimbursement eliminated all financial support for the program. Hopefully, research studies will continue to provide the growing body of evidence necessary so that policymakers cannot ignore these new forms of care delivery.

CONCLUSIONS

Lessons to take away from these research studies involve both successes of the programs and concerns regarding implementation and long-term sustainability. The most important lesson is that most people can successfully participate in home telehealth programs when the programs are appropriately designed and participants are sufficiently motivated. A local "champion" is needed to promote and motivate providers to consider using home telehealth for their patients. In our studies and in others, investigators have found a high degree of patient/client satisfaction with the programs, and often, patient participants were reluctant to give up the equipment at the conclusion of the study. Participants frequently offered to purchase the equipment at the study's end, but this was generally not a solution because the clinician at the provider end would no longer be available once research support ended. It was especially rewarding to see that the virtual visits were often the highlight of the home telehealth programs we have conducted, especially when considering initial concerns about usability and privacy expressed by prospective participants at the time of recruitment. Although there were significant concerns about available technology, particularly in the area of remote monitoring at the dawn of home telehealth applications, that is no longer an overriding issue. There are almost daily announcements in the popular and trade press (paper and Internet) of new user-friendly monitoring devices and data collection/transmission hubs that are available at consumer electronic pricing levels. Finally, we have found that hands-on use of home telehealth equipment is a major positive influence on peoples' perceptions of the new technology. Although verbal explanations, printed instructions, and video demonstrations are all useful, they all fail in altering peoples' perceptions when compared with patients actually using the programs for a short trial period, especially with patients who are initially skeptical of the potential available through the new technology.

We have found several areas of concern that have emerged from all our research studies in home telehealth. Surprisingly, few of them are directly technology related. The others are all "people" or societal issues that have to be resolved if the potential of home telehealth is to be achieved. One technology issue is the lack of universal availability of broadband access. Until recently, high cost and low bandwidth limited the communication medium between home and providers to primarily telephone. Federal policy that facilitated an increase in broadband availability and a corresponding decrease in cost, in both urban and rural areas, expands the communication options for healthcare providers (U.S. Government Accountability Office, 2009). Although access continues to improve, it is not yet truly universally available. The move away from landlines to cellular service is a related issue, particularly for remote monitoring devices. Most devices were designed to transmit data solely by landline. New device design must also include cellular transmission capabilities. The need for more unobtrusive, patient-passive remote monitoring devices is a technology-dependent concern driven by patient adherence problems often faced in both clinical and research studies. However, it should be remembered that there are still applications that can benefit from low-tech home telehealth solutions. Although the primary focus of telehealth research is on delivery mechanisms such as video, remote monitoring, and Web-based systems, a recent article featuring the telephone as a telehealth delivery model (Gingrich, Boxer, & Brooks, 2008) has stimulated discussion of this low-tech modality. In the United States, 96% of households have access to a telephone (Federal Communications Commission, 2009b), and implementing this technology requires minimal equipment, training, or technical support. The cost and universal availability and experience of the technology (the telephone) are distinct advantages of this form of telehealth.

People and societal concerns can be placed in two groups—behavioral and financial. Foremost among behavioral issues is one of encouraging and maintaining adherence to remote monitoring, particularly when used in the management of chronic disease. Regardless of how good the technology, if patients do not interact with providers by collecting and transmitting monitored information, for example, then the program becomes useless. This highlights the need for advances in both patient-passive device development and better understanding of adherence behaviors and how they may be changed. Technology anxiety, especially when dealing with computers, has also been an issue, but not as great a concern as has often been expressed, especially when working with an elderly population.

On the provider side, issues of acceptance of new technologies, the availability of more data more often, and reimbursement need to be addressed. Provider acceptance will grow as more studies demonstrate that home telehealth technologies can deliver the promises made in their behalf—improving outcomes and containing costs. Expanding the use of telehealth within healthcare delivery systems is dependent upon sustainable reimbursement of services delivered and alignment of financial incentives. Our home monitoring research provided evidence for the inclusion of home spirometry Medicare reimbursement. Although our research on home-based interactive telehealth has shown evidence of improved outcomes, Medicare does not recognize the home as an originating site for telehealth reimbursement and results in unsustainable telehealth research programs. Additional research on the effectiveness of home-based video telehealth would provide additional support for reimbursement policy.

An exception is the Veteran's Health Care System, an integrated healthcare system funded and operated by the U.S. government (Kizer & Dudley, 2009). Within this single-payer system, the financial incentive to reduce inpatient utilization exists. The Care Coordination/Home Telehealth program for veterans with chronic conditions utilizes varying levels of telehealth to reduce hospital admissions and long-term institutional care (Darkins et al., 2008). Unlike our research telehealth programs, the sustainability the Care Coordination/Home Telehealth program is dependent on its cost effectiveness to the overall Veteran's Health System, not third-party reimbursement.

Finally, the most appropriate business plan or plans for developing a profitable delivery model in home telehealth systems is still evolving. Traditional models focused on selling either devices or services to potential customers are likely candidates because they have been profitable in the past. Other approaches such as integrating device/system developers, producers, and users may emerge as the benefits, problems, and potential of home telehealth are more clearly defined.

REFERENCES

Adam, T. J., Finkelstein, S. M., Parente, S. T., & Hertz, M. I. (2007). Cost analysis of home monitoring in lung transplant recipients. *International Journal of Technology Assessment in Health Care, 23*(2), 216–222.

Bendixen, R. M., Levy, C. E., Olive, E. S., Kobb, R. F., & Mann, W. C. (2009). Cost effectiveness of a telerehabilitation program to support chronically ill and disabled elders in their homes. *Telemedicine Journal & E-Health, 15*(1), 31–38.

Bohnenkamp, S. K., McDonald, P., Lopez, A. M., Krupinski, E., & Blackett, A. (2004). Traditional versus telenursing outpatient management of patients with cancer with new ostomies. *Oncology Nursing Forum Online, 31*(5), 1005–1010.

Cady, R., Finkelstein, S., & Kelly, A. (2009). A telehealth nursing intervention reduces hospitalizations in children with complex health conditions. *Journal of Telemedicine & Telecare, 15*(6), 317–320.

Cady, R., Kelly, A., & Finkelstein, S. (2008). Home telehealth for children with special health-care needs. *Journal of Telemedicine & Telecare, 14*(4), 173–177.

Centers for Medicare and Medicaid Services. Medicare program; Payment policies under the physician fee schedule and other revisions to part B for CY 2010; Proposed rule, 33542 (13 Jul 2009).

Chlan, L., Snyder, M., Finkelstein, S., Hertz, M., Edin, C., Wielinski, C., et al. (1998). Promoting adherence to an electronic home spirometry research program after lung transplantation. *Applied Nursing Research, 11*(1), 36–40.

Darkins, A., Ryan, P., Kobb, R., Foster, L., Edmonson, E., Wakefield, B., et al. (2008). Care coordination/home telehealth: The systematic implementation of health informatics, home telehealth, and disease management to support the care of veteran patients with chronic conditions. *Telemedicine Journal & E-Health, 14*(10), 1118–1126.

Demiris, G., Finkelstein, S. M., & Speedie, S. M. (2001). Considerations for the design of a Web-based clinical monitoring and educational system for elderly patients. *Journal of the American Medical Informatics Association, 8*(5), 468–472.

Demiris, G., Speedie, S., & Finkelstein, S. (2000). A questionnaire for the assessment of patients' impressions of the risks and benefits of home telecare. *Journal of Telemedicine & Telecare, 6*(5), 278–284.

Demiris, G., Speedie, S., Finkelstein, S., & Harris, I. (2003). Communication patterns and technical quality of virtual visits in home care. *Journal of Telemedicine & Telecare, 9*(4), 210–215.

Federal Communications Commission. (2009a). *Broadband.* Retrieved 10/6/2009, 2009, from http://www.fcc.gov/cgb/broadband.html#Wireless

Federal Communications Commission. (2009b). *Recent releases.* Retrieved 10/5/2009, 2009, from http://www.fcc.gov/wcb/iatd/recent.html

Finkelstein, S. M., Lindgren, B., Prasad, B., Snyder, M., Edin, C., Wielinski, C., et al. (1993). Reliability and validity of spirometry measurements in a paperless home monitoring diary program for lung transplantation. *Heart Lung, 22*(6), 523–533.

Finkelstein, S. M., Potthoff, S., LeMire, T., Valley, K., Dahle, L., Ratner, E., et al. (2007). VALUE (virtual assisted living umbrella for the elderly) user perceptions. *Telemedicine Journal & E-Health, 13,* 182.

Finkelstein, S. M., Scudiero, A., Lindgren, B., Snyder, M., & Hertz, M. I. (2005). Decision support for the triage of lung transplant recipients on the basis of home-monitoring spirometry and symptom reporting. *Heart & Lung, 34*(3), 201–208.

Finkelstein, S. M., Snyder, M., Edin-Stibbe, C., Chlan, L., Prasad, B., Dutta, P., et al. (1996). Monitoring progress after lung transplantation from home-patient adherence. *Journal of Medical Engineering & Technology, 20*(6), 203–210.

Finkelstein, S. M., Snyder, M., Stibbe, C. E., Lindgren, B., Sabati, N., Killoren, T., et al. (1999). Staging of bronchiolitis obliterans syndrome using home spirometry. *Chest, 116*(1), 120–126.

Finkelstein, S. M., Speedie, S. M., Demiris, G., Veen, M., Lundgren, J. M., & Potthoff, S. (2004). Telehomecare: Quality, perception, satisfaction. *Telemedicine Journal & E-Health, 10*(2), 122–128.

Finkelstein, S. M., Speedie, S. M., & Potthoff, S. (2006). Home telehealth improves clinical outcomes at lower cost for home healthcare. *Telemedicine Journal & E-Health, 12*(2), 128–136.

Finkelstein, S. M., Speedie, S. M., Zhou, X., Ratner, E., & Potthoff, S. (2006). VALUE: Virtual assisted living umbrella for the elderly: User patterns. *Proceedings of the IEEE Engineering Medicine, Biology, Society Annual Conference, 28,* 3294–3296.

Frankl, S. E., Breeling, J. L., & Goldman, L. (1991). Preventability of emergent hospital readmission. *The American Journal of Medicine, 90*(6), 667–674.

Gingrich, N., Boxer, R., & Brooks, B. (2008). Telephone medical consults answer the call for accessible, affordable, and convenient healthcare. *Telemedicine and e-Health, 14*(3), 215–223.

Guest, A., Rittey, C., & O'Brien, K. (2005). Telemedicine: Helping neurologically-impaired children to stay at home. *Paediatric Nursing, 17*(2), 20–22.

Health Care Financing Administration. Medicare program; Revisions to payment policies and adjustments to the relative value units under the physician fee schedule for calendar year 1999, http://frwebgate.access.gpo.gov/cgi-bin/getdoc.cgi?dbname=1998_register&docid=page+58863-58912.pdf U.S.C. 58889 (2 Nov 1998).

Jerant, A. F., Azari, R., Martinez, C., & Nesbitt, T. S. (2003). A randomized trial of telenursing to reduce hospitalization for heart failure: Patient-centered outcomes and nursing indicators. *Home Health Care Services Quarterly, 22*(1), 1–20.

Johnston, B., Weeler, L., Deuser, J., & Sousa, K. H. (2000). Outcomes of the Kaiser Permanente tele-home health research project. *Archives of Family Medicine, 9*(1), 40–45.

Joseph, A. M. (2006). Care coordination and telehealth technology in promoting self-management among chronically ill patients. *Telemedicine Journal & E-Health, 12*(2), 156–159.

Karl, B. C., Finkelstein, S. M., & Robiner, W. N. (2006). The design of an Internet-based system to maintain home monitoring adherence by lung transplant recipients. *IEEE Transactions on Information Technology in Biomedicine, 10*(1), 66–76.

Kelly, A., Golnik, A., & Cady, R. (2008). A medical home center: Specializing in the care of children with special health care needs of high intensity. *Maternal & Child Health Journal, 12*(5), 633–640.

Kizer, K. W., & Dudley, R. A. (2009). Extreme makeover: Transformation of the Veterans Health Care System. *Annual Review of Public Health, 30,* 313–339.

Lindgren, B. R., Finkelstein, S. M., Prasad, B., Dutta, P., Killoren, T., Scherber, J., et al. (1997). Determination of reliability and validity in home monitoring data of pulmonary function tests following lung transplantation. *Research in Nursing & Health, 20*(6), 539–550.

Lorig, K. R., Ritter, P. L., Laurent, D. D., & Plant, K. (2006). Internet-based chronic disease self-management: A randomized trial. *Medical Care, 44*(11), 964–971.

Mair, F. S., Goldstein, P., May, C., Angus, R., Shiels, C., Hibbert, D., et al. (2005). Patient and provider perspectives on home telecare: Preliminary results from a randomized controlled trial. *Journal of Telemedicine & Telecare, 11*(Suppl 1), 95–97.

Murray, E., Burns, J., See Tai, S., Lai, R., & Nazareth, I. (2005). *Interactive health communication applications for people with chronic disease.* Chichester, UK: John Wiley & Sons, Ltd.

Naylor, M. D., Brooten, D., Campbell, R., Jacobsen, B. S., Mezey, M. D., Pauly, M. V., et al. (1999). Comprehensive discharge planning and home follow-up of hospitalized elders: A randomized clinical trial. *JAMA: The Journal of the American Medical Association, 281*(7), 613–620.

Sabati, N., Snyder, M., Edin-Stibbe, C., Lindgren, B., & Finkelstein, S. (2001). Facilitators and barriers to adherence with home monitoring using electronic spirometry. *AACN Clinical Issues, 12,* 178–185.

Troiani, J. S., & Carlin, B. P. (2004). Comparison of Bayesian, classical, and heuristic approaches in identifying acute disease events in lung transplant recipients. *Statistics in Medicine, 23*(5), 803–824.

U.S. Government Accountability Office. (2009). *U.S. GAO—telecommunications: Broadband deployment plan should include performance goals and measures to guide federal investment.* Retrieved 10/5/2009, 2009, from http://www.gao.gov/products/GAO-09-494

Vivian, B. G., & Wilcox, J. R. (2000). Compliance communication in home health care: A mutually reciprocal process. *Qualitative Health Research, 10*(1), 103–116.

18

Building Evidence for Practice, Training, and Policy: A Program of Research on Living Well With HIV/AIDS

William L. Holzemer

BACKGROUND

This chapter is a reflection on the past 25 years of my professional career in nursing. Having earned a PhD degree in education, I began working in nursing first at the University of Illinois in Chicago and then at the University of California, San Francisco (UCSF), starting in 1979. My research interests were shifting from educational research to clinical nursing research, so I decided to earn a bachelor of science in nursing. I completed my training from 1981 to 1985 during the beginning of the AIDS epidemic in San Francisco. I trained during a period when student nurses wore "space suits" to serve AIDS patients their lunch, while their friends were sitting on the bed with them playing cards. It was a difficult time when so little was actually known about HIV/AIDS. I observed at this time the San Francisco model of AIDS care that was being implemented by early pioneers in nursing at San Francisco General Hospital, who felt strongly that their model of care was having a significant impact upon the lives of their patients.

Upon completion of my training, I began to think about clinical nursing research in the area of HIV/AIDS nursing care and patient outcomes. It seemed to me that my university had a strong focus upon the biology of AIDS and, eventually, HIV prevention through the establishment of the Center for AIDS Prevention. However, there was little work ongoing related to the quality of life of people living with and affected by HIV and AIDS. Therefore, this became the focus of our early work. At this time at the UCSF, Dr. Marylin Dodd was doing her pioneering work on symptom management, and that became one of the core dimensions of our research.

At this time, AIDS patients were hospitalized with numerous conditions, but the most common was *Pneumocystis carinii* pneumonia (PCP). I and my doctoral student, who is now colleague and friend, Dr. Suzanne Bakken, focused our work on quality of care for people hospitalized with PCP. We published an article outlining a protocol of care for PCP (Henry & Holzemer, 1992) and began our work assessing the symptoms of hospitalized

AIDS patients. We were successful in securing two National Institutes of Health (NIH) RO1s for this work, entitled "Quality of Nursing Care of People With AIDS, 1989–1998" (RO1 NR02215 and 2RO1 NR02215). Dr. Bakken's primary interest was in informatics, and we developed a parallel of exploring nursing informatics led by Dr. Bakken (then Henry) and quality of care for AIDS patients led by myself.

Highlights from this work include the following:

- Developed an outcomes model for healthcare research (Holzemer & Reilly, 1995)
- Developed a new outcome measure entitled HIV-QAM quality audit marker (Holzemer, Henry, Stewart, & Janson-Bjerklie, 1993)
- Examined the roles of nurses versus social workers in HIV case management (Wright, Henry, Holzemer, & Falknor, 1993)
- Examined the lack of relationships between types of care planning system and outcomes of care (Henry, Holzemer, & Reilly, 1994; Holzemer & Henry, 1991)
- Described the problems of patients hospitalized with PCP (Holzemer, Henry, Reilly, & Portillo, 1995; Cosby, Holzemer, Henry, & Portillo, 2000)
- Developed a tailored measure of quality of life for people dying from AIDS (Holzemer, Gygax-Spicer, Skodal Wilson, Kemppainen, & Coleman, 1998; Wilson, Hutchinson, & Holzemer, 1997, 2002)
- Demonstrated that nurses and AIDS patients do not report the same cluster of symptoms as being important (Reilly, Holzemer, Henry, Slaughter, & Portillo, 1997)
- Provided evidence-based guidelines for symptom management for nurses caring for people living with HIV/AIDS (PLHAs; Holzemer, 2002)
- Validated a sign and symptom checklist for PLHAs (Holzemer, Corless et al., 1999; Holzemer, Hudson, Kirksey, Hamilton, & Bakken, 2001)
- Developed a measure of engagement with care (Bakken, Holzemer, Brown et al., 2000; Kemppainen et al., 1999)

This work provided me with credibility among clinicians, educators, and researchers. Of course, if you were not in direct clinical practice, you were never 100% credible, but I believe that our work on HIV symptoms and engagement with care providers was seen as clinically relevant among practitioners. This expertise, knowledge, and credibility allowed me to assume leadership roles with the Association of Nurses in AIDS Care by chairing their research committee, and the American Academy of Nursing by serving as chair of the expert panel of HIV/AIDS (Holzemer, 2002; Holzemer & Portillo, 1994). This combined work led to the opportunity to provide testimony nationally on issues such as the confidentiality of HIV testing and support for the Ryan White Care Act.

Also, at this time, I was invited to serve with one other nurse on a guideline panel with the then Agency for Health Care Policy and Research. The title of our publication was *Managing Early HIV Infection* (El-Sadr et al., 1994). This clinical practice guideline was written when the only HIV medication available was AZT and many communities were convinced that AZT was killing PLHAs. This text is well read today, where it describes the social context of HIV infection. A social worker and I spent considerable time authoring sections that demanded recognition of HIV disease beyond its biology and treatment. One significant impact that I had on this publication was to get the title changed. Everyone expected the title to be something like *The Management of Asymptomatic HIV Infection*. Our work provided evidence that upon diagnosis with HIV, psychological symptoms, such as depression, anxiety, and fear, were pervasive and that there was no phase of the HIV trajectory that was actually asymptomatic. This convinced the panel comprised mostly of physicians to change the title of the publication to *Managing Early HIV Infection*.

Within the context of our knowledge of HIV and treatment modalities, a program of research was launched and continues to this day that focuses on the quality of life of people living with and affected by HIV and AIDS. Our early work focused on understanding how mostly young men in San Francisco were dealing with the quality of life that remained for them while seriously ill with HIV infection. By 1996, when the International AIDS Conference was held in Vancouver, Canada, HIV medications had become available and the epidemic made a dramatic shift from being an acute illness with a short lifespan to a chronic illness. People with AIDS living in hospices in San Francisco and Los Angeles literally packed their belongings and went home. Many were able to return to work. Our program of research shifted to conceptualize HIV as a chronic illness with this profound change in the availability of medications.

In 1996, my colleague Dr. Carmen Portillo and I launched the UCSF International Center for HIV/AIDS Research and Training in Nursing, articulating a mission statement that focused on improving the lives of people living with and affected by HIV and AIDS (Holzemer, 2002, 2007). In the beginning of our center's work, we spent considerable energy providing workshops and training for clinicians working in HIV care in hospitals where most of the AIDS patients were located. At this time, we were successful in securing an Institutional Training Grant from the National Institute of Nursing Research (T32 NR07081) entitled "HIV/AIDS Nursing Care & Prevention." We have received the third round of 5 years of funding under this mechanism that supports four predoctoral and two postdoctoral students. Our graduate students were directly involved in all activities of our HIV/AIDS center. At this time, we also developed an advanced practice specialty combining our existing adult nurse practitioner program with HIV/AIDS care, providing one of the few programs for master's-level preparation as a nurse practitioner in HIV/AIDS care.

We continued our work on symptom management, because the side effects of the new medications were very challenging, and we began to focus upon adherence to medications. A component of our UCSF Center's activities included the establishment of the International HIV/AIDS Nursing Research Network, which has been described in the literature (Holzemer, 2007). We put a call out for interested nurse scientists to join us in San Francisco to plan our first collaborative study focusing on measuring the frequency and intensity of HIV-related symptoms. Individual investigators joined by becoming a site director and by agreeing to participate in a commonly developed protocol. Each site director agreed to collect data on a specified number of participants, usually 100, and we aggregated the data at UCSF. We have conducted three descriptive studies on symptom assessment, use of self-care symptom management strategies, and predictors of medication adherence. Our fourth protocol was a randomized clinical trial testing the effectiveness of a self-care symptom management manual compared with a nutrition manual. Each network study usually has between 8 and 12 participating sites, and participation by our international colleagues has grown over the years. Our network continues today and is in the process of conducting its fifth collaborative research project (www.aidsnursing. ucsf.edu) focusing upon a theoretical question of the relationship among self-esteem, self-efficacy, and self-compassion as they relate to self-care symptom management and medication adherence. We have published over 30 manuscripts together.

With the advent of medications for the treatment of HIV, the focus of our research continued on the assessment and management of symptoms and expanded to include the concept of adherence to medications. We secured an NIH RO1 (NR/AI04846) entitled "Outpatient Nurse Managed HIV Adherence Trial 1999–2005." We conducted a randomized controlled trial testing an intervention named CAP-IT (Client-Assessment Profiling–Individual Tailoring; Holzemer, Henry, Portillo, & Miramontes, 2000). Our nonsignificant results were similar to those of many other randomized controlled trials conducted at this time designed to test an adherence intervention (Bakken, Holzemer, Portillo, Grimes, & Welch, 2005; Holzemer et al., 2006).

This work resulted in my being invited to a policy forum held by the American Public Health Association exploring what lessons researchers working on adherence in HIV can learn from the years of adherence research ongoing in hypertension and diabetes. The interesting outcome of this symposium and publication was that the data on adherence in hypertension and diabetes were extremely discouraging–clinicians are very happy with 60%–80% adherence; in HIV adherence work, clinicians expect 95% adherence, and hence, there were few lessons that HIV adherence researchers could learn from others working in the field of adherence.

Highlights from this work include the following:

- Understanding the predictors of medication adherence (Holzemer, Corless, & Nokes, et al., 1999)
- Understanding the link between symptom severity and nonadherence (Hudson, Kirksey, Bunch, & Holzemer, 2000).
- Global nature of the challenge of symptom management and adherence in Taiwan (Tsai, Hsiung, & Holzemer, 2002)
- Role of self-care in understanding symptom management (Chou & Holzemer, 2004; Chou, Holzemer, Portillo, & Slaughter, 2004; Coleman, Ellen, Nokes et al., 2006)

During this time, I was invited to serve on an Institute of Medicine (IOM) study asking what appeared to be an important question for policy makers. In the United States, an AIDS diagnosis is reportable to public health officials, and this information is used to make funding allocations for AIDS care. Some political groups felt that we should be allocating resources based upon the prevalence of known HIV status, rather than AIDS diagnoses, because it is a precursor to the needs that will follow and may better reflect how the epidemic is moving into communities such as men and women of color. This IOM (2003) report explored this question and resulted in the publication of *Measuring What Matters*. The short answer to this complicated question was that it made no statistical difference if allocations were based on AIDS diagnoses or known HIV cases (where such data were reported) because they correlated almost perfectly. The opportunity to serve on this panel allowed me to learn about the IOM and how it conducted such comprehensive studies with the purpose of informing public policy for the president and the Congress of the United States.

During this time, I became a leader in the HIV/AIDS Network of the International Council of Nurses, Geneva, and provided consultation to them on their global policy statements. The world became acutely aware of the devastation of the HIV pandemic on families in sub-Saharan Africa—reminiscent of the epidemic that we had experienced in San Francisco some 15 years earlier. Through this work with the International Council of Nurses and my connections with other nurses working in HIV globally, in 2000 I was able to secure funding from the Secure the Future Foundation, Bristol-Meyers-Squibb, to replicate some of our work on HIV symptom management in four African nations (Botswana, Lesotho, South Africa, and Swaziland). We revalidated our symptom management/manual in Africa (for copies of manual see http://AIDSnursing@ucsf.edu) and conducted descriptive studies of the prevalence, severity, and extent of HIV symptoms in these countries for people living with HIV. This work resulted in the publication of several descriptive manuscripts on the quality of life of people living with HIV in these countries. Each country project was led by a nursing faculty member who became the spokesperson for policy work in his or her country. One of our collaborators became recognized as the government's primary consultant on the HIV stigma. We circulated over 10,000 copies of the Self-Care Symptom Management Manual during this period. Highlights from this work include the following:

- Described the HIV symptom experience of 743 men and women living with HIV infection in sub-Saharan Africa (Makoae, Seboni, Molosiwa et al., 2005).
- Explored self-reported self-care strategies used by people living with HIV in sub-Saharan Africa (Sukati et al., 2005).
- Demonstrated the link between the high burden of HIV symptoms and their negative impact upon quality of life in sub-Saharan Africa (Phaladze et al., 2005).

To many colleagues in Africa, this work introduced the concept of living well with HIV infection and the existence of many self-care symptom management strategies with the potential to improve the quality of lives of people living with and affected by HIV/AIDS. In 2000, the International AIDS Society held its conference in Durban, South Africa, with the theme "Break the Silence." The focus on the conference was on the effect of stigma on people living with and affected by HIV/AIDS. Stigma was perceived to affect access to testing, access and follow-up to care, adherence to medications, and overall quality of life. From that period forward, the global research community began to focus their attention on stigma—its measurement and impact, and interventions designed to reduce HIV stigma.

In the United States, in 2002, the Fogarty International Center at the NIH put out a call for proposals on stigma. We teamed with colleagues from five African nations and were successful in securing 5 years of funding for the study entitled "Perceived AIDS Stigma: A Multinational African Study" (R01, TW006395; 2003–2009). We worked with colleagues from Lesotho, Malawi, South Africa, Swaziland, and Tanzania. The purpose of the research was to develop an understanding of stigma and its impact through qualitative focus groups with PLHAs and nurses, to develop instruments to measure HIV stigma among PLHAs and nurses, to explore how HIV stigma impacts the quality of life of PLHAs and quality of work life for nurses through a 1-year cohort study, and to pilot test a stigma reduction intervention based upon our work to date. This project is now completed, and we have done the following in the literature:

- Described how community members think and talk about stigma as "eating plastic" (Uys et al., 2005; Holzemer & Uys, 2004; Greeff, Uys et al., 2008)
- Described how HIV stigma violates human rights (Kohi et al., 2006) and is different in urban and rural settings (Naidoo et al., 2007)

- Developed a conceptual model of triggers of HIV stigma (Holzemer et al., 2007)
- Linked the negative impact of HIV stigma to verbal and physical abuse (Dlamini, Kohi et al., 2007), failure to disclose HIV status (Greeff, Phetlhu et al., 2008), and poor medication adherence (Dlamini et al., 2009)
- Developed a validated instrument to measure perceived stigma among PLHAs (Holzemer, Uys, Chirwa et al., 2007) and perceived stigma among nurses (Uys et al., 2009).
- Reported on the contribution of perceived HIV stigma among nurses to job dissatisfaction (Chirwa et al., 2009) and their intent to migrate out of their country (Kohi et al., 2010)

This body of work is one of the most comprehensive examinations of the impact of HIV stigma in Africa that has been conducted. We developed two instruments to measure stigma that are being adopted in numerous interdisciplinary studies; we conceptualized a model of HIV stigma based upon our qualitative research findings; we demonstrated that HIV stigma, by association, impacts nurses' thoughts about leaving their profession; and we have shown, contrary to common opinion, that people on HIV medications experience more stigma than those not on medications. We believe that this last finding has important policy implications for care providers who can provide advanced counseling for their clients to expect potentially more incidences of stigma once they begin medications, as they will be more visible in clinic lines and will be taking their medications every day for life.

While this work was in process, I was invited again by the IOM to be on another study, this time focusing upon a preliminary evaluation of the President's Emergency Fund for AIDS Relief (PEPFAR) legislation. The PEPFAR provided the largest health initiative globally in our history and provided support for prevention, treatment, and care for people and families living with HIV in 15 countries, primarily in Africa. I played a leadership role on that panel as a co-chair of the care subpanel, a team leader for site visits to Africa, and a collaborating author on several sections of the final document. This report (Sepulveda et al., 2007) was authorized via Federal legislation asking the question "Should the U.S. government continue support for this project?" Our challenge was to provide a coherent response to the Congress as they contemplated reauthorization of the PEPFAR legislation. The legislation itself was filled with many controversies, such as its focus on abstinence, lack of family planning services for HIV-positive women, and other factors. I had responsibilities for writing parts of the care section of the report, although given how IOM reports are written, nothing ultimately really belongs to any of the individual authors. My contributions focused upon ensuring that the prevention, treatment, and care sections were balanced in emphasis; that HIV infection was conceptualized as a chronic illness with a somewhat predictable trajectory; and that future funding allows for the support for prelicensure training, not just continuing education, for existing healthcare workers.

Initial PEPFAR policies supported allocating significant resources to training existing nurses, physicians, pharmacists, and other healthcare workers with updated skills on HIV/AIDS prevention, treatment, and care. This policy only allowed funds to be used for postlicensure training, and these training activities quickly saturated the existing workforce by offering many continuing education programs on HIV/AIDS. In 2006, the World Health Assembly (World Health Organization, 2006) annual report provided detailed data on the need to train new healthcare workers. This report also stated that in most countries, 80% of these "healthcare workers" are nurses. My message to this IOM committee was that we needed to make a recommendation to support the training of new healthcare workers, particularly, of course, nurses. Adopting this collaborative supportive position allowed others to join in support of this concept, and finally the committee did agree to recommend that PEPFAR adopt a policy to allow the training of new healthcare workers. It is a great pleasure for me to see that in the new PEPFAR legislation, there is authorization to train some 100,000 new healthcare workers. We must now watch this process to ensure that nursing receives its fair share of these resources.

Our work has examined in depth some HIV-related symptoms and provides data for constructing evidence-based practice guidelines. We have described the prevalence of symptoms, examined the correlates of symptoms, and explored self-care guidelines for HIV-related symptoms. Our work has focused upon pain (Holzemer, Henry, & Reilly, 1998), diarrhea (Henry, Holzemer, Weaver, & Stotts, 1999), cognitive functioning (Corless, Bakken, Nicholas, Holzemer et al., 2000), fatigue (Corless et al., 2002; Voss, Dodd, Portillo, & Holzemer, 2006; Voss, Portillo, Holzemer, & Dodd, 2007; Voss, Sukati, Seboni, Makoae, & Holzemer, 2007), peripheral neuropathy (Nicholas et al., 2002; Nicholas, Kemppainen et al., 2007; Nicholas, Voss, Corless et al., 2007; Corless, Voss et al., 2008), anxiety (Kemppainen et al., 2003; Kemppainen et al., 2006), and depression (Eller et al., 2005). We tested the effectiveness of an HIV symptom management manual (Wantland, Holzemer, Moezzi et al., 2008) and we challenged the use of the term asymptomic in AIDS care (Willard, Holzemer, Wantland et al., 2009).

This program of research belongs to my colleagues and students and the people living with HIV whom we serve. We have always had a commitment to improve the lives of people living with and families affected by HIV/AIDS. Initially, there was no expectation that the findings from the research or the experiences in the field would provide a platform that had the potential to inform health policy at national levels. However, those of us working in HIV/AIDS research have learned a great deal from the community activists who took to the streets to change Food and Drug Administration drug approval procedures and questioned the concept that control groups in randomized control trials should receive placebos. The United States has demonstrated vision and foresight in its support of the domestic plan for the prevention, treatment, and care of HIV disease through the Ryan White Care Act, and internationally through the support of the PEPFAR legislation. We are proud to join other nurse scientists and nurse activists who have contributed to this work. It is not clear how directly our work has impacted health policy, but this program of research on living with HIV as a chronic illness created many opportunities to be "at the table" when these policy decisions were being formulated.

REFERENCES

Bakken, S., Holzemer, W. L., Brown, M. A., Powell-Cope, G. M., Turner, J. G., Inouye, J., Nokes, K. M., & Corless, I. B. (2000). Relationships between perception of engagement with health care provider and demographic characteristics, health status, and adherence to therapeutic regimen in persons with HIV/AIDS. *AIDS Patient Care and STDs, 14*(4), 189–197.

Bakken, S., Holzemer, W. L., Portillo, C. J., Grimes, R., Welch, J., & Wantland, D. (2005). Utility of a standardized nursing terminology to evaluate dosage and tailoring of a nurse-delivered HIV/

AIDS adherence intervention in a randomized controlled trial. *Journal of Nursing Scholarship, 37*(3), 251–257.

Chirwa, M. L., Kohi, T. W., Greeff, M., Naidoo, J., Makoae, L. N., Dlamini, P. S., Kaszubski, C., Cuca, Y. P., Uys, L. R., & Holzemer, W. L. (2009). HIV stigma and nurse job satisfaction in five African countries. *Journal of the Association of Nurses in AIDS Care, 20*(11), 14–21.

Chou, F. Y., & Holzemer, W. L. (2004). Linking HIV/AIDS clients; self-care with outcomes. *Journal of the Association of Nurses in AIDS Care, 15*(4), 58–67.

Chou, F. Y., Holzemer, W. L., Portillo, C., & Slaughter, R. (2004). Self-care strategies and information resources for HIV/AIDS symptom management. *Nursing Research,* Sept–Oct. *53*(5). 332–339.

Coleman, C. L., Eller, L. S., Nokes, K.M., Bunch, E., Reynolds, N., Corless, I., Dole, P., Kemppainen, J. K., Wantland, D., Kirksey, K., Seficik, L., Nicholas, P., Hamilton, J. J., Tsai, Y.-F., & Holzemer, W. L. (2006). Prayers as a complimentary health strategy for managing HIV related symptoms among an ethnically diverse sample. *Holistic Nursing Practice, 20*(2), 65–72.

Corless, I. B., Bakken, S., Nicholas, P. K., Holzemer, W. L., et al. (2000). Predictors of perception of cognitive functioning in HIV/AIDS. *Journal of Association of Nurses in AIDS Care, 11*(3), 19–26.

Corless, I. G., Bunch, E. H., Kemppainen, J. K., Holzemer, W. L., Nokes, K. M., Eller, L. S., Portillo, C. J., Butensky, E., Nicholas, P. K., Bain, C. A., Davis, S., Kirksey, K. M., & Chou, F.-Y. (2002). Self-care for atigue in HIV disease. *Oncology Nursing Forum, 29*(5).

Corless, I., Voss, J., Nicholas, P., Bunch, E. H., Bain, C., Coleman, C., Dole, P., Eller, L., Hamilton, M., Holzemer, W., Kemppainen, J., Kirksey, K., Sefcik, E., Nokes, K., Tsai, Y. F., Reynolds, N., Wantland, D., McGibbon, C., Davis, S. M., Rivero, M., & Valencia, C. (2008). Fatigue in HIV/AIDS patients with comorbidities. *Applied Nursing Research, 21*(3), 116–122.

Cosby, C., Holzemer, W. L., Henry, S. B., & Portillo, C. J. (2000). Hematological complications and quality of life in hospitalized AIDS patients. *AIDS Patient Care and STDS, 14*(5), 269–279.

Dlamini, P., Kohi, T., Uys, L., Phetlhu, R., Chirwa, M., Naidoo, J., Holzemer, W., Greeff, M., & Makoae, L. (2007). Manifestations of HIV/AIDS stigma: Verbal and physical and neglect abuse in five African countries. *Public Health Nursing, 24*(5), 389–399.

Dlamini, P., Wantland, D., Makoae, L., Chirwa, M., Kohi, T. W., Greeff, M., Naidoo, J., Mullan, J., Uys, L. R., & Holzemer, W. L. (2009). HIV stigma and missed medications among HIV+ persons in five African countries. *AIDS Patient Care and STDS, 23*(5), 377–387.

Eller, L. S., Corless, I. B., Bunch, E. H., Kemppainen, J. K., Holzemer, W. L., Nokes, K., Portillo, C. J., & Nicholas, P. (2005). Self-care strategies for depression in persons with HIV disease. *Journal of Advanced Nursing, 51*(12), 119–130.

El-Sadr, W., Oleske, J. M., Agino, B. D., Bauman, K. A., Brosgart, C. L., Brown, G. M., Geaga, J. V., Greenspan, D., Hein, K., Holzemer, W. L., Jackson, R. E., Lindsay, M. K., Makadon, H. J., Moon, M. W., Rappoport, C. A., Scott, G., Shervington, W. W., & Wofsy, C. B. (1994). *Managing early HIV infection. Quick reference guide for clinicians (no. 7).* USPHS: Agency for Health Care Policy & Research.

Greeff, M., Phetlhu, D. R., Makoae, L. N., Dlamini, P. S., Holzemer, W. L., Naidoo, J., Kohi, T. W., Uys, L. R., & Chirwa, M. L. (2008). Disclosure of HIV status: Experiences and perceptions of persons living with HIV/AIDS and nurses involved in their care in five Africa countries. *Qualitative Health Research, 8*(3), 311–324.

Greeff, M., Uys, L.R., Holzemer, W. L., Makoae, L. N., Dlamini, P. S., Kohi, T. W., Chirwa, M. L., Naidoo, J., & Phetlhu, D. R. (2008). Experiences of HIV/AIDS stigma of PLWA and nurses from five African Countries. *African Journal of AIDS Research, 10*(1), 78–108.

Henry, S. B., Holzemer, W. L., & Reilly, C. (1994). The relationship between type of care planning systems and patient outcomes in hospitalized AIDS patient. *Journal of Advance Nursing, 19*(4), 691–698.

Henry, S. B., & Holzemer, W.L. (1992). Critical care management of the patient with HIV infection who has *Pneumocystis carinii* pneumonia. *Heart & Lung, 21*(3), 243–249. Review.

Henry, S. B., Holzemer, W. L., Weaver, K., & Stotts, N. (1999). Quality of life and self-care management strategies of PLWAs with chronic diarrhea. *Journal of the Association of Nurses in AIDS Care, 10*(2), 46–54.

Holzemer, W. L. (2002). HIV and AIDS: The symptom experience: What cell counts and viral loads won't tell you? *American Journal of Nursing, 102*(4), 48–52.

Holzemer, W. L. (2007). The UCSF International Nursing Network for HIV/AIDS Research. *International Nursing Review, 54*, 234–242.

Holzemer, W. L., Bakken, S., Portillo, C. J., Grimes, R., Welch, J., Wantland, D., & Mullan, J. T. (2006). Testing a nurse tailored HIV medication adherence intervention. *Nursing Research, 55*(3), 189–197.

Holzemer, W. L., Corless, I. B., Nokes, K. M., Turner, J. G., Brown, M. A., Powell-Cope, G. M., Inouye, J., Henry, S. B., Nicholas, P. K., & Portillo, C. (1999). Predictors of self-reported adherence in persons living with HIV disease. *AIDS Patient Care and STDs, 13*(3), 185–197.

Holzemer, W. L., Gygax-Spicer, J., Skodal Wilson, H., Kemppainen, J. K., & Coleman, C. (1998). Validation of the Quality of Life Scale: Living with HIV. *Journal of Advanced Nursing, 28*(3), 622–630.

Holzemer, W. L., & Henry, S. B. (1991). Nursing care plans for people with HIV/AIDS: Confusion or consensus? *Journal of Advanced Nursing, 16*(3), 257–261.

Holzemer, W. L., Henry, S. B., Nokes, K. M., Corless, I. B., Brown, M. A., Powell-Cope, G. M., Turner J. G., & Inouye, J. (1999). Validation of the Sign & Symptom Check-List for Persons Living With HIV Disease (SSC-HIV). *Journal of Advanced Nursing, 30*(5), 1041–1049.

Holzemer, W. L., Henry, S. B., Portillo, C. J., & Miramontes, H. (2000). The client adherence profiling-intervention tailoring (CAP-IT) intervention for enhancing adherence to HIV/AIDS medications: A pilot study. *Journal of the Association of Nurses in AIDS Care, 11*(1), 36–44.

Holzemer, W. L., Henry, S. B., & Reilly, C. A. (1998). Assessing and managing pain in AIDS care: The patient perspective. *Journal of the Association of Nurses in AIDS Care, 9*(1), 22–30.

Holzemer, W. L., Henry, S. B., Reilly, C. A., & Portillo, C. J. (1995). Problems of persons with HIV/AIDS hospitalized for *Pneumocystis carinii* pneumonia. *Journal of the Association of Nurses in AIDS Care, 6*(3), 23–30.

Holzemer, W. L., Henry, S. B., Stewart, A., & Janson-Bjerklie, S. (1993). The HIV quality audit marker (HIV-QAM): An outcome measure for hospitalized AIDS patients. *Quality of Life Research, 2*(2), 99–107.

Holzemer, W. L., Hudson, A., Kirksey, K. M., Hamilton, M. J., & Bakken, S. (2001). The revised sign & symptom check-list for HIV (SSC-HIVrev). *Journal of the Association of Nurses in AIDS Care, 12*(5), 60–70.

Holzemer, W. L., Human, S., Arudo, J., Rosa, M., Hamilton, M. J., Corless, I., Robinson, L., Nicholas, P., Wantland, D., Moezzi, S., Willard, S., Kirksey, K., Portillo, C., Sefcik, E., Rivero-Mendez, M., & Maryland, M. (2009). Exploring HIV stigma and quality of life for persons living with HIV infection. *Journal of the Association of Nurses in AIDS Care, 20*(3), 161–168.

Holzemer, W. L., Makoae, L., Stewart, A., Phetlhu, R., Dlamini, P. S., Greeff, M., Uys, L., Kohi, T. W., Chirwa, M., Cuca, Y., & Naidoo, J. (2007). A conceptual model of HIV/AIDS stigma from five African countries. *Journal of Advanced Nursing, 58*(6), 541–551.

Holzemer, W. L., & Portillo, C. (Eds.) (1994). *Proceedings of the HIV/AIDS Nursing Care Summit*. Washington, DC: American Academy of Nursing.

Holzemer, W. L., & Reilly, C. A. (1995).Variables, variability, and variations research: Implications for medical informatics. *Journal of the American Medical Informatics Association, 2*(3), 183–190.

Holzemer, W. L., & Uys, L. (2004). Managing AIDS Stigma. *Journal of Social Aspects of HIV/AIDS, 1*(3), 165–174.

Holzemer, W. L., Uys, L. R., Chirwa, M. L., Greeff, M., Makoae, L. N., Kohi, T. W., Dlamini, P. S., Stewart, A. L., Mullan, J., Phetlhu, R. D., Wantland, D., Durrheim, K. (2007). Validation of the HIV/AIDS Stigma Instrument—PLWA (HASI_P). *AIDS Care 19*(8), 1002–1012.

Hudson, A. L., Kirksey, K. M., Bunch, E. H., & Holzemer, W. L. (2000). Symptom management and adherence in HIV/AIDS. *Medical Postgraduates, 38*(3), 67–74. [In Japanese].

Kemppainen, J. K., Eller, L. S., Bunch, E., Hamilton, M. J., Dole, P., Holzemer, W., Kirksey, K., Nicholas, P. K., Corless, I. B., Coleman, C., Nokes, K. M., Reynolds, N., Sefcik, L., Wantland, D., & Tsai, Y.-F. (2006). Strategies for self-management of HIV-related anxiety. *AIDS Care, 18*(6), 597–607.

Kemppainen, J. K., Holzemer, W. L., Nokes, K., Eller, L. S., Corless, I., Bunch, E. H., Kirksey, K. M., Goodroad, B. K., Portillo, C. J., Miramontes, H., & Chou, F. Y. (2003). Self-care management of anxiety and fear in HIV disease. *Journal of the Association of Nurses in AIDS Care, 14*(2), 21–29.

Kemppainen, J. K., O'Brien, L., Williams, H., Evans, L., Weiner, K. N., & Holzemer, W. L. (1999). Quantifying patient engagement with nurses: Validation of a scale with AIDS patients. *Outcomes Management for Nursing Practice, 3*(4), 167–174.

Kohi, T. W., Makoae, L., Chirwa, M., Holzemer, W. L., Phetlhu, D. R., Uys, L., Naidoo, J., Dlamini, P. S., & Greeff, M. (2006). HIV and AIDS stigma violates human rights in five African countries. *Nursing Ethics, 13*(4), 404–415.

Kohi, T. W., Portillo, C. J., Durrheim, K., Dlamini, P. S., Makoae, L. N., Greeff, M., Chirwa, M., Naidoo, J., Uys, L. R., & Holzemer, W. L. (2010). Predictors of intent to migrate among nurses in five African countries. *Journal of the Association of Nurses in AIDS Care, 21*(2), 134–143.

Makoae, L. N., Seboni, N. M., Molosiwa, K., Moleko, M., Human, S., Sukati, N. A., & Holzemer, W. L. (2005). The symptom experience of people living with HIV/AIDS in Southern Africa. *Journal of the Association of Nurses in AIDS Care, 16*(3), 22–32.

Naidoo, J. R., Uys, L. R., Greeff, M., Holzemer, W. L., Makoae, L., Dlamini, P. S., Phethlu, R., Chirwa, M. L., & Kohi, T. W. (2007). Urban and rural differences in HIV/AIDS stigma in five African countries. *African Journal of AIDS Research, 6*(1), 17–23.

Nicholas, P., Kemppainen, J. K., Canaval, G. E., Corless, I. B., Sefcik, E. F., Nokes, K. M., Bain, C. A., Kirksey, K., Eller, L. S., Dole, P., Hamilton, J. J., Coleman, C. L., Holzemer, W. L., Reynolds, N., Portillo, C. J., Bunch, E. H., Wantland, D. J., Voss, J., Phillips, R., Tsai, Y-F., Mendez, M. R., Lindgren, T., Davis, S. M., & Gallagher, D. M. (2007). Symptom management and self-care for peripheral neuropathy in HIV/AIDS. *AIDS Care, 19*(2), 179–189.

Nicholas, P. K., Kemppainen, J. K., Holzemer, W. L., Nokes, K. M., Eller, L. S., Corless, I. B., Bunch, E. H., Bain, C. A., Kirksey, K. M., Davis, S. M., & Goodroad, B. K. (2002). Self-care management for neuropathy in HIV disease. *AIDS Care, 14*(6), 763–771.

Nicholas, P., Voss, J., Corless, I.B., Lindgren, T., Wantland, T., Kemppainen, J., Canaval, G., Sefcik, E., Nokes, K., Bain, C., Kirksey, K., Eller, I., Dole, P., Hamilton, M. J., Coleman, C., Reynolds, N., Portillo, C., Bunch, E., Rivero-Mendez, M., Tsai, Y. F., & Holzemer. (2007). Unhealthy behaviors for self-management of HIV-related peripheral neuropathy. *AIDS Care, 19*(10), 1266–1273.

Phaladze, N. A., Human, S., Dlamini, S. B., Hulela, E. B., Hadebe, I. M., Sukati, N. A., Makoae, L. N., Seboni, N. M., Moleko, M., & Holzemer, W. L. (2005). Quality of life and the concept of living well with HIV/AIDS for people in sub-Saharan Africa. *Journal of Nursing Scholarship, 37*(2), 120–126.

Portillo, C. J., Mendez, M. R., Holzemer, W. L., Coreless, I. B., Nicholas, P. K., Coleman, C., Dole, P., Eller, L. S., Hamilton, M. J., Kemppainen, J. K., Kirksey, K., Nokes, K. M., Reynolds, N., Wantland, D. J., Sefcik, E. F., Bunch, E. H., & Canaval, G. E. (2005). Quality of life of ethnic minority persons living with HIV/AIDS. *Journal of Multicultural Nursing & Health, 11*(1), 31–37.

Reilly, C. A., Holzemer, W. L., Henry, S. B., Slaughter, R. E., & Portillo, C. J. (1997). A comparison of patient and nurse ratings of HIV-related signs and symptoms. *Nursing Research, 46*(6), 318–323.

Sepulveda, J., Carpenter, C., Curran, J., Holzemer, W., Smits, H., Scott, K., & M. Orza (Eds.). (2007). *PEPFAR implementation: Progress and promise.* Institute of Medicine. The National Academies Press: Washington, DC.

Sukati, N. A., Mndebele, S. C., Makoa, E. T., Ramukumba, T. S., Makoae, L. N., Seboni, N. M., Human, S., & Holzemer, W. L. (2005). HIV/AIDS symptom management in Southern Africa. *Journal of Pain and Symptom Management, 29*(2), 185–192.

The Institute of Medicine. (2003). *Measuring what matters: Allocation, planning, and quality assessment for the Ryan White Care Act.* Institute of Medicine. National Academy of Science, Washington, DC. [panel member].

Tsai, Y. F., Hsiung, P. C., & Holzemer, W. L. (2002). Symptom management in Taiwanese patients with HIV/AIDS. *Journal of Pain and Symptom Management, 23*(4), 301–309.

Uys, L., Chirwa, M., Dlamini, P., Greeff, M., Kohi, T., Holzemer, W. L., Makoae, L., Naidoo, J. R., & Phetlhu, R. (2005). Eating plastic, winning the lotto, joining the WWW: Descriptions of HIV/AIDS in Africa. *Journal of the Association of Nurses in AIDS Care, 16*(3), 11–21.

Uys, L. R., Holzemer, W. L., Chirwa, M. L., Dlamini, P., Greeff, M., Kohi, T. W., Makoae, L. N., Stewart, A. L., Mullan, J., Phetlhu, R. D., Wantland, D., Cuca, Y., & Naidoo, J. (2009). The development and validation of the HIV/AIDS Stigma Instrument- Nurse (HASI-N). *AIDS Care, 21*(2), 150–159.

Voss, J. G., Portillo, C., Holzemer, W. L., & Dodd, M. (2007). Symptom cluster of fatigue and depression in HIV/AIDS. *Journal of Prevention & Intervention in the Community, 33*(1–2), 19–34.

Voss, J. G., Dodd, M., Portillo, C., & Holzemer, W. (2006). Theories of fatigue: Applications to HIV/AIDS. *Journal of the Association of Nurses in AIDS Care, 17*(1), 37–50.

Voss, J. G., Sukati, N., Seboni, N., Makoae, L., & Holzemer, W. L. (2007). Symptom burden of fatigue of men and women living with HIV/AIDS in Southern Africa. *Journal of the Association of Nurses in AIDS Care, 18*(4), 22–31.

Wantland, D. J., Holzemer, W. L., Moezzi, S., Portillo, C., Willard, S., Arudo, J., Kirksey, K., Corless, I., Rosa, M. E., Robinson, L., Nicholas, P. K., Hamilton, M. J., Sefcik, L., Human, S., Rivero, M., Maryland, M., & Huang, E. (2008). A randomized controlled trial testing the efficacy of an HIV/AIDS ymptom management manual. *Journal of Pain and Symptom Management, 36*(3), 235–246.

Willard, S., Holzemer, W. L., Wantland, D. J., Cuca, Y. P., Kirksey, K., Portillo, C., Corless, I. B., Rivero-Mendez, M., Rosa, M., Nicholas, P. K., Hamilton, M. J., Sefcik, E., Kemppainen, J., Canaval, G., Robinson, L., Moezzi, S., Human, S., Arudo, J., Eller, L., Bunch, E., Dole, P. J., Coleman, C., Nokes, K., Reynolds, N. R., Tsai, Y.-F., Maryland, M., Voss, J., & Lindgren, T. (2009). Does "asymptomatic" mean without symptoms for those living with HIV infection? *AIDS Care, 21*(3), 322–328.

WHO. (2006). *The World Health Report 2006—Working together for health*. WHO: Geneva, Switzerland.

Wilson, H. S., Hutchinson, S. A., & Holzemer, W. L. (1997). Salvaging quality of life in ethnically diverse patients with advanced HIV/AIDS. *Qualitative Health Research, 7*(1), 75–97.

Wilson, H. S., Hutchinson, S., & Holzemer, W. L. (2002). Reconciling incompatibilities: A grounded theory of HIV medication adherence and symptom management. *Qualitative Health Research, 12*(10), 1309–1322.

Wright, J., Henry, S. B., Holzemer, W. L., & Falknor, P. (1993). Evaluation of community-based nurse case management activities for symptomatic HIV/AIDS clients. *Journal of the Association of Nurses in AIDS Care, 4*(2), 37–47.

19

Forging the Missing Link: From Nursing Research to Health Policy

Ada Sue Hinshaw and Patricia A. Grady

Forging the missing link is the phrase that signifies the challenging journey of nurse investigators and teams in moving their research programs into health policy. The compelling descriptions of the programs of these investigators and their colleagues, given in earlier chapters, provide evidence of how their research shaped health policy at the local, community, state/province, national, and international levels. As pioneers in building long-term research programs to guide practice, they have each individually extended their capability in advancing nursing's influence on health policy as well. All have influenced health policy and some have additionally shaped science policy.

Analyzing the experiences of these scientists, a number of general themes or issues need to be made explicit. These issues need to be used by other colleagues and must be taught as part of nursing undergraduate and graduate programs. In addition, many lessons and strategies for informing health policy have been learned during these pioneering research programs—lessons that are important to summarize in this text for the benefit of the nursing discipline and the scientific community.

This final chapter will examine the following:

- Those general issues identified across the scientific and health policy endeavors relating to the ways in which nursing research informing health policy.
- The numerous "lessons learned" by senior nurse investigators as they shaped health policy through the use of their research programs and the expertise they gained from their scientific endeavors.
- The issues identified and the lessons learned, illustrated through the examples provided by the nurse scientists in their stories of how nursing research shaped health policy.

GENERAL ISSUES: NURSING RESEARCH SHAPING HEALTH POLICY

Several general issues were identified that surfaced across the multiple experiences outlined by the authors in describing how their research programs shaped health policy. Five general issues will be discussed: (1) influence on several levels of health policy, (2) various

281

types of models that provide the context for understanding nursing research shaping health policy, (3) multiple factors besides and, sometimes, instead of research, that inform health policy, (4) long-term planning for nursing research programs to shape health policy as an important factor in scientific programs and training, and (5) influence on the general direction of the nursing profession while in addition to shaping health policy.

Levels of Health Policy

Nursing research has informed health policy at multiple levels of policy making. The long-term scientific programs of the authors indicate that most research programs shaped several levels of health policy, from local organizations to international practice and quality guidelines. Some of the authors clearly intended their research to have a local practice influence, such as with Metheny's studies of tube feeding and the proper placement of such tubes. Her research provided the science required for evidence-based practice in placing feeding tubes, and rapidly decreased the consequences and illnesses that resulted from improper placement. This had been her initial purpose for the studies and no one was more surprised than Metheny when her work had greater widespread influence through textbooks used for several health professions, e.g., nurses, nutritionists, and physicians. In addition, her scientific endeavors informed a national American Association of Critical Care Nurses Practice in 2005 and federal reports from the U.S. Food and Drug Administration. What had begun as a local issue spread to influence the practice of multiple health professionals at state and national levels. Sampselle's research program on the prevention of urinary incontinence (UI) also started as a local concern and initially influenced organizational ambulatory clinics, especially those focused on women's health issues. Collaborating with the national organization, Association of Women's Health, Obstetric and Neonatal Nurses (AWHONN), she and others repeated the interventions substantiated from the research in multiple clinics around the country and evaluated their translated effectiveness. This resulted in the evidence-based interventions being incorporated in numerous clinics across the country. Based on her scientific endeavors, Sampselle participated in national and international guideline task forces, using her expertise and her research findings to formulate new health policy guidelines at several levels of policy making.

The community level of health policy making and influence is clearly evident in the Gross and Crowley endeavors. Their focus on health promotion and prevention in early childhood resulted in the development and study of the Chicago Parent Program. A program for preschool children of low-income communities, it focused on promoting positive parenting and child mental health by concentrating on the issues of parents raising young children in low-resource environments. The success of the program is evident by its incorporation as one of the recommended interventions for Head Start in Chicago, an exciting evidence-based program that makes an investment in young children who are the future of society—an investment that will pay off for a number of years.

Aiken's and O'Brien-Pallas and Hayes' research programs have greatly influenced the U.S. state and Canadian province levels of health policy. Aiken and her colleagues have focused on the work environment of nurses and the impact of that environment on both nurse and patient outcomes. She has especially studied one factor in the environment, i.e., the adequate staffing of nurses and what that means for nurses and patients. Scientific endeavors from this program of research have provided important findings relating to the number of patients that a nurse can safely handle before patient mortality begins to increase, failure-to-rescue incidents increase, and burnout and job dissatisfaction occur for nurses. In addition, her research has shown the greater safety of patients with better educated nurses. These data have been used in crafting state laws (e.g., California) to recommend the optimum number of patients that nurses can care for at one time. Nationally, she has provided testimonies for the U.S. Congress and the Institute of Medicine (IOM) relating to these same findings. O'Brien-Pallas and Hayes describe the scientific endeavors of the team of colleagues studying health and human resource strategies for nursing in Ontario, Canada. O'Brien-Pallas and her team were awarded a major center, the Nursing Health Services Research Unit, for developing large databases from which they could provide human resource projections based on the needs of the population, including evaluated health outcomes for the population and the provider. Their work has guided many of the policies in Canadian provinces for human health resource needs. Because of her success in identifying the number of nurses needed to provide healthcare under various conditions, she has participated in numerous national task forces and given testimonies for national health policy making as well.

Naylor and Kurtzman describe the manner in which nursing research has shaped national health policy in terms of a new, well-substantiated model for healthcare: transitional care. Transitional care consists of care provided by advanced practice nurses during the period of time from discharge from the hospital to being settled in either a home or nursing facility. Naylor and her colleagues have primarily studied this model with elderly adults who are experiencing hospitalization for some medical problem. They have measured both the health outcomes for these patients and the economic costs of using such a transitional model. The economic value has been apparent mainly by keeping elderly patients from being readmitted to the hospital and having fewer consequences of their illnesses. This research program, substantiated by other investigators, has caught the attention of the American Association for Retired Persons (AARP) and is part of the healthcare reform plans in the U.S. President's 2010 budget according to the Office of Management and Budget, as well as part of congressional legislative proposals.

A fewer number of nursing research programs shape health policy at the international level. Holzemer's program of research, "Living Well With HIV/AIDS," describes how he has used his expertise in this area to influence health policy both nationally and internationally. Although the specific results of his own research were not always utilized, his expertise based on the research program placed him in a number of leadership positions with the IOM, the International Council of Nurses, and others to influence guidelines on the prevention and care of individuals with HIV/AIDS. Some of the nurse researchers mentioned earlier, such as Sampselle, have also been instrumental in forming international practice guidelines for conditions such as UI.

These examples of nurse researchers provide evidence of some of the influence that nursing research has had on the shaping of health policy at multiple levels. For a discipline with approximately 25 years of stable funding for its research endeavors, this level of informing health policy is remarkable.

Models Providing Context for Shaping Health Policy

In this section, the models referred to are those that articulate the processes or context for using research in shaping health policy. Most of the research programs in this text are guided by theoretical frameworks that explain the expected relationships among the concepts and their staging. These are different from the models relating nursing research and health policy.

Several models are outlined for moving research into health policy. Both Feetham and Hinshaw address the use of the Richmond and Kotelchuck model that consists of three components: knowledge and information, political will, and social action or new policy programs. This general model provides a context for understanding the major aspects of research and policy without itemizing the process of moving them together. Feetham also speaks of an evidentiary model that makes explicit the multiple bodies of knowledge and research needed and used to inform health policy. Shamian and Shamian-Ellen provide a more detailed model that provides both context and process. The stages of the model identify the context of what is being done, i.e., Getting to the Policy Agenda and Moving Into Action. The steps in the model outline the process of using research or knowledge to reach the endpoint of policy making: regulation, adaption, and revision of a policy and the ensuing program. Hinshaw and Heinrich use the model of Shamian and her colleagues to illustrate the establishment of the National Institute of Nursing Research (NINR) within the mainstream of scientific investigation in the United States. Block's model, addressed in Hinshaw's chapter, is an excellent example of most of the process models in health policy: agenda settings, policy formulation, policy adoption, policy implementation, policy assessment, and policy modification.

The important point in acknowledging the multiple models that address the context and processes for moving research into health policy is for the discipline of nursing to understand that such models are critical in policy scholarship. The use of theoretical frameworks for explaining relationships and stages in nursing research is well established, but the use of research to policy models needs to be just as explicit.

Multiple Factors Inform Health Policy

Numerous factors are active in shaping health policy. Several of these factors were most influential in terms of the scientific endeavors of these investigators. The recent economic climate was a major factor in reversing the telehealth programs that Finkelstein was able to institute as part of state health policy and programming. In several incidents, he was able to convince the state to fund telehealth programs only to have the funds withdrawn when the state experienced economic difficulties. The second factor involved with Finkelstein's difficulty in sustaining changes in telehealth programming and policies was the lack of reimbursement for such health interventions. In slow economic periods, it was also not possible to promote legislation for new telehealth programs. It was a different story for Naylor's transitional model of care, as legislation for reimbursement was introduced by the AARP. Two major situational factors might have accounted for the differences. Naylor's research showing significant cost savings with transitional care was substantiated by others across several disciplines. Also, she had been successful in convincing a major, large-member organization, i.e., the AARP, of the importance of the evidence-based care model. The AARP is a major lobbying organization with a very large voting membership. However, Naylor was facing a particularly difficult challenge, i.e., a change in culture in terms of offering care across settings (hospital to nursing facility to home). Reimbursement is essentially structured by setting.

Sometimes, the changes recommended by the findings of research programs were quite complex and required changes in cultures and attitudes. For example, Naylor's recommendation of transitional care requires a change in the basic structure of reimbursement for healthcare in order to cut across several settings. Evans and Strumpf confronted a similar situation with their research recommendations to change the use of restraints in nursing facilities with only limited use of such a technique. Nursing facilities were used to placing a number of elder patients in restraints of some type—it was the common practice of the day. It was necessary to change the regulations and accreditation standards governing nursing facilities, as well as to experience several media exposés in order to bring about the changes suggested by their research program.

Several other research programs were influenced by a shifting political climate in terms of scientific endeavors being able to shape health policy. Villarruel and Jemmott's research programs indicated that abstinence was not as effective a method as a safe-sex intervention for young adolescents in controlling undesired pregnancies or sexually transmitted diseases. However, at the time their research could be used to shape health policy, the political climate was not conducive to such findings being heard or adopted. O'Brien-Pallas and her team's research findings on health human resources were used and sought much more during periods of nursing shortage. A shortage of nurses brought political pressure on government policy makers to search for information and strategies for handling this major healthcare problem. When there is no nursing shortage, careful and systematic projections are less likely to be in demand. These are examples of the influence of a shifting political climate on the ability of nursing research to shape health policy.

Both Sampselle and Tilden focus their research programs on areas that are very sensitive to the public, another factor that influences public debate and health policy making. Urinary incontinence is a subject not easily discussed because of the personal and private nature of this type of condition. Thus, as important as strategies for handling this condition are, they are not apt to be the subject of public discourse except in healthcare forums. Not often will UI reach a congressional forum unless a strong champion can be identified who is willing to discuss such an intimate topic. Tilden's research program in end-of-life care is a very different type of subject, but death is not easy for individuals to discuss either. Thus, special circumstances need to occur for public debates to focus on such topics. The fact that a sizeable percentage of the healthcare dollar is spent in the last period of a person's life made end-of-life wishes of the family a major health policy issue in Oregon. Thus, the necessary debates and policy changes could occur.

Long-Term Planning to Shape Health Policy

Long-term planning in terms of nursing research programs informing health policy was limited to only a few of the investigators and their teams. It is common for research programs to be focused on providing information to influence nursing practice, but a newer concept for long-term strategic planning for results is needed to shape health policy. How is it possible to predict the future and strategically plan for research findings that could inform health policy? Health and healthcare challenges that loom on the horizon will ultimately bring undesirable consequences to society and, thus, will lead to health policy changes. It is these healthcare challenges that need to be identified in order to guide an investigator's research programs when they match the science that is being pursued by the researcher.

Aiken and her team consistently plan their research based on the work environment issues and the nursing shortage cycles for results that will be able to shape health policy in the future. The Nursing Health Services Research Unit of O'Brien-Pallas was instituted for the purpose of monitoring the human resource needs of Ontario, Canada, and developing major databases that could be used for future projections. Naylor and her colleagues' research programs have been planned during their last several investigations to provide information, such as refined economic and quality measures, to convince policy makers that transitional care can be effective and can lower healthcare costs. Only with such data might there be a stronger possibility of obtaining reimbursement for such care. These are examples of research programs that have anticipated healthcare challenges and have planned for producing data that would be valuable in shaping the healthcare debates and, ultimately, health policy.

Providing Direction for Nursing's Path

Several of the nurse investigators illustrated how their research programs provided new direction for nursing practice and resulted in changes in the attitudes of nurses and the environment. Evans and Strumpf's research program changed the entire face of nursing facilities and how elderly people were treated. Restraints have become rare occurrences, and communication and attention to specific needs are more frequent. This changes the entire environment. O'Brien-Pallas and her team have changed the variables involved in understanding and monitoring the projection and use of human resources during periods of high and low supply. Adding concepts of multiple outcomes that need to be considered within the context of the population studied has changed how human resources, such as nurses, are viewed and treated. The establishment of the NINR as described by Hinshaw and Heinrich has changed science policy and, thus, health policy by bringing new perspectives to the scientific inquiry in health. For nursing, the NINR provided a stable funding base, an important credibility to the discipline's science by its placement at the National Institutes of Health, and an ever-growing and evolving body of knowledge from which to influence practice and inform health policy.

LESSONS LEARNED

What are some of the lessons learned from the preceding chapters that can be generalized to facilitate policy change through research? Clearly, the overall significance of the problem selected for study maximizes the potential for making an impact. The greater the public health importance, the more people will be affected and the likelier any research results are to be noticed. However, beyond this, several other factors emerge from these programs of research: the value of economic outcome, the "window of opportunity," gaps in knowledge, strategies for turning nursing research into health policy, stakeholder involvement, and barriers and roadblocks.

Value of Economic Outcomes

One way to communicate clearly the possible impact of the research is to incorporate an economic model or economic indicators. Not all research studies lend themselves to this approach. The overall impact can be inferred by the significance of the problem, number of people affected, number of workdays missed, or decreased lifespan, for example. For a more compelling argument, it is often helpful to include economic indicators to demonstrate improvement on health outcomes and to tie those outcomes to cost savings to present a clear, measurable case for the benefits of change. Examples of this approach are shown in the work of Drs. Naylor and Kurtzman, O'Brien-Pallas and Hayes, and Finkelstein and Cady.

The early tests of the Transitional Care Model of Naylor et al. demonstrated improved patient satisfaction, reduced rehospitalizations, and reduced healthcare costs among the intervention group of patients compared with controls. Despite these consistently positive results, this work did not receive wide acceptance, although it was acclaimed. Adding a way to measure cost savings to the design gave a clear way to translate the positive health outcomes of decreased rehospitalizations into cost savings. Two additional steps enhanced the impact. In one study, the researchers selected a patient sample with "common medical and surgical" conditions, which represented the top 10 categories of Medicare reimbursement. Yet another study focused on the elderly with heart failure, one of the groups most resistant to treatment. Thus, the case was readily made for the effectiveness of the intervention in the most predominant and hard-to-treat elderly.

Finkelstein's approach was twofold in considering the value of economic factors. It was important to first overcome the perception that technology is expensive and would therefore increase costs and, second, to show concrete outcomes that technology actually could decrease costs. It was also important to demonstrate that patients were satisfied with care that was technologically delivered or augmented, thus overcoming the perception that machines were replacing human caregivers with the goal of saving money. The approach he used was that technology is an adjunct to enhance or complement standard care and be more cost effective. One last point made to offset the cost versus care concern was that study subjects were reluctant to give up their virtual visits at the end of the study because they did not want to lose the regular visits made possible by the technology. Outcomes included decreased emergency room visits, higher use of pharmacy delivery services, and lower use of transportation services.

Thus, by using objective, measurable outcomes, Finkelstein provided the data available for Centers for Medicare and Medicaid Services (CMS) changes in reimbursement. He also provided data to assure critics of the acceptability of this approach by including quality-of-life satisfaction data.

In a somewhat different manner, O'Brien-Pallas and her collaborators showed the cost effectiveness of appropriate use of human resources. In doing so, she used more global measures of cost such as absenteeism and retention of workforce. She did, however, link her measures to those in which the Canadian government had an interest, which enabled a more direct link to national policy. This work is in contrast to that of Aiken, who links nurse staffing to patient outcomes and patient safety.

Windows of Opportunity

Another important lesson shown by the researchers in this volume is that of recognizing and taking advantage of a window of opportunity. Convergence of factors, societal trends, changes in thinking, advances in technology, and emergence of new health issues can all lead to a window of opportunity and enhance the probability of changing policy.

An excellent example of this is the creation of the NINR described by Hinshaw and Heinrich. More nurses were doing research, the science was developing, and an IOM report was released, calling for the formation of an institute to support this type of research. The nursing community began to unify around a compelling idea. Champions were developing in the Congress and from a national political perspective; the idea of doing something visible and supportive of women was getting traction in the middle to late 1980s. The creation of the NINR was a tribute to the synergizing of all of these factors and still stands as a visible tribute to what the nursing community can accomplish as a united force.

The window of opportunity for Dinges' work hinges on patient safety and societal safety related to the effects of partial sleep on formal and informal caregivers, National Aeronautics and Space Administration astronauts, shift workers of all walks of life, and the military. His work shows the dramatic and detrimental effects that decreased or poor quality sleep can have on executive and motor function. With the increasingly compelling evidence, agencies responsible for caregiving and safety of various populations are moving toward instituting safeguards.

For the work of Naylor et al., the primacy of HMOs, health insurance companies, and the rebuilding of the CMS have set the stage for receptivity of this work, but the effort being put into healthcare reform has opened a wide window of opportunity. Congressional hearings have been held, which have provided a platform for presenting the Transitional Care Model and its promise of higher quality of care with cost effectiveness.

For Stanley Finkelstein, the window has opened with the coming of age of many new technologies that can be utilized in the healthcare arena. This is coupled with the increasing population of mobile, independent adults with chronic illness versus those previously largely in hospitals or extended care facilities. In addition, our population is more widely dispersed geographically, raising access to care issues that may be better addressed by telehealth technologies. Societally, there is greater recognition of the health disparities that exist in our midst, and many of the new technologies may be a way to reach many of these underserved rural and urban populations.

Evans and Strumpf also benefitted from a window of opportunity that reflected larger global as well as local and societal trends. Social movements such as the Civil Rights and Women's Movements as well as the Cold War, with its "containment and control" of social and political themes, led to calls for freedom, autonomy, and humanism in our country. Against this background was the aging of the population and the recognition that care of the elderly, including those in nursing homes, was not optimal. In 1985, a clarion call for help was issued throughout the gerontology community, identifying the overuse of restraints in the elderly as a major problem and asking for help. The community became activated; the IOM report on Quality of Care in Nursing Homes was released; The National Citizens Coalition for Nursing Home Reform became active in pushing for reform; and the Nursing Home Act was passed in 1990. The Nursing Home Act included among its rights for patients the right to be free from restraints. This was the same year that Evans and Strumpf were funded to carry out their first clinical trial, which provided the data to support freedom from restraints. What a perfect window of opportunity!

Gaps in Knowledge

It is important to determine what gaps in knowledge the research is intended to fill when a problem for study is identified, and subsequently, it is important to assess what can or cannot be said from the research findings. Because good research studies often generate as many new questions as they generate answers, the process of developing a program of research is essentially an iterative process, with later studies building on the earlier ones. Assessing the gaps for planning future studies is often a byproduct of efforts to implement findings into practice or policy. The answer to the question "If this is not convincing, what else is needed to convince them?" may be the gaps in the knowledge and the subsequent studies required to accomplish the goal of translating research into practice and policy.

This iterative process can be clearly seen in the work of Naylor et al. and Gross and Crowley, as well as Metheny and Melnyk. In underscoring the importance of research to establish evidence-based practice, Melnyk clearly speaks to the iterative nature of the process. Once something works, she points out, it is important to evaluate and fine tune the approaches in order to make them truly evidence based. Deborah Gross also employed this approach in her research with early childhood parenting and health issues. Metheny's work demonstrates a systematic approach to solving a problem and letting the results guide future studies. In order to provide an evidence base for parenteral tube feeding, she took her work from bedside to bench and, finally, to practice over the course of her program of research. Starting with auscultation, the traditional method of testing for feeding tube placement, Metheny and her team systematically evaluated various methods for ascertainment of placement. At one point, she needed to switch to an animal model in order to study aspiration. Because she determined that bilirubin concentrations in feeding tube aspirates were helpful in predicting location, Dr. Metheny et al. also developed a bilirubin test strip that could be used at the bedside.

Strategies for Turning Nursing Research Into Health Policy

There are many different models for shaping health policy, as described by Hinshaw, and a variety of ways that research can become a foundation for health policy, as described by Grady. A number of different and successful strategies were used by the investigators in this volume, and they are described in elegant detail. Linda Aiken speaks of doing "policy-relevant research," where the greater the public health issue addressed, the more likely the research results will influence health policy. Evans and Strumpf considered this when they took on an issue germane to the aging population, one that was growing in importance because of changing population demographics. Villarruel and Jemmott began their research in HIV/AIDS prevention in teenagers at a time when the disease was increasing dramatically, was becoming a chronic disease, and had begun disseminating throughout the general population, with teenagers and young adults at particular risk.

Connecting and working with the media are other strategies that were helpful in many instances. For Virginia Tilden, the interest of the leading state newspaper, *The Oregonian*, in dying provided an important venue for stories that underscored the usefulness of her team's research findings. This ultimately provided for a national forum that led to other opportunities and other publications featuring this ground-breaking research. This is a strategy that is increasingly accepted as an important adjunct to professional journal publications in order to reach broader audiences who may be instrumental in catalyzing policy change.

Providing testimony to the Congress, other federal agencies, the IOM, or advocacy groups is another approach that can lead to policy change. Having credible research results on substantive areas of interest can provide a very persuasive argument to any of these groups and enables them to consider making recommendations (or laws in the case of the Congress) that are evidence based. Examples of this strategy are seen in the works of Naylor, Aiken, Dinges, Holzemer, and Evans and Strumpf.

National and community policy change can also be effected through working with local groups or local chapters that feed into national organizations. Gross' successful research work to improve parenting and decrease negative behaviors, which was carried out in early childcare centers in Chicago, was recognized by the commissioner of the Chicago Department of Children and Youth Services. She and her team were asked to test their program in the Early Head Start Programs for possible implementation across Chicago. They were successful, and implementation took place. This program is now being adapted elsewhere across the country.

Another example of national and community policy change was provided by the work of Villarruel and Jemmott, who, cognizant of the importance of the window of urgency in HIV/AIDS prevention, marketed their successful intervention to the CDC, which incorporated it into their education videos for HIV prevention. Thus, they have made it available to a national and even global audience.

Adoption of research findings into national guidelines that carry the imprimatur of major organizations or agencies is another way to reach the level of policy. Two good examples of this include the work of Carolyn Sampselle being adopted by the AWHONN and the work of Evans and Strumpf being incorporated into routine care of the elderly. Metheny, with the incorporation of her work into textbooks, has altered what was considered routine, safe state-of-the-art care of patients with feeding tubes.

One of the most direct ways to change policy is through legislation. Aiken's work has resulted in policy changes in California related to nurse–patient ratios, and legislation is pending in both Houses of Congress to make Naylor's Transitional Care model of care delivery reimbursable through the CMS. Evan and Strumpf's work with the Congress and the Committee on Aging led to changes in policy in HealthCare Financing Administration (HICFA), the forerunner of CMS.

At some point, individual researchers can become so identified with an area that they are able to facilitate changes in policy simply by their participation as a thought leader in an arena not directly connected to their data. Bill Holzemer embodies this spirit with his work in global and local communities in the fight against HIV/AIDS. Other examples include O'Brien-Pallas with regard to human resource utilization in Canada and Melnyk as a prime mover for evidence-based practice.

Stakeholder Involvement

Stakeholder involvement is most often key, if not essential, in making this transition from research to policy. Stakeholders are those individuals or groups who have the most to gain or lose around the issue of interest. It is useful to cast a broad net when thinking about who are the stakeholders and being more inclusive wherever possible. In particular, stakeholders offer varying perspectives and bring a real-world aspect to the research endeavor that is essential to translation into other venues. They are also likely to have a variety of contacts and networks that are outside the scope of most researchers. A good example is that of the middle-aged to older adults, who comprise the membership of AARP and to whom the issue of Transitional Care of the Elderly is of particular importance.

It is important to start including stakeholders early in the process so that they will have a vested interest in the project. Naylor, Tilden, and Finkelstein all provide interesting examples of stakeholder involvement.

Barriers and Roadblocks

It is useful to learn what barriers others have encountered and to consider what barriers might be lurking on the horizon, for those are issues that can derail or slow down progress, resulting in frustration and sometimes preventing incorporation of findings.

A frequent theme mentioned was that of "myth busting" or overcoming notions that, although incorrect, were quite entrenched. Evans and Strumpf encountered this with the use of physical restraints in the elderly; Tilden, with end-of-life decision making; Villarruel and Jemmott, with overcoming the notion that young male teenagers would not be receptive to altering intimate behaviors; and Finkelstein, with dealing with the ideas that technology would be too expensive, too difficult for patients to manage, and too impersonal to provide satisfaction with care. Each of these researchers dealt successfully in overcoming the myths, using somewhat different approaches.

The need to change entrenched traditional methods and practices also provides a challenge for those wanting to incorporate new ideas and policies. Melnyk addresses this extensively as she underscores the need to provide evidence for practices that may be the convention but are unproven; Naylor mentions overcoming the silos of care that she encountered throughout the system; and Aiken has addressed this by trying to demonstrate the relationship between nurse–patient ratios and patient safety, and between educational and experiential levels of nurses and patient safety. Attempting to translate these outcomes into policy has been challenging.

Finally, communication and dissemination of results are critical to influencing policy. How to communicate, when to communicate, where to communicate, and to whom are the critical factors. Most of our contributors have addressed this explicitly. Getting the information to the most important audiences is the goal, and getting the information to those individuals who can make a difference or to whom it will have the most impact is key. That may be the Congress, national organizations, and community organizations, all of these are reflected throughout the chapters in this book. Dissemination alone is usually not enough to make change. Linking to systems that are already in place for implementation can be useful. Sometimes a broker may be necessary to bridge with the community, members of the Congress, or regulatory agencies. This is an area where advocacy groups and community leaders may be especially helpful.

CONCLUSION

As nurse investigators and their teams have forged the link from nursing research to health policy, many general issues and "lessons learned" have been experienced. Analyzing the numerous journeys of the scientists has advanced understanding of the context and processes that facilitate and/or constitute barriers to informing health policy with nursing research.

The issues raised and the lessons learned from these early successes simultaneously provide examples and building blocks for advancing nursing science's ability to inform health policy. The idea that nursing research transforms into policy becomes a reality when examining these scientific endeavors. This transformation foreshadows the natural evolution of the future, which would link nursing research to health policy. The collection of these scientific endeavors and policy experiences confirms that nursing research has an integral position in formulating public health policy.

Index